Questions
&
Answers
in the Practice of
Family Therapy

Edited by

Alan S. Gurman, Ph.D.

*Associate Professor,
Department of Psychiatry
University of Wisconsin Medical School*

Brunner/Mazel, Publishers • New York

SECOND PRINTING

Library of Congress Cataloging in Publication Data
Main entry under title:
Questions and answers in the practice of family therapy.

  Includes bibliographical references and index.
  1. Family psychotherapy. I. Gurman, Alan S.
[DNLM: 1. Family therapy—Examination questions.
WM18 P895]
RC488.5.Q47   616.89′156   80-22460
ISBN 0-87630-246-0

Published by
BRUNNER/MAZEL, INC.
19 Union Square
New York, New York 10003

MANUFACTURED IN THE UNITED STATES OF AMERICA

PREFACE

The developmental history, if you will, of a book, especially the initial impetus for its creation, is rarely described to its readers. Indeed, it is often quite difficult for a book author or editor to identify the formative events in the evolution of his or her volume, particularly its early stages. In contrast, *Questions and Answers in the Practice of Family Therapy* has come about through a series of very concrete actions and events.

When, in 1978, ownership and publication of the *International Journal of Family Counseling* was taken over by Brunner/Mazel, its name was soon changed to the *American Journal of Family Therapy*. Soon thereafter, Dr. Richard Sauber, editor of the *Journal*, invited me to be the Section Editor of a Research and Clinical Exchange department, to appear as a regular feature of each quarterly issue of the *Journal*. The aim, scope and purposes of the Exchange were explicitly defined: readers were invited to submit, to the Section Editor, brief, focused Questions involving practical issues in the conduct of family therapy, or in the teaching or research investigation of family therapy. The Section Editor, serving as a kind of broker, would then solicit a family therapist who was a recognized expert in the area in question to prepare an equally straightforward, concise Discussion of the issue raised by the reader.

The material appearing in the Exchange in the first year of its existence received such widespread positive reactions from the *Journal*'s readers that Bernie Mazel, publisher of the *Journal*, suggested to me that I might use the same format to create a book-length manuscript. As is evident, I found the idea very attractive.

Thus, the basic rationale for this volume, as for the Exchange (which continues independently of this book), was twofold. First, it was then, and still remains, clear that the professional literature on the practice of marital and family therapy has no shortage of ambitious and stimulating discussions of the theories and principles of treating families. Far less frequently, the literature presents, in everyday conversational language as would be used in informal collegial discussion, down-to-earth discussion of the handling of common clinical issues, problems and decisions. The second, and related, rationale was that the accumulated practical wisdom of experienced family therapists, born of years of clinical work, had a great deal to offer both beginning and advanced clinicians, but that a good deal of this wisdom had, at least in public contexts, remained unarticulated. Thus, the strategy for the present volume was to bring to bear explicit statements of how seasoned family therapists actually *think* and what they actually *do* in common clinical situations.

Original contributions were sought from practitioners with widely varying theoretical orientations, who, as a group, were known to work in a broad range of clinical settings. (A small number of contributions have been reprinted from the Research and Clinical Exchange section of the *American Journal of Family Therapy*.) Each contributor was invited to compose his or her own Question and a succinct Discussion. Contributors were free to select a topic area of their choice. It was assumed, and the actual content of this volume confirms, that this self-selection process would produce the discussion of an array of clinical matters that would be representative of the kinds of day-to-day issues and problems faced by the practicing family clinician.

The contributions to this volume have a general temporal organization, progressing from issues of engaging couples and families in treatment, to treatment planning, to resistance to change, to common mid-phase matters and the treatment of special disorders, populations and problems, to termination. As the reader may readily note, a number of the contributions might have been located, with good reason, in other sections of the book, e.g., a contribution dealing with the management of resistance with a particular clinical population might have been placed either in a section dealing with resistance to change or in a section focused on the clinical population in question. In the end, arbitrary editorial judgment was used to decide what was the most prominent theme in a contribution, and the piece was placed accordingly. A related editorial judgment, made at the outset, was that the majority of the most salient clinical issues in family therapy apply across different treatment methods, i.e., are not specific to particular "schools" of family treatment. Moreover, it was decided that family clinicians would profit from learning how therapists of theoretical orientations other than their own address many of these issues. Hence, no sections of the book deal exclusively with matters that are unique to a particular "school" of therapy.

It is hoped that the present volume offers the beginnings of a new dimension to the published literature on the practice of family therapy. The contributions were intended to be both practically informative and, in some instances, provocative. Hopefully, as a group, they are sufficiently thought-provoking to lead the reader to examine carefully his or her own assumptions about the process of clinical change in families, and to stimulate the reader to articulate his or her own thinking, if only privately, about *what* he or she does in family therapy, and *why*.

Finally, I want to express my appreciation to Richard Sauber, from whose idea for the Exchange this volume evolved, and to Bernie Mazel, who has fostered this process so enthusiastically.

Alan S. Gurman
Madison, Wisconsin
January,1981

CONTENTS

SECTION II
Patient Selection and Treatment Planning

SECTION III
Resistance and Countertransference

SECTION IV
Treatment of Severe Disorders

SECTION V
Separation, Divorce and Remarriage

SECTION VI
Special Areas and Issues

PART A: Multigenerational Issues

SECTION VII
Termination of Family Therapy

SECTION I

Engaging Families in Treatment

1. Convening the Family: Guidelines for the Initial Contact with a Family Member

Question:

Convening the family is the first crucial step, and often one of the most difficult ones in family therapy. The therapist wants to establish positive rapport with the contacting family member and, at the same time, set the stage for the subsequent family meeting. With what attitude and preparation should the therapist approach this initial contact? How can the therapist most effectively gather information about the family's problem from this person? What kind of resistances are likely to be encountered in requesting the family's presence and how can they be successfully addressed? Finally, what specific conditions must be agreed to in order to properly arrange a family evaluation?

Discussion:

When a family member first contacts a therapist, the call can be viewed both as an individual cry for help and a message of distress from the individual's family. The contact usually occurs in the form of a telephone call or a face-to-face meeting. A therapist's goal here is to establish a positive relationship with the family member and to explore the possibility of bringing in the rest of the family for an evaluation. Because of the exploratory nature of this contact, it should be brief, limited to no more than 15 or 20 minutes. The message communicated should be, "I am interested in helping you with your problem. In order to get the proper start, we'll need your family here to accomplish this."

Therapists should attempt to take their own phone calls or to be present at the initial intakes with contacting family members. Appointment secretaries or nonfamily-oriented intake workers may be likely to overlook the importance of arranging a family evaluation or may not be trained to deal with the resistances that may arise when this request is made. Therapists who work in an agency or institution

5

that is organized along traditional, individual lines will need the support of their supervisors and administrators to conduct family evaluations. The intake process, as well as logging and billing procedures in these settings, often impede therapists' attempts to convene the family; therapists ought not to proceed until these issues have been administratively resolved.

Gathering Information

When a family member begins to describe his problem, the therapist should listen sympathetically. He should also pay attention to the interactional aspects of the problem. For example, if a husband says, "I'm not getting along with my wife," or, "My wife and I are having a terrible problem with our teenage daughter," or even, "I've been awfully depressed and haven't discussed this with anyone in my family," he is already introducing interpersonal elements of the problem. The therapist may take note of this issue and return to it later, when he explains the importance of including the other family members in the evaluation. If the person describes the problem only in personal terms, e.g., "I've been suffering from severe headaches and my family doctor tells me it's my nerves," the therapist may inquire if anyone else in the house is aware of this problem and how they have responded to it. This reframes the problem in interactional terms, and allows the therapist to find out who else lives in the house and how they may be involved in the problem.

While the therapist wants to convey his interest in the contacting person's concerns, he must be careful to avoid eliciting sensitive feelings or opinions about other family members, or personal painful secrets that would make it difficult for this person to return and speak openly with other family members. If the therapist senses that too much is being said, he may gently suggest that these issues might be better discussed at a later time, when more trust has been established and more constructive solutions seem possible. This approach to information gathering thus allows the therapist to establish the role of other family members in the presenting problem and at the same time protects the integrity of all family members and the therapist's future relationships with them.

Dealing with Resistances

Family members present certain characteristic resistances to the idea of bringing others in their family to an evaluation session. One of the most common type are questions about the rationale for this request. They want to know why it is necessary and how it will help them with their problem.

It is worthwhile to give some attention to this question. Many family therapists believe that there are specific indications for convening a family for evaluation and treatment. Clarkin et al. (1979) present their selection criteria for family therapy and a helpful bibliography on this subject. Other therapists believe that it is useful to evaluate the person along with other family members, regardless of the circumstance, and that to begin therapy in any other way handicaps the therapist (e.g., Haley, 1976).

It is beyond the scope of this discussion to adequately debate this issue; therapists, nonetheless, ought to be familiar with the pros and cons and formulate a position of their own. This author's position is that it is useful to meet with other family members in an initial evaluation whenever possible, and that it is not potentially destructive to the contacting person's family relationships. Both ethical and strategic considerations enter into this viewpoint. Family members are committed to each other in their relationships by virtue of deep existential ties, or loyalties (Boszormenyi-Nagy and Spark, 1973), which supersedes acquired antagonisms or emotional cutoffs between them. The therapist should not overlook these relationships as potential sources of help in the treatment. Family relationships also engender an organizational structure that defines how the family members perceive themselves and relate to others. Working directly with these relationships may allow the therapist more leverage to effect paradigmatic change (growth) rather than the reversible changes that often occur when the homeostatic forces that maintain family psychopathology cannot be dealt with directly.

If the contacting family member has questions about the rationale for bringing in his family, the therapist should try to answer him directly and honestly. He may reply, "When one family member is in pain, we often find that other family members are in pain as well. Bringing everyone in can result in more people receiving benefit from the treatment," or, "When one member of the family is having a problem, we find that it helps to get the opinions of other family members about how to solve the problem. People who know and care about each other often have a lot to contribute to each other."

Another common type of resistance to convening the family is the fear of how other family members would respond to this request or to discussing sensitive or potentially painful issues openly. The contacting person may protest, "My parents could never stand to talk about these things. They would be too upset to discuss them!" or, "My children would be devastated if they discovered that I had emotional problems. What would they say if they learned that their mother was seeing a psychiatrist?" The request may also generate skepticism: "My husband would never agree to come in. He doesn't believe in psychiatry, and thinks I'm silly to come here." Therapists must recognize the deep-seated protective feelings that lie behind these responses and help the contacting person to deal with these feelings in a supportive manner. Therapists can reply, "Perhaps you are underestimating your parents' own need to discuss these problems. The opportunity to talk here might be a relief for them," or, "It might be helpful for your children to discover that their mother is a person, too, and can hurt. Kids often appreciate that in later life, when they become parents," or, "Would you be willing to ask your husband to come here? He might agree if he discovered that you were convinced that it would be good for both of you."

Logistical problems often arise in the first contact with a family member that complicate therapists' attempts to arrange a subsequent meeting with the family. Finding a convenient time for everyone to meet, arranging transportation and coping with financial and occupational pressures are all issues that the contacting person must undertake along with his or her family. Therapists, on the other hand, can facilitate this process by scheduling their hours flexibly, being aware of convenient transportation facilities to and from the office, and being willing to provide employers with medical releases that will allow family members to attend sessions that occur during work hours. Therapists must acknowledge that arranging a family interview does indeed involve sacrifices on everyone's part, but that these sacrifices may prove to be worthwhile if gathering the family together helps to resolve the problem more effectively.

In many cases, though the therapist deems it advisable, the contacting family member chooses not to invite his family to the next session. Therapists differ as to how they proceed in this situation. Some believe that it is destructive to see the person without first evaluating the family system, and they will refer the person to someone else. Other therapists agree to see the person individually, assuming either that the family may be brought in at a later time, or that they can effect change in the family system indirectly by working with one family member. Therapists must consider each of these situations on an individual basis; however, they should never agree to see the person without the family when this decision could have serious negative consequences, such as when symptoms erupt in a small child or when psychosis or suicide threatens the lives of any family members. *One wishes for therapists the wisdom to know when family participation is a necessity, the courage to press for it when it is, and the humility to take what they get.*

Specifying Conditions

When the therapist does obtain the agreement of the contacting family member to bring in his family, he must be careful to specify who should be present at the next session, and at what date and time. In many situations, these conditions are not made explicit, and the family may fail to return with a key member, or they may come at the wrong time, etc. Therapists do best to repeat their agreement with the contacting family person and to request confirmation once the details have been settled with the family. Specific dates and times can be offered here. By utilizing these and previously mentioned guidelines, therapists can best gain the confidence of the contacting family member and insure the likely participation of other family members in the subsequent evaluation.

References

Boszormenyi-Nagy, I., and Spark, G. *Invisible Loyalties: Reciprocity in Intergenerational Family Therapy.* New York: Harper and Row, 1973.

Clarkin, J. F., Francis, A. J., and Moodie, J. L. Selection Criteria for Family Therapy. *Family Process,* 1979, *18,* 391-404.

Haley, J. *Problem Solving Therapy.* San Francisco: Jossey-Bass, 1976.

ROBERT GARFIELD, M.D.
Assistant Professor and Director
Master's of Family Therapy Program
Department of Mental Health Sciences
Hahnemann Medical College & Hospital
Philadelphia, PA

2. Dealing with Common Resistances to Attending the First Family Therapy Session

Question:

A family was referred to me by a therapist who met with the family previously for two sessions. This referral raised some important questions for me regarding whom to include when starting family therapy. The information received from the referring therapist is as follows:

The family consists of a 56-year-old father, 54-year-old mother, and an oldest son, age 32, who is a hospitalized schizophrenic. There are also three other siblings—a male 28, a female 27 and the youngest, a female 20. These siblings live outside the family home but in the same geographical vicinity. The family was referred for therapy ostensibly because the parents, who have barred their schizophrenic son from the family home, are ineffective in enforcing this rule when he is out of the hospital. Moreover, the parents evidently give mixed messages and have on occasion subtly encouraged their son to come home. Most important is the fact that in the last session with the referring therapist, the son slapped his mother across the face.

I called the family home to make an initial appointment for the father, mother and schizophrenic son and talked with the father. On the day we were to meet, the father and son arrived without the mother. The father stated that the mother refused to attend the session because of the slapping incident, and moreover, that she was too emotionally fragile to attend sessions. The son was initially angry about his mother's absence, but later in our meeting agreed with the father's wishes to continue with father-son meetings in order to "improve our communication and have a safe place to talk with one another." I agreed to see them on this basis, but now I am feeling uncomfortable with this arrangement. My questions are as follows: How do you decide which family members to include in a first family therapy session? What do you do when only a part of the family arrives for a session? How do you get missing family members to attend when it appears that they are uninterested and/or unmotivated to participate?

Discussion:

It must be emphasized that you are asking whom to include in beginning family therapy when it is important to assess the family system. Who is included after you understand the system is another matter. In answer to your first question, the case you present is an excellent illustration of why, as a matter of policy, it is invaluable to insist that all family members attend a first session, even (or especially) if they do not currently live in the household. The referring therapist ought to have attempted to set this precedent. Some psychotherapists might take the stance that family therapy is not indicated when the patient is likely to become overwhelmed by negative affect to the point of assaulting a parent. The experience I have had with such patients, however, is that the schizophrenic offspring rarely becomes so overwhelmed *when other siblings are included in the sessions*. The presence of all family members is paramount and serves the following functions:

1) The focus, and thereby some pressure, are removed from the identified patient by initially defining the problem as involving every family member.
2) The identified patient is provided with the opportunity for support and validation from other siblings.
3) The therapist is afforded the opportunity to observe how the entire system functions, permitting more precise assessment of the nature of the problem.
4) The likelihood that a family member would unwittingly (accidentally) sabotage therapy can be decreased. Also, the therapist is in a better position to ascertain who in the family has the most vested in the status quo.
5) It is well known that when an identified patient's symptoms remit, another family member may become symptomatic. Inclusion of non-labeled siblings serves to prevent this from happening.
6) Nonpatient siblings sometimes form alliances with the therapist which can facilitate engaging all family members in the process of therapy.
7) The identified patient's "disturbed" behavior may seem congruent when observed in the whole family context. This can be invaluable

information for staff who work with the identified patient using other treatment modalities.

8) The presence of nonpatient siblings may diminish guilt and defensiveness on the part of parents, who all too often are adjudicated as "schizophrenogenic" by hospital staff and then treated accordingly.

Although it is speculative on my part, I would guess that had all siblings been present the patient would not have slapped his mother. For it appears to me, that father and son each had a stake in the mother's absence. I think the son bailed the father out by taking the responsibility for the mother's absence by slapping her and thereby providing his father with a "real" reason for excluding the mother. Please note that father and son wanted "a safe place" to communicate. Did they mean "safe" because of the therapist's presence or because the mother was absent, or both? The father and son were in collusion; the son acted out his own as well as his father's feelings. In the process, he protected his mother from risking therapy and provided both parents with an added bonus, mainly, an incident the marital couple could probably agree upon. When all family members are included in a first session, collusion to extrude other family members is more difficult to accomplish.

In this referral you were caught in a very common trap. You accepted the father's word that the mother refused to attend sessions and that her absence was appropriate. It is unwise to accept second-hand messages of this sort, for most often they are projections and/or distortions. You will find more often than not, that the "unwilling" family member will attend sessions if requested by the *therapist*. It is also not unusual for the unwilling family member to become an ally of the therapist. In this case, I would not have seen the father and son alone. Rather, I would have sent them home, making clear that I wanted to meet with the entire family, i.e., all siblings and the mother, and I would have told father-son that I would take responsibility for calling each of them. This results in presenting each family member with responsibility for his or her own behavior regarding attendance and makes collusion to exclude someone more difficult.

This does not completely answer the general question regarding what to do when some family members fail to show for a first or subsequent appointments. Some family therapists will work with whomever is willing to attend sessions. Their rationale is that the family system can be altered by influencing any part of the system. I believe that this is a matter of clinical judgment and will depend upon what you know about the specific family, when in the course of therapy this happens, how you assess the reasons for not showing, etc. However, at a first meeting in which all family members have agreed to attend, I would not see the family if one member does not show.

As for the question of how you get "unwilling" family members to attend sessions, this can sometimes be an arduous task, especially for the therapist who was trained in individual psychotherapy and who embraced family therapy as another viable treatment modality. In consulting with such therapists, I find that many feel ambivalent about the idea of phoning family members. Some therapists express that to do so feels like soliciting business or pleading with a patient to come for treatment. Also, phoning involves taking responsibility that should be the patients', and this runs counter to the way most psychotherapists are trained. I believe that this dilemma stems from thinking in terms of individual psychodynamics rather than systems. Specifically, the concepts of motivation and responsibility are not meaningful when the patient is the entire family. What does "responsible family" or "motivated family" mean?

I view therapists' reluctance actively to engage all family members in sessions as analogous to novice therapists' apprehensions about audiovisual recordings; most often, this is more the therapist's problem than the patient's problem. Teachers of psychotherapy know only too well that refusal for permission to videotape is most frequently provoked by the therapist's ambivalence. It is likely that the therapist's ambivalence about actively engaging all family members in sessions would be resolved by a paradigmatic shift in thinking from individual psychodynamics to systems. When the therapist calls, family members may certainly be resistant, and sometimes therapists unwittingly participate in the opposition by operating on the assumption that the family members must somehow define the problem as a family problem. Such an assumption is unnecessary and is likely to be communicated to the family member. This can provoke opposition because, in the clients' eyes, there is no family problem.

To answer your last question, let's discuss typical kinds of opposition one runs into when one calls family members in an effort to engage them in sessions, and how a therapist might deal with these.

1) "There is nothing wrong with this family or anyone in this family except (the labeled patient)." This is probably the most common reply when a therapist tries to get the whole family together. And it is pointless to argue the issue. I usually ask the family members whether, if it were possible, they would be willing to help their sibling, or mother

or father. This usually elicits an affirmative response. I then simply tell each person that his attendance at sessions will help me to help the patient and ask if he is willing to attend. If the family member is hesitant, I add something to the effect that he is a very important member of the family, that he knows a great deal about his family from his own unique perspective, and that, therefore, no one else can supply this perspective. It is rare to draw a "no" after this. In the few instances when this happens, I ask if he would be willing to come only once.

2) "I do not live in this family anymore." (Included here also would be, "I'm no longer part of this family" or "I have a family of my own.") Generally, I never argue the point; I usually agree and then redefine the stated circumstance as precisely why this person's presence at family sessions would be invaluable. For example, I might say, "The fact that you now have your own family means that you are the one person in a position to have a more objective view of your family than any other family member, and therefore, your presence would be invaluable."

3) "I'm too upset (angry, etc.) and I can't handle it." This is somewhat more difficult to deal with because the family member might be accurate. I would ask this family member what he/she thinks would happen in a session. Frequently, the therapist is in a position to allay some understandable fears, e.g., that expression of anger or hurt feelings would be hurtful and upsetting to another family member or to oneself. The reassurance that such expression is not expected and indeed might even be unwise is frequently sufficient to enlist attendance. The therapist does not lose any ground with this statement because it is rare that someone will volunteer something which they are reluctant to reveal. A therapist's sanction to withhold emotionally laden material or expression is disarming and is more likely to facilitate disclosure.

4) "How will talking about the problem in a family meeting help?" I would reply to this, "It may not help directly, but it might help me figure out what might be done that will help. But it will be more difficult to do this unless everyone attends the meeting."

5) "I hate them and refuse to come." Therapist: "Thanks very much for being so candid; you already have helped *me* because I had no idea that you felt that way." This usually elicits a response which leads to some dialogue. For example, when an angry adolescent persisted in refusing to attend sessions, I replied, "I was warned by your parents that you would be unreasonable but I told them that I understand young people and that if you were asked in a nice way, I would be surprised if you would refuse to attend." This adolescent complied, I

think, because I let him know that I knew his parents asked him in a way designed to provoke a negative response and also to flaunt that his parents were wrong. Sometimes telling a family member that he/she will probably be talked about, and that this offends the therapist's sense of fairness, will be sufficient to enlist cooperation.

6) "Why should I do something for them; they never did anything for me." Although this sounds like a simple refusal, when verbalized in this manner it is an invitation to the therapist to supply some face-saving reason for the family member to refrain from acting out the hurt feelings evident in this response. In this instance, a general strategy would involve reframing attendance "for your benefit and not your family's." To accomplish this will require engaging the person in a dialogue.

I want to emphasize that in general I do *not* like phone contact and am loath to talk with individual clients or family members on the phone once therapy has started. But it is far better to make this effort in starting therapy so that assessment and decision making can be based on firsthand information and direct observation rather than hearsay, collusion, etc. The precedent the phone calls set is easy to break.

It should be evident that the strategies discussed above have one common thread: Nothing is asked of family members other than attendance at a first meeting. The beginning family therapist might be apprehensive that nothing will happen when the family arrives for the first meeting, i.e., that reluctant family members will not talk about anything relevant. Herein is the beauty of working from a systems framework, because the interaction and process are important, not the content which family members choose to reveal. Moreover, the very fact that a family member protests about attending sessions indicates sufficiently strong affect, so that it is highly unlikely that this person will remain silent or fail to interact with others. Paradoxically, when several family members protest about attending sessions, it is more warranted for the therapist to be apprehensive that too much will happen too quickly. What one does once one has succeeded in engaging all family members in the first session is what family therapy is about.

SHELDON STARR, Ph.D.
*Chief, Family Therapy Training
and Education, VA Medical Center;
and Clinical Associate Professor
Department of Psychiatry and Behavioral
Science, Stanford Medical School
Palo Alto, CA*

3. Involving Resistant Family Members in Therapy

Question:

How can I get all the family members to be present for therapy? This is a question commonly asked regarding family treatment. The reluctance of the family to have all members present for therapy is often the manner in which the therapist experiences the first resistance to treatment. This resistance takes the form of members' absenting themselves from initial meetings, which tends to render the therapist ineffective. The difficulty can occur because the person making the initial contact has identified him/herself as the problem, or has been labeled "the problem" by other family members or social agencies. At times the other family members, for a multiplicity of reasons, refuse to participate in therapy. It then becomes the responsibility of the therapist to develop methods to gain access to the entire family and effectively begin the treatment process. The question remains: How can one gain access to the entire family without resorting to seeing members separately?

Discussion:

The personal philosophical orientation of the therapist is the main factor in involving all family members in therapy. This is more important than technical expertise or elaborate strategies. This means that the therapist must have a firm commitment to and understanding of a family systems model. The therapist must be firmly convinced that treatment cannot proceed unless all members are present and that therapy with anything less than the complete unit will be considered ineffective or irresponsible. This family orientation needs to be strongly conveyed to the person making the initial contact. If the therapist is not in control of this process, treatment will most likely be difficult.

Resistance will often be met at the initial phone conversation as the caller frequently asks to come to the first visit alone, and then have other members attend succeeding visits. This request needs to be handled firmly by refusing to meet the couple or family unless all the members you request to attend are present. This is necessary to avoid setting up a coalition with, or eliciting "family secrets" from, a single family member, which can have the effect of corrupting treatment. Seeing the person alone has the effect of perpetuating the myth that he/she is the problem, and thus continues a major family resistance.

To reiterate, most therapists who experience difficulties in this are not firmly committed to a family approach, and this is sensed by the family in the initial phone contact. The therapist must believe that it is all right to lose a family in treatment and refer them elsewhere rather than see isolated parts of the group. Some therapists are unconsciously more comfortable with an individual approach and breathe a sigh of relief when the family unit balks at treatment.

Many referral sources and agencies conceptualize problems in terms of individual dynamics, which makes it necessary for the family therapist to reframe the entire problem. The initial phone contact is the time to start redefinition of the problem as a family issue and to request that the family come in for at least the initial session. Often this request by the therapist is sufficient, and with a little urging the entire family will attend.

The manner in which the initial referral is handled can significantly affect the therapeutic outcome. When family members refuse to attend, an inquiry needs to be made as to the reason for the reluctance. At times it may be a resistance in the caller, while at other times resistance is found in other family members. The person making the request may only assume that other members would refuse to attend and needs to be urged to contact other members. Close questioning may reveal a covert defensiveness, that the caller does not want other members present. Each resistance, such as time problems, fears of involving other members and concerns about family secrets, needs to be dealt with in a supportive manner. This might mean reassurance that every secret need not be revealed. Often the initial caller needs to be urged to have a family meeting and confront other family members with the need to meet together. Sometimes the therapist may have to call other family members directly, though it is usually more effective to have the family rally itself for the visit rather than have the therapist take on the responsibility of calling individual members. Another method is an "impotence ploy" in which the therapist discusses his/her inability to assist the family unless all are present.

If resistance is pronounced at the initial phone encounter, the therapist can request the entire family to be present for at least one initial interview. It can be stated that the visit is for the therapist to better get acquainted with the family. Most families will accept a single visit to discuss the problem. This initial visit now becomes quite critical as the therapist must, in one session, assess the situation and determine how to involve the family in continuing treatment. In this initial session the therapist must make some emotional connection with each member to include all in the therapy. This means imparting a sense that they are all part of the family unit and that each, at least in some way, is affected by the problem and can aid in the solution. The family resistances need to be elicited and systematically dealt with for the family to wish to return. Once again, the commitment of the therapist to the family model is imperative since many resistances may seem quite reasonable to one trained in individual therapy.

A common resistance is the statement that the child or adult with the symptom is the sick one and that other family members are not involved in the situation. Often heard are, "I'm the one who is depressed, not my husband," or, "The school said my son is the problem, not me," or, "I could never talk with my wife present." In my experience, these individuals have some awareness of their complicity in the problem and further secrecy only clouds the issues. When the reluctant members appear for the first session, it is important to enlist their support for the process and stress their involvement for treatment to continue. Many times the resistant members will attend when asked to come in to protect their "interests." The therapist can let the family know that if only one member attends, a skewed view of family experiences is presented, since it represents only one viewpoint. The need for all members to be present is stressed to preserve "fairness."

An effective strategy is to ask members to be "family recorders" and help the therapist to understand the problem fully. They can be requested to take part as resource persons to allow all diverging views to be expressed. This approach enables all members to participate, while circumventing their fears of having "caused the problem." As therapy progresses, the participants begin to feel more comfortable and to contribute more willingly, accepting more responsibility for involvement. It is important to avoid coercing the family to accept systems concepts prior to dealing with resistances. This may mean accepting the family's definition of the problem until affinity can be approached.

Other strategies are necessary to involve a significantly resistant member. These can include a request for the resistant adolescent or adult to attend sessions, while being under no obligation to participate. The paradoxical technique of telling the resistant member not to talk, to read a book or just be present in the session, places no direct pressure on the person to contribute. It may take as long as eight sessions, but eventually fears can be allayed, leading to full participation. I have noted that silent members are closely attuned to the therapeutic process, and when a sensitive area is broached, they often forget their defensive stance and join in the process. A further strategy is to request the adolescent to become a "cotherapist" and "help" his/her parents with "their" problem. Thus, a therapeutic alliance can be forged to gain entrance to the reluctant family.

The resistant family is guarded and anxious and a prematurely interpreting therapist can frighten them from therapy. One commonly noted resistance appears when a family agrees by phone to have all members present, but at the initial interview one or more members are absent (often the critical people). It is important for the therapist to refuse to see this partial family and to cancel the meeting until all members can be present. In some resistant families, a home visit for the family to meet the therapist may prove beneficial. In this visit, family concerns need to be explored, and family support enlisted. The firm sense by the therapist that only an interview with the entire family is effective is primary. This position, which will not be compromised, may seem rigid, but it conveys both a strong commitment to the family approach and a concern for the well-being of the entire family.

MARTIN H. BAUMAN, M.D.
Assistant Clinical Professor of Psychiatry
Family Therapy Section
Langley-Porter Neuropsychiatric Clinic
University of California Medical School
San Francisco, CA

4. Engaging the Father in Family Therapy

Question:

One of the frequent problems I have encountered in family therapy is the failure of the father to become involved in treatment. Mothers usually request services and arrange appointments. Husbands reportedly cannot attend sessions for a variety of reasons: having to work, being out of town, or not believing that the family has a problem. What can the therapist do if the father does not attend family therapy sessions?

Discussion:

Fathers play an important role in family therapy attendance and outcome. Shapiro and Budman (1973) found that the father's attitude toward treatment is pivotal in determining whether a family remains in treatment. They concluded that "unless the father is positively involved, the treatment is likely to fail."

Cases in which the father is resistant to treatment are likely to have the following family structure: an overinvolved or enmeshed relationship between the mother and the child identified as the patient, an underinvolved or detached relationship between the father and the child, and a corresponding underinvolved relationship between the father and mother. In strategic family therapy with such a family structure (Haley, 1976), the first therapeutic goal is to increase the degree of involvement between the father and the child. The next therapeutic goal is to increase the involvement between the father and the mother. If such goals are accomplished, then the degree of involvement between the mother and child is likely to be reduced to a more appropriate level, thereby reducing the symptoms maintained by the overinvolved mother-child relationship. The father is pivotal in accomplishing these goals. His noninvolvement would severely handicap treatment progress.

Even in cases where the father is not living in the home due to divorce or separation, his involvement in family treatment is believed to be important (Leader, 1973). In such cases, the continuing conflict between the estranged parents and the lack of involvement between the noncustodial parent (typically the father) and the child usually are major factors responsible for the continuing maladjustment of the child or family (Kushner, 1965; Wallerstein and Kelly, 1977).

The engagement of a resistant father can be one of the more difficult problems in family therapy. Shapiro and Budman (1973) found that such engagement was a consistent problem encountered by beginning family therapists in their training program. The most effective time to deal with this problem is probably at the intake stage, when the family initially requests services. At this time it should be stressed that all family members attend the initial evaluation session. If such an expectation is clearly communicated, then the family will be more likely to comply (Hoehn-Saric et al., 1964). If resistances to the father's attending the evaluation are encountered, they are more easily handled at this time than later. For example, one of the most common reasons given for the father's inability to attend is that he cannot take time off from work. After this is explored, an appointment time consistent with the father's work schedule can be offered. In dealing with such resistance at the intake stage, it is important to convey the message that the father's attendance is crucial to the family's benefitting from clinical services.

If the family does not comply with the expectation that the father attend, then the reasons for noncompliance should be explored early during the evaluation session. In one such case, I asked the mother, "Your husband was unable to attend?" after making introductions. She replied that she had divorced her husband the previous day. She began talking about her marital problems, and then related these to her son's behavioral problems which prompted her to seek treatment. By initially asking about the father's absence I was able to elicit important dynamic material early in the session and to keep the child's behavior problems in the perspective of the underlying marital and family problems. As with most other cases I have encountered, the father's absence was an important diagnostic sign which was profitable to explore.

After exploring the reasons for the father's absence, I typically emphasize the importance of his involvement by asking the mother, "How can we arrange the next session so that he can attend?" This question poses a challenge to many mothers, especially those who are ambivalent about their husband's being involved in the treatment. In many cases the mother will take the initiative to see that her husband attends the next session. His failure to attend would be further dynamic material to explore. Such failure usually means that the mother does not want her husband to attend so that discussion of important marital and parental issues can be avoided.

If the father fails to attend following this intervention, I then consider making the suggestion that I contact him myself to invite him to attend. In making this contact, I am aware that a noninvolved father is likely to feel threatened by my relationship with his wife and children. He may feel that I am allied with other family members against him. To minimize the impact of such suspicions, I generally tell such a father that I would like to know his views of his child's problems so that I can better understand his child and family. I appeal to his role as an expert, and downplay his having a role as a patient.

My goal in contacting the father is to persuade him to attend one session. In one session, hopefully I will engage his active involvement, or at the very least, I should obtain his tacit permission for treatment to continue. To accomplish this, I usually try to keep this session as nonthreatening to the father as possible, by actively listening to his views and by keeping the focus on the child's problems. I keep in mind that once engaged, the father will be more open to dealing with important dynamic issues.

References

Haley, J. *Problem-Solving Therapy*. San Francisco: Jossey-Bass, 1976.

Hoehn-Saric, R., Frank, J. D., Imber, S. D., Nash, E. H., Stone, A. R., and Buttle, C. C. Systematic preparation of patients for psychotherapy: I. Effects on therapy behavior and outcome. *Journal of Psychiatric Research*, 1964, *2*, 267-281.

Kushner, S. The divorced, noncustodial parent and family treatment. *Social Casework*, 1965, *10*, 52-58.

Leader, A. L. Family therapy for divorced fathers and others out of the home. *Social Casework*, 1973, *54*, 13-19.

Shapiro, R. J. and Budman, S. H. Defection, termination and continuation in family and individual therapy. *Family Process*, 1973, *12*, 55-67.

Wallerstein, J. S. and Kelly, J. B. Divorce counseling: A community service for families in the midst of divorce. *American Journal of Orthopsychiatry*, 1977, *47*, 4-22.

THOMAS GAINES, JR., Ph.D.
Assistant Professor
Department of Psychiatry
University of Texas Health
Science Center
San Antonio, TX

5. Involving the Reluctant Father
   in Family Therapy

Question:

> In the last few years, my agency has become committed to the
> family therapy approach for treating the emotional and behav-
> ioral problems of children. This means that we want to involve
> the whole family in therapy sessions. Unfortunately, we some-
> times find it difficult to get fathers to participate. We have tried
> various approaches to involving reluctant fathers, with only par-
> tial success. Sometimes we proceed without the father if the prob-
> lem is urgent. We could use some suggestions or strategies for
> dealing with the reluctant father.

Discussion:

You have identified one of the central practical issues in family therapy—how to get fathers to participate in family sessions. In the father's
mind, there may be many "good" reasons not to participate. (Just as
in the past there were "good" reasons why therapists kept him out!)
For example, he may view the problem as the child's, not his own. He
may believe that mother should handle the kids' problems. The time
of the sessions may be inconvenient, the thought of going to a "shrink"
scary, or the idea of displaying the family's dirty linen repugnant.
Furthermore, his wife may have her own reasons for being certain that
he would never go to family therapy—for example, because he is never
involved with the children and doesn't understand their problems;
because nobody would talk openly around him; and because he may
try to impose his solutions on the family. My point is that there may
be powerful resistance on the part of *both* parents (as well as the
children) to the father's participation in family therapy.

 The first hurdle for the family therapist in dealing with this issue
is a conceptual one, namely, to view therapy as beginning, not with
the first session, but with the initial phone call from a family member,
often the mother. In an agency, the first "therapist" who encounters
the family is usually the person who schedules appointments. If the

agency is committed to working with the whole family, then the appointment scheduler should convey this policy in a matter-of-fact way to the caller. Similarly, agency staff should make referral sources clearly aware of this policy. In my experience in a youth services agency, when the telephone intake staff member treated the father's participation as "automatic," there was little resistance. I have had the same experience in private practice when I handle the initial call myself. Any fudging about "wanting" to have the whole family, or explaining that everyone in the family is part of the problem, tends to lower compliance. On this last issue of explaining the entire-family policy, the father is probably scared enough without his wife telling him that the agency says he is part of the problem and must attend the meetings. In sum, I think the most important strategy for involving fathers is simply to have an unambivalent policy on the issue and to convey this policy clearly and nondefensively to parents at the first therapeutic contact, usually on the telephone.

What if this does not work? Let's say that mother calls back with the news that her husband refuses to come. Normally, my advice is to refuse to work with the family until mother can get father to participate. My usual assumption is that the mother has enough power over her husband to persuade him to join her in therapy—if she chooses to exercise this power. Her unwillingness to press the issue may signal her own ambivalence about getting the kind of help that might change the family system. In this case, to allow her to control the terms of therapy would undermine the goals of therapy. In a general sense, my view is that the *family* is withholding a key member, and that the therapist is often wise to stand firm and wait out the family's resistance. This strategy seems especially appropriate for chronic problems around which the family has been stabilized for a long time, since postponing intervention is not apt to be dangerous and the family is forced to confront their level of motivation for serious change.

In an acute emergency situation, e.g., the possibility of family violence or suicide, a different approach may be needed if father will not attend the first session. One approach I may take is to telephone the father and make a personal appeal to him as an important member of the family without whom my hands will be tied in helping the child. This strategy often works. Alternatively, I may schedule the first therapy session and place the burden on mother to get her husband there; but in this emergency situation I am willing to conduct the first session without the father if he refuses to attend. These approaches are also useful in nonemergency or chronic cases if the therapist decides not to take the hard-line of refusing to see the family without the father's presence.

What if the family, despite my most ingenious efforts, shows up for the first session *sans* father? The therapy now centers around getting the father to the next session. I think it is a mistake to convey the sense to the family that we will muddle along without father if we have to. Once again, there are a number of different approaches one might take, depending on the specific family. One approach consists of using the therapeutic alliance established in the first session as leverage in persuading the mother to work much harder to move her husband. In fact, both parents may have been waiting for the mother to get a sense of what the therapist is like before committing themselves to therapy. If the mother thinks that the therapist is OK, then she may get serious about involving the father. Similarly, after one session without him, the father may realize that the die is cast (the mother may have been threatening therapy for years) and that he had better represent his own interests in the sessions. A second, complementary approach is to telephone the father after the first session with a special invitation like the one mentioned above. With one family, when I learned from the mother that the father had expressed fears of being verbally attacked in front of his children, I offered to meet once with him and his wife alone; if he didn't like what happened or if he still feared being attacked, then he was free not to return. He came and stayed.

Suppose that despite these strategies, the father remains *in absentia* for the second session, with no prospect for ever joining the therapy. Now we have a therapeutic crisis. I would be very reluctant to continue therapy under these circumstances. If the presenting problems are chronic and the family is reasonably stabilized, then I would be likely to terminate therapy, with the invitation to resume when the whole family was willing to participate. On the other hand, if the problems are acute and health threatening, or if the family is very unstable (e.g., parents are on the verge of a break-up), then I would continue to work with the family. One of the central issues for discussion with the mother would be whether she wants to stay married to a man who will not help the family during a severe crisis. On this point, Jay Haley once described a case in which the reluctant father was heavily implicated in the serious problems of his adolescent daughter. Haley's strategy for involving the father: The therapist directed the mother to tell her husband that she would divorce him if he did not attend the next session. He showed up with his tie on straight and his suit neatly pressed. This example may appear extreme and risky, but Haley points out that the stakes were high.

To conclude, I want to emphasize that the key to involving reluctant fathers in family therapy is the therapist's (and the agency's) expectation that fathers will participate. Stated differently, when the therapist believes that of course the father will attend (although it may take a little persuading or pressuring), then that therapist is apt, in my view, to have little problem with absent fathers. Conversely, therapists are likely to have difficulties in this area if they are timid or inconsistent in demanding fathers' presence. *The therapist's control over who participates in family therapy sessions is the* sine qua non *of successful outcome.* It would be nice if we had good empirical data to support this last statement, but even without such data I think that this is as close to being a therapeutic axiom as we have in our field. Be firm.

WILLIAM J. DOHERTY, Ph.D.
Assistant Professor
Department of Family Practice
University of Iowa
Iowa City, IA

6. Involving the Peripheral Father in Family Therapy

Question:

Frequently the request for therapy comes by way of a phone call or walk-in by the mother, who is terribly concerned about her child or children. Or it might eventuate from a referral from school, court or medical personnel. When an appointment is offered and the mother is told it is necessary for the entire family to attend the initial session, it is not unusual for her to respond, "My husband won't come."

How does the therapist intervene to insure the father's attendance? Once the father does agree to come, and arrives, how can his resistance to participating be overcome? What if he agrees to come, and then the rest of the family arrives without him?

Discussion:

When a wife tells me her husband will not come, I immediately reiterate my earlier statement that it is essential. There can be no equivocating if the therapist is to be perceived as being sufficiently knowledgeable and powerful to be of help. I'll explore why she thinks he won't come and initially deal with the concrete reason she presents. If it is, "He is too busy," I will ask when he is likely to be available and offer to set the appointment at his convenience, even if it is an unusual day or hour, for the first session only. If her answer is, "He is not interested," or, "He has no time for shrinks," or, "He thinks I should handle the children's problems," and she remains adamant about his unwillingness to attend, I am likely to assume she has a vested interest in excluding him, and that this is apt to be a dynamic family pattern. At that point, my next move may be to ask her permission to contact him directly. Such a request has yet to be denied, although sometimes it requires a good deal of persuasion.

A phone call to the husband usually proceeds as follows:

Th.: Mr. X, this is Dr. K. As you may know, your wife has contacted

27

me for an appointment to discuss her concerns about your son, Jerry. She tells me you are quite busy, but *I am sure you are also interested in your son's well-being* (school work, health or whatever the presenting problem appears to be) and I wanted you to know *how important your participation is.* As a matter of fact, I will not be able to be of much assistance without your input and collaboration.

Mr. X: Well, it will be difficult, but if we can find a suitable time, I'll try to manage. . . . Yes, of course I care about my son!

This reaching out to the father in a way that supports his commitment to his child, which at some level he has, and that establishes the father's importance, thereby including him in the family and building his sense of self-esteem, is hard to resist. It is much more likely to succeed at least in arousing his curiosity about the caller, and possibly beginning to enlist his cooperation, than is an approach that attempts to pressure or shame him into coming in. This "seduction" can be used by therapists of either sex and tends to be irresistible when used in the service of engaging or re-engaging the peripheral father in the family and its treatment. Whitaker (1973) put it succinctly, "If you don't seduce the father in the first interview, you've had it." Such an intervention also sets the groundwork for utilizing therapeutic double binds later, if necessary.

When this kind of family arrives for the initial session, I welcome them and ask everyone to introduce him/herself, telling me their name and age and what they do, that is, kind of work or grade in school. We proceed around the circle, usually with my asking the person on one side of me to begin, so that no power issues surface too quickly. In having everyone speak in the first 10 minutes of the session, I have an opportunity to hear the voice tone and observe the way in which they present themselves orally. It also provides the family with a chance to settle in gradually and get acclimated. Meanwhile, they sense that this is a place where everyone will have a turn to talk and be heard and the therapist can scan how each reacts to all the others' self-introductions. Next, in order to engage the father in the therapy and reinforce my earlier communiqué about my perception of his importance, I will probably say, "Mr. X, can you tell me what brings you and your family here today?" (By contrast, when the "peripheral father" is not a factor, I will raise this question without directing it to anyone special, and assess who answers first as part of the diagnostic data being collected.)

Rapidly, the children take notice that someone in authority is turning to Dad for some information and considers what he thinks to be worthwhile. If he has been extruded from a mother/son or mother/children coalition, this directed intervention begins to disrupt the pattern of mother being pivotal. If he has been passive and ineffective, it forces him to be more active. If Mom plunges in to answer, one can say, "I know that you are glad your husband arranged to come and since you wanted him to be involved, let's hear what he has to say first. Then we'll all want to know your thoughts on the subject." Here, the therapist is doing some restructuring of the power balance while identifying with mother's spoken wish to have her husband do more. One is supporting the positive side of her ambivalence, the wish for her husband to be a more involved and concerned father and husband who shares responsibilities, while being aware of the other aspect of her ambivalence, the desire to keep him peripheral so that she can criticize him for his neglect and maintain her control of the children and her niche as ostensibly favorite parent.

Usually I'll be sitting by this time between the mother and the identified patient, so that both will feel the rudiments of an alliance with me. And I'll be facing the father, showing genuine interest in his comments. Most men, especially those who have been denigrated by their wives and disparaged or disobeyed by their children, defrost with the flattery of attentive listening and respect for their ideas and feelings. In behaving this way, the therapist is also modeling a different way of relating which hopefully will gradually have a ripple effect as others test out the possibility of emulating it.

If Mom begins to get uncomfortable and starts to complain about how overburdened she is, that she practically raises the kids alone, that her husband is too busy or too disinterested, the therapist should sympathize with how difficult this must be for her and compliment her on what a fine job she has done, alluding to whatever accomplishments are obvious and the positives in the family that have been described. The therapist must avoid fighting with Mom or seeming to compete with her, since to topple her strength is to undo the glue holding the family together without yet being able to replace it with a healthier cohesive form. At this juncture I will usually say something about the good prospect for Dad's beginning to pitch in more, thereby relieving her of some of this huge burden, in a way reflecting back that exactly what she seems to be asking for may happen. By being empathic with this part of the mother's cry for help in handling the problems, I diminish the risk of alienating her while continuing to seduce Dad into deciding there will be some benefit for him in attending these sessions. One cannot dethrone the Queen (mother) while putting the exiled King (father) into the other seat of power. It requires skillful maneuvering

since, if the father does not become engaged in the therapy in the first
session, he is not like to return (Le Fave, 1980), and if the mother is
antagonized, she will refuse to come back. Thus one begins to shape
a new, delicate balance quickly, hoping both will be sufficiently intrigued and will derive enough of a realization that their deeply entrenched and unsatisfactory patterns might be disrupted in therapy
to really make a positive difference in their lives, that the therapist
is indeed a powerful enough expert or healer to help them find a better
way to fashion their lives and the relationships within the family
system. If all goes well, by the end of the session I indicate, if it is true,
that I hope they will decide to enter treatment as a family unit as I
think there is a good chance we could accomplish quite a bit together
and ask if all are willing to agree to further sessions. If they are
uncertain, I will tell them to discuss it among themselves and ask Dad
when the next day it will be convenient for him to call me and let me
know their decision. About 95% of the time he follows through and the
answer is in the affirmative.

When everyone has agreed to come for the initial session, and then
they show up minus Dad, I indicate that this is contrary to our agreement and I wonder aloud how this could have happened, conveying at
the outset my expectation that commitments made are bonafide contracts and people are responsible for keeping their word. I will usually
see them briefly, focusing on Dad's absence. This emphasis is heightened by adaptation of the gestalt technique of using an empty chair
for the missing father. I ask them whether he really is a member of
this family, and if so, what his absence means to them. We consider
what it means to be a member of a family unit and how it feels when
any member of the group decides not to be involved. I may use an
analogy to a football team that forfeits if one player does not show up,
or to an orchestra that does not sound whole unless each instrument
required for a symphony is represented, depending on which kind of
metaphor the family will grasp best. Then I will describe my role as
coach or conductor, indicating that I will only be able to do my job if
all are present. I have them talk to the absentee father in the empty
chair; they may express hurt, anger, understanding or futility, or plead
with him to care. Then I'll suggest they go home and share what has
transpired with him, offer another appointment telling them that it
will not be held unless father comes along next time. He invariably
does, even if only to tell his side of the story—and usually because
they tell him he was missed so much and is important to them.

It does help immensely if the therapist has made peace with his/her own personal and professional fathers and believes they were/are important.

References

Le Fave, K. Correlates of engagement in family therapy. *Journal of Marital and Family Therapy*, 1980, *6*, 75-81.
Whitaker, C. *The Technique of Family Therapy.* Ackerman Memorial Address, Family Institute of Philadelphia Annual Conference, 1973.

FLORENCE W. KASLOW, Ph.D.
Professor, Department of Mental Health Sciences
Hahnemann Medical College
Philadelphia, PA

7. Involving Latency and Preschool Children in Family Therapy

Question:

How can one minimize the problems and maximize the benefits of including latency and preschool children in family therapy sessions?

Discussion:

1) Have an office layout and play materials which make it possible for family members to work all together at once or in separate subgroups.

I shall describe an ideal work area even though most family therapists will not have the means or motivation necessary to incorporate many elements of it into their own office space. This ideal arrangement includes separate areas for discussion, play, observation and time-out. See diagram below.

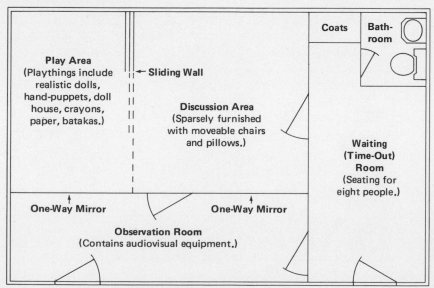

The discussion area should contain little except pillows big enough for sitting on and chairs light enough to be easily moved around. The play area should be separated from the discussion area by a sliding wall which can vary the degree to which the two spaces are hidden from one another. The play area should contain only play materials whose use is likely to be intelligible to both adults and children. For example, it should have dolls and hand puppets which represent typical family members rather than darts or trucks. It is easier for everyone to understand what it might mean when a child smashes the mother puppet into the father puppet than when he bangs two trucks together. The observation room should have audio and video equipment which can be operated both from that room or remotely from the play or discussion areas. The time-out space should be cut off visually and acoustically from the other spaces. Many waiting rooms can serve this purpose. This complex of spaces allows for everyone to work together in one space but also permits various combinations of physical, visual and acoustic isolation of family subgroups.

2) Have a versatile cotherapist.

Two therapists can form a powerful unit when working with all family members together but can also lead and coordinate separate activity in subgroups. Ideally, each therapist has skill working one-to-one with children and adults but can also conduct groups containing individuals of all ages. It is essential that these therapists can help all family members feel engaged and understood.

3) Offer explicit ground rules, especially about limit-setting.

The following rules are recommended:

a) That everyone cooperate to prevent physical injury.
b) That the parents are responsible for the protection and discipline of young children except when these children are in different spaces from the parents. In that case, the therapist who is with the children is responsible.
c) During the session, no one ever has to answer any question put to him/her. "I don't want to answer," or, "I don't know" are always acceptable responses.
d) During the session, no one ever has to follow any therapist suggestion except those which are specifically directed at maintaining safety.

e) After the session, no one is to be punished for anything said or done
during the session.

It is important that whatever ground rules one uses are stated explicitly in a language comprehensible to anyone over the age of three.
It is also important that the goal of the session(s) be explained.

*4) Try to actively engage the children in whatever diagnostic explora-
tion or treatment objectives are being pursued.*

If the therapist is exploring history, latency children can be engaged
by asking them to play out for the therapist events they have heard
about or can remember. Such children are likely to transmit richer
historic information through play than through verbal description.
Two types of play may be used. Children can play psychodramatically:
They can set up and act out scenes using family members to play
themselves or others. Children can also portray past events by using
dolls or hand puppets. Before asking children to use toys to depict
history, one might say: "*Real play* is using toys to show things just the
way they happened; *make believe play* is using your imagination. Right
now I would like you to stick to *real play*." Children can play and
rehearse such performances in the play area with one therapist, while
complex data of the remote past are collected from parents in the
discussion area. Later, when all get together, the children can play
their scenes for the parents and the parents can portray for the children
a few key events from the past which might be useful for the children
to see.

When therapists are exploring the patterns of current interaction,
it is essential for them to engage simultaneously all family members
who live together. Generally the whole family is given a task which
the therapist observes in order to determine the dysfunctional elements
of family conduct and structure. The family may be asked to plan a
picnic together, to discuss among themselves the presenting problem,
or to get on the floor and play a game that involves everyone. It is
essential for the therapists not to join in this sample of family interaction.

When therapists are exploring how each member of the family sub-
jectively experiences the family, children can be actively engaged by
using family sculpting, kinetic family drawings or make-believe with
dolls or hand puppets. Such play should be highly directed by therapists. One might say: "These are the members of a family just like
yours. Show me what they do." One should avoid: "Here are toys that
you can play with."

When the therapeutic objective is for the family to understand itself better, the effects are stronger if the children as well as the adults gain in awareness of their history, the current interaction and their separate subjective experiences. The therapists can offer historical insight by retelling the family history in a story which shows both grown-ups and children how their current predicament is the result of events and forces from the past. The therapists can help family members become aware of how they interact by playing back short segments of videotape or by asking a family member to get behind the one-way mirror. The therapists can enhance empathic awareness of one family member for another by asking them to switch roles with one another, a technique which many latency age children can manage.

If the therapeutic objective is to transform family conduct and structure through the use of directives, it is valuable to have the whole family involved in order to see and shape the impact of such instructions on family behavior. When a directive is given to be carried out at home, it is more effective if every family member is present to be given a specific chore in the overall family task.

When a therapeutic objective is to use the therapists as models for identification, the presence of all members is helpful in order for therapists to show how a parent might treat a child, how a child might treat a parent, how grown-ups can disagree constructively about children, etc.

This discussion was designed to offer suggestions for use with most of the family therapy approaches which prevail today, except for those which purposefully avoid the active inclusion of children.

RICHARD CHASIN, M.D.
Assistant Clinical Professor of Psychiatry
Harvard Medical School
Assistant Clinical Professor of Child Psychiatry
Boston University School of Medicine
Faculty, Family Institute of Cambridge
Cambridge, MA

8. Helping Parents Get Resistant Adolescents into Family Therapy

Question:

Very often my first patient contact is with a dismayed parent who calls about the behavior of an adolescent in the family. Often prompted by events at school or a minor infraction of the law, the parent reports a variety of management problems and concludes that the adolescent and/or the family needs help. Once it appears that an appointment needs to be set up, the parent then reports that there is no way to get the "reluctant" adolescent in for treatment. The usual complaint is, "He won't come," or, "He's bigger than I am," or, "He'll run away." The parent often comes across as helpless and overwhelmed. Are there strategies or techniques available for getting the rebellious or defiant adolescent to join the family in treatment, or at least to get him or her in as part of a family evaluation? What should one say to the parent on the phone and what stance should one take about seeing the family without the adolescent?

Discussion:

While there are clearly no hard and fast rules for bringing reluctant adolescents into an evaluation or therapy program, a number of relevant issues often arise which can lead to specific therapeutic interventions.

Experience has taught that the crucial period upon which the success or failure of an intervention depends, such as the one under discussion, occurs with the initial phone call. Particularly when the identified patient is an adolescent, it is often useful for the therapist to make the appointment with the family directly, rather than involving a third party such as a secretary or clerk. It should be made very clear to the parent that all members of the family are to attend; assistance can be offered by assuring that as a parent he or she can insist on a son's or daughter's attendance.

Some family therapists would not meet with a family who showed up without all members present when the initial telephone agreement stipulated such attendance. I disagree with this position because it sets up a dogmatic stance on an issue that may underlie much of the family's pathology. Without a thorough knowledge of the dynamics underlying the absenteeism, it seems premature to set such a rule. If the parent had sufficient control of the situation to get the youngster to the session, chances are the family would not need to come in, in the first place. But often, there are other motivations for "leaving" the identified patient at home.

One family frankly admitted that it was a relief to have the family together for a discussion without the disturbing influence of the identified patient. They felt that they could talk more easily and share their frustrations more openly without the hostile and provocative responses of their oldest boy. It is apparent that, at least in some cases, family members are ambivalent about whether they want the identified patient at the family meeting initially.

Another situation which often contributes to the reluctance of an adolescent to attend a meeting has to do with subtle sabotage by one or more family members, usually a parent, due to a fear of 1) an alteration of a delicate family balance caused by the press of a variety of marital or other family issues, or 2) the adolescent making public an embarrassing event or family secret. For example, in one family it became apparent that the father had rather mixed feelings about his daughter coming to the sessions; while he wanted help for her and the family, he feared she would reveal that he had struck her on several occasions after losing his temper. His guilt and embarrassment at his own behavior led him to deliver mixed messages about the need for his daughter's attendance at the session. Other issues such as alcoholism, incest and a variety of unspoken family fears can also contribute to a parent's collusion with an adolescent son or daughter. Such fears often relate to a reworking of family relationships following the increased autonomy of the maturing adolescent and the resulting impact on the parents' marriage. As long as the focus remains on the adolescent, these other issues cannot easily be dealt with.

There are two simultaneous techniques that need at least to be considered given this situation. The first is to ask what family function is being served by the adolescent's absence. This may take a session or two to explore but the focus should stay with the issue of the absenteeism in an effort to diffuse the family's resistance. A detailed explanation of this process in the therapy of schizophrenia has been presented by Sonne et al. (1962). So while the therapist agrees to see the family without the adolescent, on a limited basis, the focus on the family's maneuver and its meaning is emphasized. Second, if the therapist feels that there is a clear manipulation going on, with a resulting power struggle between the parents and the therapist, then more direct actions need to be undertaken. This situation arises when 1) it is clear that the parents want the therapist to take over the parenting and the responsibility for the adolescent during the sessions, at which time they will become competitive, angry, and will join the adolescent against the therapist; 2) a crisis of sufficient magnitude is developing that a family meeting needs to occur for some prompt decision making; or, 3) the family's resistance cannot be shaken by other methods.

One technique which can be very effective is for the therapist to refuse the parent role altogether and to firmly but supportively tell the parents that it is crucial that *they* get their youngster to the meeting. They are told that success depends on how far they want to go to reach these ends. With apparent seriousness, the extreme is stated, "If need be, you can arrange for an ambulance with a police escort." Without being sure whether or not the therapist is serious, the parents get the point that they have the power as adults to act and that there are specific methods at their disposal should they wish to use them. Next, some practical suggestions are given along with support, for example: "Remember he/she is only 15 years old"; "If need be, a neighbor or family member could assist in getting the youngster into the car"; "You could pick up the youngster right from school and avoid a late return from the school bus," etc.

The parental response is frequently the same, "But we don't want to get him/her here by force, we want him/her to want to come in." One response to this paradoxical ploy (Selvini-Palazzoli et al., 1978) is, "First things first; you have stated that it is important for him/her to be here, so as competent parents you need to decide how to get him/her in. We shall worry about the next issue later." An appointment time is then rather abruptly arranged, leaving the responsibility and the decision making to the parents.

If the issue of family resistance has been touched upon, and if some rapport and sense of support have been offered, in the vast majority of cases the reluctant adolescent is found in the waiting room along with his or her family at the appointed hour. In addition, in most cases no heavy-handed force has been required. Surprisingly, while hesitant, shy and somewhat uncertain, the youngster, previously described as a 6'5" fullback, is often slight of build and very cooperative and helpful in the family session. What was required was 1) an undermining of the family's resistance and 2) a statement by the therapist that takes the parents' expressed wishes for the adolescent's attendance at face value.

As an additional point, it can be helpful not to mention anything about the youngster's previous absence or anything about the difficulty in getting him/her to attend. Such comments often embarrass or criticize. Rather, the session might begin by welcoming all members, bringing people up to date on what had occurred in previous meetings, if any, and continuing with the therapeutic process. By beginning the session in another direction, the therapist diffuses the resistance and focuses on other more fruitful areas of discussion.

References

Selvini-Palazzoli, M., Boscolo, L., Cecchin, G., and Prata, G. *Paradox and Counterparadox*. New York: Jason Aronson, 1978.

Sonne, J. C., Speck, R. V., and Jungris, J. E. The absent member maneuver as a resistance in family therapy of schizophrenia. *Family Process*, 1962, *1*, 44.

LAWRENCE FISHER, Ph.D.
Associate Professor
Department of Psychiatry
University of California, San Francisco
Medical Education Program
Veterans Administration Medical Center
Fresno, CA

9. Convening the Family for Experiential Family Therapy

Question:

> Within an existential/experiential family therapy model, who and how many family members need to be present for therapy?

Discussion:

Anyone familiar with the history and development of family therapy is aware that opinions range widely on who and how many members of a family must be present to make family therapy work. As Gurman and Kniskern (1978) commented in their recent review of marital and family therapy:

> Given the division of opinion within the family field noted earlier with regard to who should be treated in systems therapy, a most important issue that must be addressed in future research involves identification of the conditions under which two-generational (parents and children) and one-generational (marital dyad) therapies maximize outcomes for both the IP and the system-as-a-whole. To date, not a single study has addressed this matter of major theoretical and practical significance.

Thus, at this time, there exists no scientific basis for determining who should be present. Any rules can only come out of theoretical assumptions and clinical experience. I will give some rules of thumb which I have found useful and in line with experiential theoretical assumptions. Furthermore, I hope to sensitize therapists to the variety of subtle real life nuances that interplay in the clinical situation, resulting in variations of these general rules.

From an experiential perspective (e.g., Whitaker and Keith, 1981), I view the change process in family therapy as usually starting from the *inter*personal *experience* that one has in the therapy room. I assume that the larger the relevant interpersonal world one collects in the room, the greater the chance of making an impact that might resonate throughout the system and touch the individuals within it. The basic rule is: Get as many people into the therapy room as you can! Always push for the largest number of people possible. For example, having four complete generations in the room allows a much greater opportunity to create change or movement in the system than working with parts of one or two generations. I have never seen a negative result from too many people or generations.

The importance of large numbers has been noted by many theorists. From a diagnostic view, one has an opportunity to see patterns that might not be apparent with fewer people present. Laing (1979) has said that the greater the number of family members present, the greater the chance of the therapist seeing the "basic rhythms of the family dance and assessing the current cacophony," and Bowen (1976) writes, "This distant drumbeat is often obscured by the noisy insistence of the foreground drumbeat, but it is always there, and it tells its own clear story to those who can tune out the noise and keep focused on the distant drumbeat." Our experience is that this "distant drumbeat" becomes amplified louder and louder as one increases the number of family members present.

It is easier to clarify and change patterns in the larger system and then work with the subsystems and perhaps, if necessary, the individuals involved. Often, changing the large system dysfunction clears up subsystem problems. Thus, for example, I would rather deal earlier with a repetitive three- (or more) generational pattern of divorce, and only later deal, if necessary, with specific sexual dysfunction with a couple in a given generation. Working on the three-generational divorce motif might, in this example, clear up the dyadic sexual dysfunction and make further intervention around this issue unnecessary.

Another disadvantage of working with subsystems is that by starting with smaller systems you often form loyalty bonds which make it later impossible to expand upwards into larger systems. Common problems in this regard are seen when an individual therapist tries to switch to family therapy or when a family therapist working with a parent-child dyad later asks the other parent to join.

Although I will always push for as large a system as possible, I almost always have to settle for some compromise with the family. This is because family members are hesitant to make themselves vulnerable and will, on some level, fight to keep their pain out of the therapeutic setting. There have been many rules of thumb for pointing out how to make this compromise. These vary from: "Start with everyone living under the same roof" to, "Start with everyone who gets initially defined as being part of the problem," to, "Start with two complete generations." We think that in general these rules make sense and to a large extent overlap. It is best to begin with complete generations. We would perhaps more easily compromise on breaking the sibling generation than on breaking the parental generation. Both parents *always* seem critical to working in family therapy, while occasionally it seems possible to start without a married child or one living far from home. However, there is a significant literature on the "absent member maneuver" which postulates that even the absence of a seemingly innocuous member of the family system is often a way of the family short-circuiting the therapy process.

If viewed as a game of poker, the decision of the therapist to require specific family members to be present is equivalent to "at how much to set the ante" when starting the poker game. In order to allow the family to participate in the "game" of family therapy, the "ante" can't be so high as to cause them to "fold" (such as requiring that all members of four generations meet for therapy every week). At the same time, it is not worth the therapist's, or the family's, time to "play" if the stakes are so low that no amount of playing would really create significant change. The therapist can usually "up the ante" in a crisis situation because of the family's vulnerability and obvious need for help. For example, a mother and father brought their 17-year-old daughter into our office because of their concern about her increasing alcoholism and sociopathic behavior. She had two recent run-ins with the legal system that really activated her parents' anxiety. The parents did not even hesitate to respond to our request to have their other two children living up to 500 miles away join us for a three-hour family session early the following week.

Occasionally, the ante is set at the minimum level that the therapist feels is necessary for therapy to succeed and even this might be too high for the family. For instance, a family might balk at the demand for an asymptomatic daughter to join in the sessions. I feel it is better to lose some families rather than feel that I have to work with every case that contacts us. Inability to engage a family in therapy on our terms is not a treatment failure. Rather, it is the result of an intricately negotiated process with the family on the appropriateness and necessity of therapy at that given time. To change requires the family taking a risk: Their fear is that things might change for the worst. At a given time in the family's life cycle, their refusal to accept our terms might merely mean that they are not desperate enough to risk change. I feel that it is better to not attempt therapy that doesn't have a reasonable chance of succeeding. If and when the family wants to risk change enough, they will then meet our terms.

Specific Issues: Age and Distance

Perhaps the most frequent objection that the family raises is not to include members who are "too young" or "too old." Concerns vary from, "The children shouldn't hear this; it'll make them upset," to, "My mother is too old; she'll have another stroke." There are many reasons to include everyone, particularly the very young and very old.

From a tactical point of view, as I said earlier, it is much easier to start with a larger group and get smaller than vice versa. Including the children allows a much wider range of options in actual family therapy work. These include using the children as cotherapists, directing interventions to them, making indirect interpretations to the children about the family or parents that they can't deny, etc.

Including the children is often helpful diagnostically. For example, a covert fight between Mom and Dad would be missed except for the keen observer who saw the sibling conflict as mirroring the parents' fight.

Existential/experiential therapy places a high premium on the experience in the therapy room. In fact, the experience of the family as a whole, as a complete unit, seems to me to be a curative factor in family work. For example, the couple cannot deny their anxiety about being parents and the irreversibility of that fact if their three-month-old baby is in the therapy room. Existential anxiety over death can't be blocked out or denied by a couple pretending to be quarreling courting adolescents if we force them to confront the reality of their impending old age by demanding that their two grandchildren be present in the therapy room.

Young children also are often aware of key family secrets that are relevant to therapy. If you can provide them with enough of a feeling of safety in the therapy room, children will tell you what's really going on in the family: father's affair with his secretary, or mother's daily nips at that bottle in the hall closet. This spontaneity and honesty, our right-brained side, usually gets supressed as we get older and more socialized. Families who come to therapy seem to have blocked out this free, spontaneous dimension of experience to an even greater extent. In effect, the children alone become the repositories of the family's freedom and aliveness. If one can nurture and reinforce this dimension in the children, they can serve as a model for the family during and after therapy.

One might respond to the family's concerns that the children are too young to hear about their problems by suggesting to them that on some level they probably know it anyway or, that it is better they find out about it now. Much family therapy literature has commented on the deleterious effects of secrets on family workings. I have never seen a situation in which the exposure of secrets has, in the long run, been detrimental to the family. This doesn't mean that every specific detail must be explored. In a case of rape, for instance, the physical details don't have to be discussed in front of the seven-year-old, but the child certainly knows already of "Mommy's hurt." Further discussion and/or experience of this incident as it relates to the current interpersonal world of the family would not be harmful to the child. An answer such as, "Your attempts to protect your child from pain are admirable, but in the long run they won't help the situation," is a reasonable response in this case. Another dynamic in this issue is that children often feel responsible for the horrors that befall their parents. In this particular example, talk of "Mom's rape" and what really occurred could, if done in the right way, significantly reduce the child's hypertrophied sense of guilt. This dynamic is seen commonly in cases of divorce in which children often feel they caused the split-up.

A word or two about elderly family members. I don't know of a case in which the physical or mental health of an elderly person was injured by the family therapy process. Many times when one reaches an impasse in therapy, it is helpful to bring in the grandparents to break up this logjam. For example, in a family in which the therapist is unable to facilitate growth in the mother-daughter dyad, the presence of mother's mother might add the necessary monitoring and amplifying experience to free up the system and allow for future therapeutic growth. The therapist should make a particularly significant effort to include the parental (who are sometimes elderly) generation of a couple without children. It seems to us that, often, much of the experiential affect that is necessary for therapy is bound up in the families of origin until the birth of children. The presence of a new generation gradually helps transfer affect and involvement into the family of procreation.

Distance and time are frequently mentioned as objections to keeping the full family from being present in therapy. One or more essential members may live outside of an easy commuting area to the therapist's office. A general rule I follow is to seriously encourage the family to ask the essential family members to be present, even if this means that family members living far away will have to lose time from school or work and endure some economic hardships in traveling to therapy. Often, the members who live nearby will resist asking distant relatives to come to therapy, only to find that the relatives, perhaps feeling left out of being helpful to a hurting part of the family, would be quite willing to attend. Thus, it is important to have the request extended, no matter how unlikely the possibility of compliance seems even to the therapist. This is especially true if it is a member of the minimum two-generational unit.

Another alternative to consider is the use of telephone receiver amplifiers. A distant relative can call long distance and the phone can be attached to an amplifier that allows his or her voice to be heard and him or her to hear the others in the family. Although the telephone call is not as significant as having the person present, the symbolic act of participation via phone can sometimes complete the family patterning necessary for therapy to be effective.

Summary

Some basic guidelines for determining how to deal with the issue of who needs to be present for family therapy to work have been given. In my model, the therapist should push the family to bring as much of the interpersonal anxiety as is possible into the therapy room. This is directly related to increasing the number of family members present. A negotiated compromise is inevitable, with the therapist conceding attendance based on theoretical assumptions, clinical intuition and past experience. What constitutes failure is not losing the case but rather conceding so much that there is not even a realistic chance for therapy to work. Only if and when the family accepts the ante offered by the therapist can the game of family therapy begin.

References

Bowen, M. Theory in the practice of psychotherapy. In P. Guerin (Ed.), *Family Therapy: Theory and Practice*. New York: Gardner, 1976.

Gurman, A. S. and Kniskern, D. P. Research on marital and family therapy: Progress, perspective and prospect. In S. Garfield and A. Bergin (Eds.), *Handbook of Psychotherapy and Behavior Change*. Second edition. New York: Wiley, 1978.

Laing, R. Invited address at the Annual Conference of the American Association for Marriage and Family Therapy, Washington, D.C., October 1979.

Whitaker, C. A. and Keith, D. V. Symbolic-experiential family therapy. In A. Gurman and D. Kniskern (Eds.), *Handbook of Family Therapy*. New York: Brunner/Mazel, 1981.

STUART R. SUGARMAN, M.D.
Assistant Professor
Department of Psychiatry
University of Connecticut
School of Medicine
Farmington, CT

10. Establishing a Therapeutic Alliance in Family Systems Therapy

Question:

In Bowen's family systems therapy with one family member, it is important that the therapist does not engage the patient in a dependent relationship. In other words, the therapist should stay outside the emotional system of the patient, should not be triangled into it; yet, he or she has to be able to connect with the patient so that the latter will continue to come for therapy. How do you accomplish this difficult task?

Discussion:

In family systems therapy, the task is always to connect with the family system rather than with the individual patient. This means that the therapist must try to bring into the context of the family system whatever information is obtained from the individual patient. This is accomplished by not responding to the information as such but by putting it back into the family system. In doing so, the emotional process operating in that particular family can become more quickly apparent to the therapist than if he or she responded to the content of the individual's information. In addition, this technique will enable the therapist to recognize circuits of family behavior patterns without ever seeing the entire family.

The art of connecting with the patient lies in choosing the issue most important for the patient, and then connecting with that issue on a cognitive rather than an emotional level. There are a few basic principles to consider in accomplishing this task.

The first is the decrease of anxiety. Therapeutic measures that reduce anxiety will enable the patient to approach his or her problem more successfully. There are several methods for doing this. Since the narrow focus on the individual patient often causes anxiety, which then reinforces the symptom—a typical vicious cycle which is hard to break—the therapist should defocus the symptom by bringing it into context with the patient's emotional family field. This can be accomplished by asking questions such as: Are you the only one in your family—including the extended family—who has problems with this particular issue? How do other family members deal with this issue? What's the rule in your family about how one should deal with this issue or similar issues? By doing this, the focus of interest will be removed from the patient and extended to the larger family system. This process is usually followed by a decrease in anxiety in the patient, due to removal of the pressure to look within him or herself for all the causes of the problem and all the answers to it. With the decrease in anxiety comes an increase in objectivity about the problem, an objectivity which can then lead to new insights and understandings which open the door for change. This decrease in anxiety is also experienced by the patient as relief, a circumstance which certainly facilitates a therapeutic alliance.

Another way of decreasing anxiety is to set the symptom in a larger frame of time and context, by asking questions such as: When did you have more of the symptom? When did you have less? What was the difference in the circumstances? What other events are usually going on in your life when you have a more intense symptom? What is going on when you have a less intense one? Do you see any similarities in the circumstances? Are there any patterns to the process?

Another technique for decreasing the anxiety concerning the symptom would involve the use of behavioral desensitization techniques. What may be the most important and basic technique of decreasing anxiety is for therapists to relate to patients and their symptoms in a non-anxious way. There are two elements which are extremely important in this technique. The first is that therapists should not worry about either the patients or their symptoms; the second is that therapists should be careful to be aware of any possible aversive reaction of their own to the symptom. Both of these circumstances will result in the therapists' feeling an urgent need to change the symptom immediately. This pressured attitude usually increases the patients' anxiety and thereby works against the therapy.

The second principle to consider in connecting with the patient on a cognitive level involves the therapist's goal of enabling the patient to be as independent and self-reliant as possible. The family systems approach has a definite educational component. In this therapy, patients can gain understanding of the therapeutic process itself. They can even learn the technique of "defocusing" or "enlarging" the focus or "objectifying" the problem by asking themselves questions similar to those asked by the therapist. This contrasts sharply with other family therapy techniques, such as strategic therapy, in which the therapist makes interventions or gives paradoxical prescriptions which patients must follow blindly without understanding the therapeutic process. The educational process in a family systems approach leads to an educational alliance which rests on a cognitive rather than an emotional level. This therapy, therefore, is an educational process rather than a purely therapeutic one in which a doctor treats a patient. The consequence is that patients will become increasingly independent of the therapist, exploring and learning more on their own. They will be grateful to the therapist for the teaching, but will be no more dependent on him/her than students are on their teacher. They will become students who have learned whatever they could learn and are moving into the world.

However, it is important to note the difficulties in this cognitive approach. If the therapist expands the focus too fast from the patient and symptom without coming up with broader patterns that make sense to the patient, the patient might feel the therapist is not really interested in his or her problem and, therefore, not helpful. As soon as the therapist helps the patient to see some patterns, the patient becomes fascinated by the process and will usually be eager to learn more about it.

One major concern many people have with a family systems approach is the way of dealing with a patient's feelings, which is often seen as being cold or lacking empathy. Since family systems therapists relate to emotional issues in an objective way, they treat feelings as they treat symptoms: They do not respond to them directly, thereby encouraging the patient to express them, but set them into the context of the emotional family system. This certainly does not mean that feelings should be ignored, but that therapists should be able to go beyond the feelings. The issue of how to deal with feelings is one of the most important differences between family systems therapy and other therapies. In family systems therapy, therapists do not stay with the emotional symptom by putting it into a feeling concept such as low self-esteem, anger, guilt, etc. They will acknowledge the emotional symptom, then set it into a larger context such as an interactional pattern between significant family members. They will ask questions such as: How does your family react to your feelings? Is there anything they do that influences them? If anything does influence them, how can they make you feel better? Is anyone in your family aware of your intense reaction? All these techniques are not an avoidance of the feelings by the therapist; they are defocusing techniques which are meant to decrease anxiety and enhance a learning process. A final and cogent point is that this technique requires, from the therapist, a low level of anxiety about these emotional issues. If the therapist handles the above mentioned techniques skillfully, the patient will perceive the therapist not as being cold or indifferent but rather as being objective.

In summary, we would say that methods which can facilitate the therapeutic alliance by decreasing anxiety are the following: placing the individual within the context of his emotional system, enhancing the learning process of the patient, and translating emotional concepts into interactional patterns.

URSALA DAVATZ, M.D.
Fellow in Family Systems Therapy
Georgetown Family Center
Washington, DC

11. Symptom/Patient Defocusing in Family Therapy

Question:

In working with families in which there is a clearly identified patient, I frequently attempt to explore the extent to which the patient's problems are tied to the relationship system that surrounds the patient. When it is clear to me that the patient's symptom functions to maintain the relationship system's homeostasis, I will directly attempt to modify that system so that it no longer requires the patient's problem as a homeostat.

When I attempt to shift the focus from the patient's symptom to the (or a) relationship system in the family, for either diagnostic or therapeutic purposes, I frequently encounter considerable resistance from family members. Working with families with a child identified patient, I often find the parents respond to my attempts to explore their relationship with statements like, "We are not here to talk about our marriage. The problem is our son." In treating couples in which there is a clearly identified patient, I have had trouble shifting the focus from the presenting problem to the relationship between the partners. With one couple, every time I tried to shift the focus from the wife's obsessive/compulsive behavior to her feelings about her relationship with her husband, either the husband or the wife refocused the discussion on her symptoms.

I would appreciate any ideas you might have about how to shift the focus of therapy from the identified patient and/or the presenting problem to the relationship system in which the patient/symptom is embedded.

Discussion:

You are talking about the problem of transactionalizing the symptom—a very common and difficult maneuver (particularly with pseudomutual, united-front systems) in family therapy. I will present and

discuss the *symptom/patient defocusing operation**—a therapist operation (a series of linked interventions with a particular goal) designed
to shift the focus from the identified patient or the presenting problem
to the relationship system with minimal family resistance. The basic
principle or concept behind this operation is that it continually links
the exploration of the pertinent relationship system to the presenting
problem. More specifically, it relates the investigation to the system's
effort to successfully resolve or handle the presenting problem. This
principle rests upon a conceptualization of the family members, particularly the parents and/or marital dyad, as the primary agents for
solving the presenting problem. Concomitantly, it is based upon a
definition of the therapist as a consultant to the distressed relationship
system.

Patient/symptom defocusing involves at least four major stages, each
of which generally involves a variety of micro-interventions. The first
stage, *problem identification*, sets the stage for the rest of the operation.
In this stage, the family therapist identifies the (or a) presenting problem from the perspective of one family member—the entry person. In
selecting the entry person, the therapist should choose a family member who is part of an important dyad in the family and who cares about
and has a powerful response to the identified patient's problem. In
certain situations, such as marital therapy with a symptomatic spouse
(see Example 2), the entry person may even be the identified patient.
This stage usually entails a number of micro-interventions that specify
the exact nature and course of the presenting problem. Although this
stage focuses primarily on the entry person's perspective, it is also
useful during this stage to examine, at least partially, the other family
members' perspectives on the presenting problem. This examination
facilitates selection of the entry person. The following types of intervention characterize this step:

What do you see as the problem?
Exactly, what do you think is wrong with you, Lisa?
So, you think that Tim's drug problem is the major reason that
you're here today.

---

*The concept behind this therapist operation was initially developed through extensive
observation of family therapy conducted by Dorothy Horn, M.S.W., and Sol Levin, M.D.,
at the Department of Psychiatry, McMaster University Medical School, Hamilton, Ontario, Canada. Subsequently, the operation has been extended and refined in my work
at the Center for Family Studies.

The second stage of the defocusing operation, *reaction identification*, identifies the entry person's emotional reaction to the presenting problem. In this stage, the therapist can focus alternatively on the entry person's cognitive reaction (understanding, interpretation, etc.) to the presenting problem. However, this stage as well as the entire operation has the greatest impact when the therapist targets the emotional reaction. During this stage, it is very important to spend enough time empathically clarifying and heightening the entry person's experience of his/her emotional reaction to the presenting problem. This step builds an empathic gangway into the family system and involves the following sorts of intervention:

How did you feel about your daughter's refusal to talk?
What feelings did you have about losing your job?
It made you sad to hear about his stealing?

In the third stage, *sharing query*, the therapist begins the transactional part of the operation. Typically, it involves at least two microinterventions. The first is asking the entry person whether he/she does or can share his/her reaction to the presenting problem with anyone. The second identifies the person (relevant other) with whom the reaction is either shared or not shared. The relevant other should be someone who is or should be important to the entry person and the identified patient. Usually with a child identified patient, the entry person will be one parent and the relevant other will be the other parent, whereas in the symptomatic spouse situation the entry person will be the patient and the relevant other will be the other spouse.

If the entry person acknowledges sharing his/her reaction to the presenting problem with someone who is of minimal diagnostic interest or relevance (a sibling, friend, etc.), the therapist should ask directly about the relevant other who is or should be significant. The following examples typify the sharing query step:

When you're feeling down about Joan's school problems, is there anybody whom you share those feelings with?
Is there anyone whom you can tell your feelings about your son's stealing?
What about sharing them with your husband?
Did you ever let your wife know what losing your job meant to you?

The fourth and last stage, *relationship exploration*, investigates the communication or sharing process within the family relationship system. To remain consistent with the other steps in this operation, the exploration should be confined to an examination of the way in which the entry person shares or does not share his/her emotional reaction to the presenting problem with the relevant other. In response to the stage three sharing query, if the entry person acknowledges not sharing his/her reaction with the relevant other, the therapist should examine the communication block in that relationship with interventions like the following:

What stops you from sharing these feelings about your son with your husband?
What do you think would happen if you let your wife know how sad you really are about Susie's illness?
Why didn't you tell her how worthless it made you feel?

If the entry person, in response to stage three, acknowledges sharing his/her reaction to the presenting problem with the relevant other, the therapist should explore the communication process, in very specific and detailed terms. This examination may reveal an effective and appropriate communication process, which may reflect the family's health and problem-solving ability. On the other hand, it may reveal a superficial and ineffectual communication process that the family is attempting to conceal behind a united front. The following types of interventions are useful in examining the communication process:

Tell me exactly what happens when you tell her about these feelings.
So, you try to tell him, but he doesn't really seem to grasp the depth of your hurt.
After he says he's sorry that you feel that way, where does that leave you?
Does it help when you tell her?

The fourth step completes penetration of the family relationship system and permits exploration of a critical (to the etiology and/or maintenance of the presenting problem) dyad in that system. That the exploration confines itself to communication about one member's reaction to the presenting problem, gives the exploration a certain "face validity" or relevance to the dyad. Tying the exploration to the presenting problem reduces the likelihood that family members will question the appropriateness of the exploration. In contrast, if the examination were not confined in this way, if it focused on general, nonproblematic aspects of the relationship ("Do you two communicate with each other?" "Do you get along with each other?"), it would generally increase resistance.

Despite this topical confinement, if a dyad member questions the exploration ("I don't see what how my wife and I communicate has to do with Ann's problem"), a useful therapist response set up by the circumscribed, problem-centered exploration is, "I think it is going to be very hard for the two of you to solve or deal with this problem if you can't or don't communicate your feelings and thoughts about it to each other." Such a response implies a positive conceptualization of the family members as the primary agents for solving the presenting problem. This conceptualization functions as a health- and competence-promoting "demand characteristic."

The defocusing operation can be used as a diagnostic probe to assess the emotional communication process in significant family dyads. It can also be used therapeutically to gain access to the "inside" of a dyad in order to facilitate change. The primary purpose of this operation is to gain access to the relationship system without eliciting unproductive resistance. Which additional operations the therapist chooses to use once the dyad has been accessed depends on both the therapeutic task at hand and the information gained during the defocusing operation.

The following transcript examples illustrate this operation as applied to family (Example 1) and marital (Example 2) therapy situations. Parenthetical notations indicate stage transitions. For brevity's sake, some of the stages exemplified below are more condensed than they would be in a normal therapy situation.

Example 1

Therapist: Mrs. Smith, what do you see as the major problem that brings you here today? (*problem identification*)
Mother: Our problem's with Janie. She just won't do anything we ask her.
Therapist: What happens when you ask her to do something?
Mother: She refuses. She either insults us or just walks away.
Therapist: So, she gets abusive or acts as if you don't exist.
Mother: Right. As if I haven't been talking to her.
Therapist: How does it make you feel when she does that? (*reaction identification*)
Mother: I don't like it.
Therapist: What exactly do you feel—sad, hurt, mad?
Mother: I guess hurt. Frustrated too. It's like a slap in the face from someone whom you care about.

Therapist: And, you feel like you can't do anything about it. You're helpless.

Mother: Yeah, it's so frustrating that nothing gets through.

Therapist: When you're feeling hurt and frustrated, like nothing gets through to her, is there anybody whom you can talk to about how upset you feel? (*sharing query*)

Mother: Well, sometimes, I talk with my friend, Sheila.

Therapist: What about your husband? Can you share those feelings about Janie with him?

Mother: Yes, sometimes.

Therapist: What happens when you tell him how you feel? (*relationship exploration—process*)

Mother: He tells me not to worry.

Therapist: Does that help?

Mother: Not really.

Therapist: What would be helpful from him at those times?

Father: She wants me to get as upset as she is.

Therapist: Why don't you find out if that is what she really wants from you?

Father: Isn't that what you want from me?

Example 2

Therapist: What seems to be the problem? (*problem identification*)

Husband: Well, my wife is so perfectionistic that she can't leave anything alone until it's absolutely perfect. She spends hours fixing her hair, drives the kids crazy fixing their hair and clothes, and sometimes she won't let me go until she's picked every speck of lint or dirt off what I'm wearing.

Therapist: What do you think about what your husband said?

Wife: He's right. I'm obsessed. It all has to be perfect.

Therapist: What's it like for you when you can't leave something in a less than perfect state? (*reaction identification*)

Wife: It's awful. I just have to fix it.

Therapist: You feel like you have to make it perfect. What feelings do you have then?

Wife: I'm not sure. Maybe scared.

Therapist: As if something terrible would happen if you left it alone?

Wife: Yeah, that's it.

Therapist: When you're feeling scared, is there anyone whom you can talk to? (*sharing query*)

Wife: No, not really.

Therapist: You can't tell your husband how you feel?

Wife: Well, he's got enough to worry about, with his job and all. He works very hard and isn't home a lot.

Therapist: So, you don't want to burden him. What do you think would happen if you did, if you let him know how scared you feel? (*reaction exploration—block*)

Wife: I don't know. I don't want to burden him.

Therapist: You're assuming that he'd feel burdened. Why don't you check that out with him right now and see if you're right.

Wife: Would you feel burdened if I told you how upset I get sometimes?

Husband: I don't know. It depends on how you tell me.

WILLIAM M. PINSOF, Ph.D.
Associate, Center for Family Studies
The Family Institute of Chicago;
Department of Psychiatry and Behavioral Sciences
Northwestern University Medical School
Chicago, IL

12. Avoiding Dropouts in Couples Group Therapy

Question:

There is interest at the large family service agency where I work in making more use of group therapy for couples. The problem is that, even though we are drawing from a substantial pool of couples seeking treatment, we have had great difficulty keeping such groups going. Frequently several couples will drop out in the first three or four sessions of a group, or will attend irregularly, leading to further dropouts and a demoralized "group" of one or two remaining couples. The first four couples groups we tried basically never got off the ground. Although such groups would help us enormously in reducing waiting times, there is probably a good chance that the program will be scrapped unless things go better in the next one or two tries. I would really appreciate any suggestions you might have about getting such groups going and keeping them going.

Discussion:

I can suggest several ways of approaching the problems which you are having at a direct clinical level. I think before applying solutions at that level, however, you really should examine the issues at an organizational-systems level. You've got to ask yourself what support exists within the agency for the application of couples groups. Over the years group therapy of all sorts has had notoriously low valence and has been viewed as second-rate treatment. Although there may be interest at your agency in such groups, and people may know in their heads that developing this program would reduce waiting times, is there really *support* for the program? If the answer is no, then before doing anything else, you had better educate providers about the value and efficacy of group therapy for couples. If this is not done, couples arrive at the group as latent dropouts. A referring provider who doesn't know much about couples group therapy or who views it as a poor alternative to other treatment approaches will (perhaps unintentionally) bias couples against this modality. Unless you can drum up at least moderate support among the other therapists, your program will never get off the ground.

Now, supposing that you are able to educate and interest other providers, what next? Along with my colleagues at the Harvard Community Health Plan in Boston, I have developed a pregroup preparation and screening approach, which has reduced our couples group dropout rate to nearly zero (Budman and Clifford, 1979).

This approach, the Couples Communication Workshop (CCW), is based upon the fact that the best predictor of future behavior is present behavior.

Before a set of couples groups begin (generally we treat enough couples to begin two groups simultaneously), we have a 1½ hour CCW. The CCW usually includes eight to 12 couples and three therapists. For the most part, couples have been seen by another staff member or by one of the CCW leaders three or four times conjointly prior to the workshop.

We introduce the workshop by explaining that it is offered in order to give people a sense of the type of experiences that they may expect as part of a couples group. We believe that the CCW allows people to see if they would feel comfortable as part of such a treatment group, and it also gives us a sense of whether couples group treatment would be the most useful modality for them. Finally, if they do go on to join a couples group, this workshop will be good orientation and preparation.

The CCW is made up of three exercises:

1) Each couple pairs up with another couple. These "quartets" then introduce themselves to one another. After about 15 minutes couples rejoin the larger group and are asked to introduce one member of the couple with whom they just met to the whole group.

2) Couples are asked to think about one of their typical arguments (for some couples where the issue is an inability to argue, we suggest that they think about their typical aborted argument). Then the couples return to their quartets (see #1 above). Once in these smaller groups we ask the couples one at a time to role play their argument. The other couple functions as observers. Once a couple is into its argument we will make a variety of interventions with the help of the observing couple. We may ask the observers what they see going on between the arguing partners, or we may substitute one of the partners from the observing couple and request that that person help bring the argument to a resolution. At other times, if the couple is unable to

argue, the observers may "alter-ego" and express the feelings which the other couple are unable to express. Each couple functions as both arguers and observers and the exercise is processed and discussed. This part of the CCW takes about 40 minutes.

3) The last exercise of the workshop is a whole group exercise. The entire group imagines that they are neighbors living in the same area. The therapists direct them to "plan a large neighborhood party (dinner, picnic, etc.)." The group is given 20 minutes for this task.

At the conclusion of the third exercise we discuss some of what has gone on, explain that we will get back to people shortly (in a week or so) about the group, and ask them to think about whether or not they have interest in being part of a couples group.

The three exercises we use have evolved over a five-year period of trial and error in doing these workshops. The first exercise allows participants to feel a little less anxious about being part of a group. They meet one other couple and so know someone in addition to their spouse. The second exercise, to some degree, simulates interactions in a couples group. In such a group couples express and demonstrate their conflicts with other couples observing and/or intervening. If a couple cannot do this in the workshop because they are too inhibited, or because they wish only to reveal such issues to a therapist, they probably won't do well in the group. The final whole group exercise gives people some sense of what it is like to be part of a large group with a task.

Although our couples groups themselves are *not* highly structured, the CCW clearly is. This is not a problem. We explain to patients the differences between the group itself and the CCW in regard to structure, and this seems to suffice.

We have had great success in using the CCW as a preparation and screening. Of the nearly 100 couples who have attended workshops and begun groups, only *one* has dropped out. Several reasons contribute to the utility of this preparatory and screening approach. From the perspective of the couples, they know what they are buying into before the group begins. If it is apparent to them from the workshop that this is not an approach they feel comfortable with, or if they believe that such treatment will not be helpful, they can choose not to join a group. Thus, dropouts occur *before* the group ever begins, rather than hindering the process of the starting group.

From the perspective of the therapist, the workshop is also of great value. For one thing, some couples absolutely will not fit in a given group for one reason or another. We have, for example, screened out couples where one partner was much too disturbed to be a member of a group, or where a given couple was so different from the others that the fit would have been a very poor one. The CCW also helps the therapist in that, when the group does begin, patients are less anxious and better prepared to work. Although we often assume that patients know what to do in psychotherapy, this may not be the case. Couples rarely have clear ideas about group therapy and the CCW educates them.

From what I have stated above, it should be apparent that a great deal more should go into starting a couples group then just setting a date and getting the referrals. By laying good groundwork and preparing both your colleagues and your patients, you enhance the likelihood of a successful program.

Reference

Budman, S. H. and Clifford, M. Short-term group therapy for couples in a health maintenance organization. *Professional Psychology*, 1979, *10*, 419-429.

SIMON H. BUDMAN, Ph.D.
Staff Psychologist
Harvard Community Health Plan
Instructor in Psychology in Psychiatry
Harvard Medical School
Boston, MA

13. Encouragement in Family Therapy

Question:

What is the importance and role of encouragement in family therapy? I have observed that, while many clinicians diagnose deficits and liabilities, others emphasize the importance of recognizing assets, resources and potential. How can encouragement be systematically used in family therapy?

Discussion:

Encouragement is often identified as the most important technique available to the therapist. If we recognize that most interpersonal problems are the result of discouragement, then the obvious antidote is encouragement. Discouragement is a result of negative influences in the family, such as high standards, overambition, negative expectations and pessimism. When someone in the family moves into a superior position and communicates to the other members of the family as if they were inferior, this communication of high standards—"My Dad never did it that way"; "We don't do things that way"—produces discouragement (Allred, 1976).

In the same way, overambition expressed—"That's pretty good but I know you can do better"—discourages. These statements, though often said with good intentions, are destructive in the communication system of the family. They lower self-esteem and feelings of worth and lessen the desire to cooperate and work with other members of the family. Discouragement is a common factor underlying psychopathology or failure to function.

Encouragement is the process of enhancing individuals' self-esteem and self-confidence, thereby increasing the self-concept and freeing them to be less defensive and more able to work with other members of the family.

The therapist needs specific *encouragement skills*. These skills include the ability to:

1) Listen attentively and hear content, feelings and intentions
2) Respond empathically to the whole message

3) Focus on strengths and resources
4) Help persons see their perceptual alternatives
5) Focus on efforts and contributions
6) Identify discouraging beliefs
7) Encourage commitment and movement

Encouragement is not only a philosophical position, it is a series of concrete skills. The first encouragement from the therapist occurs by attending closely to each family member's communication and indicating clearly that each one is heard. By indicating universalities and similarities in beliefs and feelings of the varied members, the therapist helps to create a feeling of belonging and acceptance.

The collaborative relationship, in which the therapist and all members of the family work together as equals, is also encouraging. As the goals of each family member and the therapist are aligned, everyone is valued for his or her full and equal participation in the process.

One of the most significant encouragement procedures occurs during the diagnostic phase. Instead of only focusing on psychopathology and liabilities, the therapist is equally interested in each person's strengths, assets and resources. The therapist who encourages is a "talent scout," identifying the assets which will enable family members to deal more effectively with the challenges of living, including family relationships.

Thus, the therapist will look for and affirm any positive movement, involvement or attitude. This requires a different kind of diagnostic thinking. The therapist must be able to see the positive side or element in what appears to be negative. The trait of stubbornness can be considered determination. The trait of anger can indicate involvement.

The encouraging therapist is involved in helping each member of the family become aware of his or her strengths and how to use these assets for personal and family growth.

One of the most encouraging things the therapist does is to help members of the family be aware of choices. It is very encouraging to recognize that, regardless of the situation, the members of the family can choose to function differently. They do not have to insist on fighting (a cooperative activity, because they must both agree to fight); instead they can learn to cooperate in more positive ways. A full awareness of the power of choice can be quite encouraging.

The therapist's hypotheses about individuals' purposes and symptoms are encouraging in that the tentativeness—"Could it be. . . ?" "Is it possible. . . ?"—places full responsibility for confirmation on the individual.

Empathy is also encouraging in that it goes beyond mere reflection of feelings. While it is good to know that your feelings are understood, it is more empathic and encouraging to hear your beliefs, intentions and purposes are understood. A deeper level of empathy occurs when the therapist not only acknowledges—"You're feeling like no one cares"—but goes further—"It seems like there's no use in trying." "Is it possible you give up to keep us from being involved with you?"

As the members of the family increase their feelings of self-esteem and worth, they are more ready to cooperate and work with each other. They become encouraged by their new ability to identify each other's strengths.

The therapist's personal belief that each person has the capacity to change is also encouraging. By being accepting, supportive, confrontive and never overambitious, the therapist demonstrates encouragement.

Reference

Allred, G. H. *How To Strengthen Your Marriage and Family.* Provo, Utah: Brigham Young University Press, 1976.

DON DINKMEYER, Ph.D.
*President, Communication and
Motivation Training Institute
Coral Springs, FL*

and

DON DINKMEYER, JR.
*Doctoral Candidate,
University of Florida
Gainesville, FL*

SECTION II

Patient Selection
and Treatment Planning

14. No Treatment as the Treatment of Choice

Question:

Most, if not all, the major theoretical contributors to family therapy talk on and on about how their own methods are the "right" ones. Some of them, but not many, will, if pushed, more or less specify the kinds of problems or families for whom their method is most useful. I'd like to hear from someone, who doesn't have a special theoretical axe to grind, about when *no therapy* is the treatment of choice.

Discussion:

The question contains a preliminary complaint against most major theoretical contributors to family therapy and ends with a specific question as to when *no therapy* is the treatment of choice. It is of interest that this pertinent observation about family therapists and the answer to the pointed question are indirectly related.

Family therapy is included within the broad field of psychotherapy and has much in common with other psychotherapeutic techniques. Jerome Frank notes six features common to all successful therapies: 1) an emotionally charged, confiding patient relationship; 2) a rationale or myth which explains the cause of the distress and a method of relieving it; 3) new information about the sources of the patient's problems and possible alternative ways of dealing with them; 4) strengthening the patient's expectations of help through the personal qualities of the therapist, enhanced by his/her status in society and work setting; 5) provision of success experiences which heighten the patient's hopes and also enhance his/her sense of mastery, interpersonal competence or capability; and 6) facilitation of emotional arousal, a prerequisite to attitudinal and behavioral change.

All of these six factors require active participation on the part of the therapist; most importantly, the therapist should be genuinely enthusiastic and convinced of the capabilities of his/her approach. The therapist's attitude heightens the patient's hopes and commitment to treatment. Thus, the tendency of family theoreticians to talk on and on about how their own methods are the right ones makes them better therapists and gives their patients a better chance of success. However, statistics may show no higher rate of success than for an equally enthusiastic therapist using a different theory and technique.

Thus, my first response to the question of when no therapy is the treatment of choice is when the therapist is not enthusiastic or not convinced about the superiority of his/her particular method. Outcome studies on the effectiveness of conjoint family therapy that examine the effect of factors (patient, therapist, technique) show that variations in these factors do have an impact on the result.

My second criterion for when no therapy is the treatment of choice is when the initial family evaluation indicates a lack of motivation for change in significant members of the family. For example, I saw a teenage boy and his parents during an initial diagnostic family evaluation. The presenting problem was that the boy was doing poorly in school, showed no interest in studying and might not graduate from high school. Two older brothers had left home and were making their own way in California. It was clear that the younger brother planned to follow them once he became of age, whether he graduated from high school or not. He was not interested in treatment, but would come so as not to upset his parents. The parents were nice, middle-class, hardworking people, who got along beautifully together, but were being severely criticized by in-laws because the children's school records were poor and there would be no college graduate from the family. They were willing to consider that something was wrong and were willing to enter family therapy if, in any way, it would help the son become a good student. They were told that no therapy was the treatment of choice at the end of the diagnostic interview.

A criterion for no *family* therapy is when the marital relationship is so filled with violent feelings and sexual problems that exposure of young children to it would be destructive to their normal psychological growth and development. It is necessary to be aware of normal childhood phases of development that need to be protected from premature or overwhelming stimulation. The problems may need handling by marital or individual therapy.

Another reason for not recommending family therapy is based on the recognition that children are individuals in their own right and do not merely react to what the parents are doing to them. Sometimes the child's individuality initiates the parental distress. Treatment of the child by a child psychiatrist may be indicated and not family therapy.

Another possible situation where family therapy might not be appropriate is when there is a destructive secret (infidelity, homosexuality, child or wife beating) that is not allowed to surface in the family group and impedes therapy. Individual sessions with the holder or holders of the secret may lead to results not possible in a family grouping.

I am sure that there are other reasons for a no treatment prescription, but I will name but one more obvious one. This is the *folie à deux* family. Here the original psychotic individual has to be separated from the chameleon members of the family so that he/she can receive individual therapy and the other members be allowed to return to normal.

PETER A. MARTIN, M.D.
Clinical Professor of Psychiatry
University of Michigan
Medical School
Ann Arbor, MI

15. Including Children in Marital and Family Therapy

Question:

I'm quite confused by all the different opinions I've heard expressed about when children should be included in marital and
family therapy. It seems obvious to me that if a child or adolescent
is the identified patient, then he or she should be present during
therapy sessions. But not everyone would agree with me on this,
since it seems that behavior therapists who work with families
often deal only with the parents and hardly talk to the identified
patient child. It's even less clear what the therapy role of children
should be when an adult (parent) is the identified patient, or
when a couple explicitly asks for help with their marriage. Are
there any good *general* clinical rules I could consider following
in making these decisions, without having to adopt rules that are
tied to just one theoretical model?

Discussion:

As is often the case in the sciences, the way in which a question is
asked shapes one's understanding of a problem and dictates the answer
one receives. In this instance, the issue in question is attendance of
family members at psychotherapy sessions. The question is asked in
terms of when children should be *included* in sessions, yet it could as
well be put in terms of when children should be *excluded* from sessions.
Each key word suggests different orienting assumptions about family
therapy, and decisions based on the questions are certain to influence
the way in which therapy is conducted.

Most family therapists, even from highly diverse theoretical models,
consider the nuclear family unit (two generations, parents and children) to have particular psychological salience. This belief is based
upon both their experience with treating families and the obvious
consideration that, in our culture at least, the nuclear family is the
unit which has the most frequent and most intimate contact with each

70

other. Such a belief dictates, for most, the overriding rule that all members of the nuclear family should attend sessions, unless a decision to exclude certain members is made based on some particular circumstances. For these therapists the issue is exclusion rather than inclusion and it is from this perspective that I will offer guidelines for practice.

The therapist's decision, as is the case with all decisions regarding therapy, can be guided by research findings, theory or personal experiences that appear to be applicable to the family in question. For me, none of these sources of wisdom offers definitive rules to guide my practice. Specific theories of therapy offer suggestions for followers of that school of therapy, but for most therapists, myself included, these guidelines are not satisfactory. Research, too, is of limited usefulness. In the most thorough review to date of research on marital and family therapy, Gurman and Kniskern (1978) found that no study has investigated directly the issue of exclusion or inclusion of children in marital or family therapy. Their review of research has indicated, however, that overall, increasing the number of family members in attendance at therapy sessions has positively influenced outcome. This has been true of fathers and mothers, although not yet investigated with other family members. Such findings, although of interest, are not sufficient to guide practice.

Personal experience then is perhaps the source of guidance most used for the shaping of practice. Unfortunately, it is difficult to transpose one therapist's guidelines, reflecting as they do specific therapist and treatment variables, to practical guidelines for another therapist. I will try, however, to describe the variables which I consider prior to making a decision about excluding particular family members and will also mention the ways in which I use these variables to help reach a decision.

Let me say at the outset that it is my preference and practice to begin therapy by seeing *at least* the entire living unit of the person or relationship identified as symptomatic or dysfunctional. In the typical American family this is the mother, father and all their children. It also includes others who live in the household, whether grandparents, aunts, uncles, foster children, etc. In addition, first order relatives are included even if they do not reside at the same address (e.g., separated parents). The decision to exclude children is made based on the following dimensions, whether for the first session or for later sessions. These variables are interactive and all need to be considered as a group rather than in isolation.

1) Who or which relationship is identified as symptomatic?

If a child or a relationship involving a child is identified as the problem, I insist initially that all children be present. It is my experience that the exclusion of a problem child invites family resistance and the exclusion of nonidentified children reifies the "differentness" of the identified patient. As a rule, when a child is the identified patient, I continue to see all children with the parents throughout therapy, or exclude all children at once from therapy sessions. Any other composition seems to confuse generational boundaries and isolates certain members.

When a parent or marital relationship is the identified patient, I am more inclined to move toward exclusion of the children or even to allow the first session to involve parents only. Many parents resist the involvement of children in their problems and would refuse to bring them to the first session. A session with an understanding therapist focused on these concerns will often overcome their fears and allow for children to be involved. After a few family sessions, the decision to treat the marital unit alone can then be made if indicated.

2) What is the presenting problem?

In most cases the specific presenting problem will not influence the decision to involve children from therapy sessions. In general, however, I do not insist on the presence of children, if their presence will require a parental disclosure which is unacceptable to the parents. For example, infidelity, sexual dysfunction or arrests are frequently not seen as acceptable topics for conversation with children present. Attempting to force the issue with parents, prior to establishing a relationship with them, even if the children are needed for solution to their problem, is almost certainly doomed to failure. It is my experience, however, that no topic needs to be kept from children and that secrets are seldom kept in a family.

3) What are the ages of children?

For the initial session, I do not believe that the age of children is an important variable for determining exclusion. Many family therapists exclude preverbal children, but I find that, despite their potential for disruption, they provide the opportunity for more rapidly engaging a family in therapy. Adolescents often resent coming to therapy, perhaps seeing their involvement as potentially regressive. Although I often allow adolescents to drop out later in therapy, I insist upon their attendance at early sessions.

4) Who suggests exclusion of children?

Is it up to the family to determine who needs to attend or is it up to the therapist? On this issue, family therapists also seem to be in general, if not unanimous, agreement that the final decision should remain the therapist's. As information accumulates during the treatment process and an understanding of the family develops, the therapist can, if indicated, alter his/her decision about who attends. Initiative to alter membership at sessions may come from either the therapist or the family. I consider a suggestion by a child that he/she not attend further sessions more seriously than a parent's suggestion that the child be excluded. The level of differentiation indicated by a child's direct request is taken to be partial evidence of the valid nature of the request.

5) How many sessions have been held?

As a general rule, in later stages of therapy a move on the family's part to exclude children from sessions is considered as more likely to be an attempt at further growth or change, rather than as a homeostatic maneuver. The reverse is true in early stages of therapy.

6) Is the therapy moving satisfactorily?

I seldom consider reducing the number of family members attending sessions when the therapy is stalemated or barely progressing. Rather, I feel these situations call for increasing the number of family members present. If, however, therapy has helped the family change and things are going well, I am likely to view a family-initiated change as their taking increased responsibility for their lives and honor the request.

These variables and their effects on treatment outcome should provide researchers with numerous topics for investigation. Until that work is done, however, they can provide a loose framework for clinician decision making. Consideration of these variables has been helpful to me in determining the best treatment composition for many families. In cases when I am unsure of the best composition, and there are many such families, I have learned the hard way to include too many members rather than too few. For me, it has always been easier to reduce the number of family members who attend than to increase the number. With particularly large families or severely disturbed ones, I have found it preferable to include a cotherapist rather than to exclude members. It is probably the case, however, that particular types of therapy (e.g., behavioral family therapy) are not as affected by exclusion criteria.

Reference

Gurman, A. and Kniskern, D. P. Research on marital and family therapy: Progress, perspective, and prospect. In S. Garfield and A. Bergin (Eds.) *Handbook of Psychotherapy and Behavior Change* (second edition). New York: Wiley, 1978.

DAVID P. KNISKERN, Psy.D.
Associate Professor
Deptartment of Psychiatry
University of Cincinnati
College of Medicine
Cincinnati, OH

16. Including Non-Blood-Related Persons in Family Therapy

Question:

Many families referred for family therapy have a history of prior treatment or ongoing contact with other agencies or professionals. In some instances family members, extended family or friends play a quasi-therapeutic role. This input often may be counterproductive to family therapy. What can the family therapist do to either "wean" the family from these sources of help or to utilize their influence in the family treatment process?

Discussion:

Family problems are frequently presented that clearly involve persons outside the immediate family group, such as extended or geographically distant family, school counselors or teachers, welfare workers, probation officers, health professionals, family friends, neighbors, co-workers, prior and current therapists, and various others. The presence of this network of "helping others" can make it difficult to decide who are the real family vis-à-vis the presenting problem. In making this decision, the family therapist must rely upon a broad concept of the family that includes as part of the family system many who do not live in the immediate family group. It is not that therapists need to work directly with everybody, but they must at least include in their therapeutic planning all of those who have participated significantly in defining the family's problem and their attempted solutions. This expanded concept of the family as a system is essential in developing therapeutic strategies and interventions.

Whenever a family therapist enters a family, it is like entering the theater in the middle of a play. Already a plot has been created, the play entitled, the set designed, and the actors are in motion. In the background the critics are making their judgments, perhaps resulting in minor or major changes in the production. In working with families, the therapist is also entering an ongoing production, one that has been created and influenced by the family's interactions with themselves and with others. Traditionally, many therapists have limited their concept of the family to combinations of the immediate and extended family and to past generations. This somewhat limited definition does not adequately recognize that many families come into therapy having had help from other therapists' counselors and social agencies. All families have had advice from friends, neighbors and relatives. To the extent that this input influences the course of the problem and the family's attempted solutions, the "helping others" must be considered a part of the family and its resources. It is essential, therefore, to include in the concept of the family unit undergoing treatment all those with whom the family is interacting relevant to the presenting problem.

This broader conceptualization of the family goes beyond traditional and legal definitions of the family. The family as an open system has shifting and fluid boundaries and these must be acknowledged and monitored by the family therapist. The family's understanding and awareness of the input of these helping others must undergo modification in order for the family to change. The family therapist must help bring about this modification in a constructive fashion that makes full use of the strength these helping others are to the family. Above all, the family therapist must avoid an adversary position. These goals may be accomplished in a variety of ways, including 1) direct intervention, 2) including the others as part of the unit undergoing treatment, or 3) including them as a part of the professional treatment (either through consultation or actual participation in the therapy). This expanded concept of the family and the resulting opportunities for therapeutic management give the family therapist significant and powerful leverage for change.

Some case examples may illustrate the application of these techniques. Recently the inpatient service of a mental health center referred a patient who seemed unresponsive to hospital treatment. He had recently been hospitalized for what was described as a sudden change in his behavior from a happy, competent person to a morose, suicidal person who would sporadically insist he was dead and refuse to move. This behavior was apparently triggered by the death of his brother and the desertion by his wife after 18 years of marriage. The family, consisting of a mother, sister and brother, emphatically took the position that the identified patient needed help. Yet when they agreed to appointments, they would not keep them. It was revealed that the family's best friend was actively advising them on the treatment of the patient, particularly the need for continued hospitalization. Her position was that he must be incurably mentally ill since he had

had time to get over his brother's death, and since any normal man would have been glad this wife had left. She advised the family to ignore outpatient family therapy treatment. It was further revealed that this woman had played a significant role in the family's transition to this country some years ago and remained a close friend and advisor regarding appropriate American behavior.

The therapists invited the family friend to come in and help them with this most serious problem. In this meeting, it became obvious that the family trusted her implicitly; they would make no move or decision without her input and management. The family therapists continued asking her help in what she had diagnosed as an unsolvable situation. By joining with her and respecting her role in the family system, it became possible to arrange to see them all in family treatment. The therapists were able to reframe her diagnosis of chronicity into a more hopeful one and thus to initiate family change. By moving with her power and entering the family through her, treatment continued to an eventual successful outcome. For treatment to be conducted, it was necessary to involve the friend as a functioning part of the family unit.

In a slightly different situation, a family asked to be seen for a problem concerning their nine-year-old daughter. Her presenting problem was described by the family as anorexia. The child had not eaten solid foods until age six. Since that time she had selected a diet of peanut butter, fruit, pancakes, cereal and french fries. Major differences between the parents concerning the handling of the problem were obvious. Mother viewed the problem as essentially coming from father's harshness, and father blamed the mother's softness. While discussing these family diagnoses, it was discovered that the mother's best friend was still "anorectic" after some years of individual treatment. The friend was actively involved with the mother in a collusive triangle against the father. Her position was that the condition would run its own course, and that, if the mother interfered or frustrated the girl in any way, it would totally ruin her for life. She was saying in part, "Do not make the mistakes my family did . . . you know what happened to me."

Some six years of this advice in the context of a close and supportive relationship had left the family with little capacity for action or change. It was apparent to the therapist that any intervention that ran counter to this input would result in failure. By taking the position with the parents that this was an "atypical anorexia," and that it did not follow the usual pattern, the therapist was able to join the friend in her alarm. This relabeling or rediagnosis allowed for the design of interventions acceptable to the mother's "anorectic" friend. The therapist through this strategy used the loyalty and support of a close family friend to resolve a parental impasse (of which she was a part) and to allow a shift to less extreme and competitive positions.

From a somewhat different perspective, an adolescent male of 14 was referred for family therapy by a placement agency. The other family members were a mother and sister. The parents had been divorced and the father was now deceased. The boy refused to come for treatment, as did his older sister. In interviewing the mother, it became apparent that this family was being seen by a number of therapists. On a weekly basis, the son was being counseled independently by a probation officer and a school counselor. The mother was being counseled by the school principal, as well as being advised by a physician at work.

The interview with the mother revealed that many contradictory and even destructive messages were being given to the family. The probation officer thought that the mother was the boy's problem and considered family therapy a violation of his diagnosis. The school counselor thought the youth was quite psychotic and in need of long-term hospitalization. The counselor saw his role as supporting the boy in order to mitigate the influence of the probation officer and the mother's ally, the school principal. The counselor also thought that family therapy was an avoidance of the real problem of psychosis. The school principal, supported by the mother's co-worker, thought the problem was the "impossible boy" and advised her to take immediate steps to have him placed outside the home. The principal saw family therapy as a denial of the boy's basic badness and an insult to the mother. This complicated set of authoritative advice and side-taking commentaries by various agents of therapeutic treatment and community agencies is not uncommon. In some instances, there may be even larger numbers of "helping others" involved. This network of helpers cannot be ignored. They must be dealt with in a way that does not precipitate angry, rejecting reactions and a resultant flight from treatment.

In this instance, the therapists talked with each one of the helping professionals, agreeing with them individually as to the seriousness of the situation. Together they reviewed the fact that past attempts by others had not worked. The therapists invited the various professionals to meet and to go back to square one to see if perhaps something could be done to unscramble the mess caused by others. All agreed. In the meeting the therapists listened to all sides, sympathized with each point of view, and accepted the helpers' need to help and their resulting frustrations. Much like with a family, the initial blaming and pointing soon lost its punch and communication improved. The continuous sabotage which had characterized previous attempts at resolving the family's problems abated. The family therapists were now perceived as the primary therapists. Continuing consultations with each professional were necessary to maintain these changes and to keep everyone constructively involved or uninvolved in the therapy.

These examples do not begin to exhaust the possibilities. Helping others can be included in the family therapy in an almost infinite number of ways. Some require the direct presence of others, even to the extent of their being part of the therapy team; others do not. The clinical issues in each family interact with the therapist's style and determine the particular level of involvement. However one conducts family therapy, one must take into consideration the fact that with all families there has been some kind of significant involvement by others attempting to help. This involvement may be formal or informal, past or present, but it always plays an important role in maintaining, escalating or even creating the problems for which the family is seeking treatment. The family therapist must be able to work creatively with this involvement, not fight it, but incorporate it strategically as a part of the family therapy treatment. To exclude the network of helping others from active consideration in therapy minimizes the possibility of change, heightens the risk of losing the family and avoids taking advantage of a major family strength.

HAROLD A. GOOLISHIAN, Ph.D.
Professor, Department of Psychiatry
University of Texas Medical Branch
Galveston, TX

and

HARLENE ANDERSON, M.A.
Faculty and Program Coordinator
Galveston Family Institute
Galveston, TX

17. Concurrent Marital and Individual Psychotherapy

Question:

A lot of marriage and family therapists warn us about the dangers of seeing one spouse in individual psychotherapy concurrent with seeing that person and his/her spouse in conjoint couples therapy, and I'm familiar with all the usual arguments against such a practice. For once, I'd like to hear someone take a stand on when such an arrangement is to be *preferred*, not just tolerable.

Discussion:

Systemic thinking does not mean a rigid adherence to always working with the total physical system—in this case, the couple. Rather, the systems approach implies an attitude on the part of the therapist which always takes into consideration the whole system (interpersonally), not just separate units in their intrapsychic dimension. When the system does not work, its constituent parts must be considered so that they can eventually work together as a whole or so that the original system is discontinued. For this, the system may have to be "taken apart."

In three general sets of circumstances it is usually preferred to see one spouse alone concurrent with seeing that person and his/her spouse in conjoint therapy. These are when: 1) unresolved anger interferes with constructive interaction; 2) sexual problems of one are not understood by the other; and 3) one spouse is inflexible regarding values. Two things should be noted regarding these three circumstances. First, seeing one member of the system individually and his/her spouse in conjoint couple therapy must be considered a temporary situation—until the problems in the areas mentioned are resolved individually. Second, this arrangement is preferred only because of the obstacles to effective communication which these problems create.

Unresolved Anger

Conjoint sessions become a waste of time when the anger accumulated through the years does not allow one or both spouses to move from the past and to focus on action for improvement. The first two or three sessions with the couple should tell the therapist if conjoint sessions are to be continued. The members of the system should be separated for therapeutic work when the clients are unable to stay in the present, when they generalize complaints, when they shift the focus from one item to another without resolving anything or, finally, when they keep interrupting each other, and the therapist is unable to alter these patterns. All these manifestations of anger and built-up resentment are triggered by the mere presence of the real or distorted cause and target of these feelings, namely the spouse. They cloud perception and create an unnecessary risk in the therapeutic process.

The risk is that the session becomes another round in the many hurtful, useless and reinforcing fights to which the couple are so accustomed. Paying money to continue the familiar pattern of fighting may have only one benefit: to shift anger to the therapist; but since the couple perceives the sessions as unproductive, the most frequent outcome is termination of the therapeutic contact. By giving the most angry spouse a chance to discuss things privately, progress can be made towards altering perceptions, and, in the conjoint sessions, the progress made individually can be applied and tested.

The refusal to follow this arrangement explains the failure of many marital therapy cases. It is easy to attribute the failure to patient resistance when the family therapist is the one who is rigid in his/her method of clinical work.

Sexual Issues

The sexual dissatisfaction of one spouse is often based on the lack of sexual interest of the other partner. This lack of interest may have deep roots which predate the current relationship (Araoz, 1980). Frequently, there is a basic ignorance of sexual matters which may be embarrassing for the "ignorant" spouse. By providing individual sessions, many misconceptions can be cleared, many questions answered, and the therapist can use his/her authority to encourage the spouse to consider sexual matters differently.

When Mr. Z. complained about his wife's lack of sexual interest, Mrs. Z. became tense and uncomfortable, refusing to talk. In individual sessions she confessed her fears, ignorance and negative reactions to sexual matters. In the conjoint sessions a sexual moratorium was agreed upon to give Mrs. Z. time to work on her sexual attitudes while the couple concentrated on other areas of their relationship. After a few weeks Mrs. Z. was able to handle the discussion of sex more securely, and the couple made good progress in their sexual relationship.

Value Inflexibility

The third set of circumstances which requires that one spouse be seen individually while the couple is in conjoint therapy takes place when one spouse has a rigid, unbending attitude towards the other *based on principle*. The "principle" aspect is important when strong feelings about religious issues, morality, social rules and so on distort one spouse's view of his/her partner. To get around this situation, the therapist must focus on the "inflexible" spouse to help widen his/her perceptual angle. In other words, the "inflexible" spouse must be helped to view his/her partner along other variables than the issue in question.

Mrs. Y., a very religious woman, could not share this area of her life with her atheistic husband but insisted on bringing up religion in her conversations with him. In individual psychotherapy, she was able to recognize his own nonreligious goodness, rather than focusing on the formal religiosity as she had done before. She came to understand what she was missing in her perception because of her preestablished viewpoint. After realizing that her religious values were also serving as personality defenses, she was able to accept her husband less judgmentally and was ready to work at the real psychological issues in the marriage.

Conclusion

Because factors below the level of awareness are at work in marriage, it is necessary to evaluate how much these factors affect the communication of the couple before proceeding with conjoint sessions. Many subconscious elements can be handled conjointly, but as long as there are basic distortions of perceptual or developmental origin, rational communication is practically impossible (Araoz, 1974). To insist on conjoint sessions under these conditions is to lose sight of the problem-solving aspect of marital therapy which demands creative flexibility from the therapist.

Progress could be made in such cases only by a method which by-passes logical thinking, such as hypnosis (Araoz, 1978). However, hypnosis is not to be used indiscriminately. For the therapist not trained in hypnotic techniques, the preferred modality is seeing one spouse in individual therapy concurrent with seeing the couple in conjoint sessions.

References

Araoz, D. L. Marital transference. *Journal of Family Counseling*, 1974, *2*, 55-63.
Araoz, D. L. Clinical hypnosis in couple therapy. *The Journal of the American Society of Psychosomatic Dentistry and Medicine*, 1978, *25*, 58-67.
Araoz, D. L. Clinical hypnosis in treating sexual abulia. *The American Journal of Family Therapy*, 1980, 8(1), 48-57.

DANIEL L. ARAOZ, Ed.D.
President, Academy of Psychologists in
Marital, Sex and Family Therapy
C. W. Post Center—Long Island University
Greenvale, NY

18. Circularity: A Preferred Orientation
   For Family Assessment

Question:

The terms linear and circular are now being used more and more often when discussing family interaction. Comments such as "but that's linear thinking" and "the hypothesis should be circular" are becoming commonplace. Systems-oriented clinicians prefer circular concepts and suggest that many of the advantages of family therapy result from a theoretical orientation emphasizing circularity. It is also suggested that intervention strategies may be more effective when circular rather than linear concepts are used in the assessment.

Just what is being referred to in the use of these terms? What are some of the differences between linearity and circularity? Why are circular concepts better? How does a circular orientation actually influence a therapist's enquiries when assessing a family?

Discussion:

When therapists sit down with a family they are confronted with a massive amount of information. The amount of data available increases exponentially with each additional family member in the interview. Therapists must somehow organize these data if they are to avoid becoming overwhelmed and thoroughly confused. The major method of doing this is by selective attention, pattern recognition and hypothesis generation. Pattern recognition is particularly important. By compressing raw data into patterns, complex information is simplified and becomes more manageable. The terms linear and circular refer to two basic (content-free) types of patterns that may be recognized.

Thus, these terms reflect contrasting approaches in making connections between events. In the context of family assessment, linearity and circularity refer to different conceptual orientations to identifying patterns to make sense of the information presented about the life of a family.

One major difference between linear and circular patterns lies in the overall structure of the connections between elements of the pattern. Linear patterns are limited to sequences (e.g., A——→B——→C) whereas circular patterns form a closed loop and are recursive (e.g., A——→B——→C——→A . . . etc., or, A⇌B, B⇌C, C⇌A). A less obvious but more significant difference lies in the relative importance usually given to *time* and *meaning* when making the connections or links in the pattern. Linearity is heavily rooted in a framework of a continuous progression of time. Linear explanations depend on careful differentiation of specific links which follow in a causal sequence. Notions of energy and force are often implied with linearity. Circularity, on the other hand, is more heavily dependent on a framework of reciprocal relationships based on meaning. Circular explanations depend on the relevance that elements have for each other and how a change in one implies a change in the other.

With circular conceptualization the progression of time (past——→present——→future) is deemphasized. The time focus is primarily on the present. This does not imply that aspects of the past and future are not included in a circular pattern or hypothesis. When identifying circular patterns or generating circular hypotheses, the relevant block of time is "collapsed," as it were, onto a flat plane of the present. With everything brought into the present, more attention can be focused on the interrelationships based on information and meaning. Although both linear and circular patterns of conceptualization are helpful, circular explanations are more useful in understanding mental events (Bateson, 1979) whereas linear explanations are better in understanding physical events. In clinical practice, these contrasting approaches make a difference in how data (regarding past family events) are collected and used in the interview. A therapist with a linear orientation would focus more carefully on details of time sequences; a therapist with a circular orientation would attend more to the present meaning of these past events, particularly in relationship to the meaning of other events.

Linear and circular explanations may be regarded as hypotheses at different levels of logical type. (Strictly speaking, as such, they should not be directly compared to one another. Bateson points out that the opposite to linear is nonlinear and the opposite to circular is lineal.) Because circularity, if anything, is at a higher level (of logical type), it represents a more complete explanation and therefore carries more "truth." Thus, circular concepts have a distinct advantage. Given a certain type of basic data, linear sequences (e.g., A——→B, B——→C, or C ——→A), may occur *within* a circular pattern (A——→B ——→C ——→A ——→B, etc.) but not vice versa. For instance, it is linear to say, "When Johnny hits

Sally, she cries," or, "When Sally cries, mother comforts her." It is circular to say, "When Johnny hits Sally, she cries and evokes mother's support which angers Johnny who hits Sally, etc." The circular explanation is systemic and is preferred by systems-oriented therapists not only because it is a more complete description, but also because it offers more alternatives for therapeutic intervention. The therapist limited to linear hypotheses would intervene to stop Johnny's behavior, whereas the systemic family therapist may target Johnny, Sally or mother, or the whole circular pattern itself (e.g., with a paradoxical prescription).

A preference for circularity influences the therapist's interviewing style in the assessment (and therapy) process. When conducting a family assessment, it is important to recognize that a process of enquiry exploring *descriptive* characteristics (e.g., "Is mother unhappy?") tends to be linear, whereas an enquiry exploring *differences* (e.g., "Who gets sad the most?") tends to be circular. It is less useful to know whether father is affectionate than to know whether there is a difference in his affection recently compared to before, or whether there is a difference in his affection towards his daughter from that towards his wife. If father is *most* affectionate with his eldest daughter now, he must be *less* affectionate with his wife.

To identify a difference is to necessarily define a relationship between whatever is being compared. A relationship in this sense implies reciprocity. If mother gets her way *more* than father, father necessarily gets his way *less* than mother. Reciprocity, in turn, implies circularity. This application of the basic notion of differences (as a deeper way of knowing—in Bateson's new epistemology) is one of the most brilliant contributions of the Milan group in refining family interviewing techniques (Selvini-Palazzoli et al., 1979). By orienting the enquiry around differences, the therapist elicits more relevant data and does so more efficiently, than by obtaining linear descriptions. The types of differences that may usefully be explored in a family assessment include differences between individuals (e.g., "Who gets angry the most?"), differences between relationships (e.g., "What is the difference between the way mother treats Sally compared to how she treats Johnny?"), differences between times (e.g., "How did she treat him last year compared to now?") and various combinations or permutations of these.

In assessment, the systems-oriented therapist attends selectively to reciprocal relationships and the redundancies of circular patterns. When linear sequences happen to be recognized, the therapist continues to search for the missing links among relevant data to complete a circular loop. For instance, it may be readily apparent in the interview that there is a linear pattern of: wife approaches——→husband withdraws. An enquiry focusing on missing connections may reveal that in bed, when husband approaches——→wife withdraws. Taken together, these sequences reveal a symmetry that has a different meaning and offers a more complete understanding than when each is considered separately.

The core notion of homeostasis in family systems is, of course, a circular concept. If a problem is chronic, it is assumed that it has come to serve a homeostatic function for the system. The therapist tries to generate a global hypothesis of family functioning which is circular, self-perpetuating and includes the "problematic" behavior. This circular hypothesis helps the therapist select a target for the therapeutic intervention. Although this discussion is focused on assessment, it is interesting to note that circular phenomena tend to change by transformation whereas linear phenomena change by altering antecedent causes (some of which may be inaccessible).

One final comment. Circular patterns and concepts are useful tools because they simplify large amounts of complex data. However, one must always remain wary of the intrinsic limitation of all procedures that simplify—a great deal of valuable data is inevitably overlooked and lost.

References

Bateson, G. *Mind and Nature: The Necessary Unity.* New York: E. P. Dutton, 1979.
Selvini-Palazzoli, M., Boscolo, L., Cecchin, G. and Prata, G. Hypothesizing, circularity, neutrality: Three guidelines for the conductor of the session. Unpublished manuscript, Centro per lo Studio della Famiglia de Milano, 1979.

KARL TOMM, M.D.
Associate Professor and Director
Family Therapy Program
Division of Psychiatry
University of Calgary
Calgary, Alberta, Canada

19. Establishing Treatment Contracts in Family Therapy

Question:

During the years of my professional growth, I have been exposed to a variety of theoretical models and a myriad of techniques and clinical procedures that I have used with individuals, couples and families. Expanding my theoretical and clinical scope has operated like a double-edged sword. On the one hand, I now think of persons holistically, as part of an ongoing biochemical, psychosocial system, and ecologically, affecting and being affected by many past and current factors, whereas my early training emphasized the intrapsychic world of a single person and his/her historical, primarily family, context only. Just as I deemphasize diagnostic classification of clients (not "patients"), I no longer think in terms of a single etiological cause, buried in one's past, but of a system which has evolved to where it is now, and which is being maintained by reciprocally reinforcing interpersonal relationships and/or biochemical factors. Nevertheless, each person does have a history which colors his/her perception and interpretation of events, creates emotional reactions and leads to behavior which may or may not be adaptive. Essentially, this is a cognitive-behavioral systems approach (Steinfeld, 1980). It is the client's responsibility to do something about his/her physical, psychological or spiritual predicaments, i.e., seek some help; it's up to us to take it from there.

All this gives me much to think about as I work with clients, and makes work exciting as I continually learn more and refine my theoretical approach and practical skills. But knowing more is also confusing. I now realize how little I know, as opposed to years ago when I believed psychoanalysis, or psychoanalytically oriented psychotherapy, had all the answers (just as I thought my therapist did). Further, having a holistic family systems model makes assessment much more complex. Finally, I have to decide, along with the client, at what level to intervene—mind, body, spirit; with what emphasis—affect, cognition, behavior; with whom—one person, marital dyad, the entire nuclear family, a subgroup; at which point in the therapeutic process; with which techniques; and for what purpose. In essence, developing and implementing a treatment plan which is ethical have become much more difficult. By "ethical" I mean one which is both effective and efficient, whereby the client gets as much as he/she gives so that a fair exchange exists between the client and the therapist (Haley, 1976). The question, then, is how can a systems-oriented, holistic therapist work comfortably, usefully and responsibly in daily clinical practice with clients who bring complex problems in living to him or her?

Discussion:

This sort of question has led me to develop a model of therapy which, to date, addresses itself to some of the above issues. But, I must confess, others still remain unresolved. Nevertheless, some things have become clear at this time, although past experience tells me that in a year or two these seemingly clear issues might be quite muddy indeed.

My Role as Therapist

1) I'm there to help clients change in some way, and to earn my livelihood. I am not there for the purpose of being comfortable, having a warm, empathic relationship with another person, sharing human experiences, exploring the human condition, etc., except insofar as these facilitate change in behavior, feelings and attitude.

2) I am responsible for inducing these changes: (a) I cannot blame the client for being resistant or difficult to work with, etc. (b) If therapy fails, I have made a poor assessment, have used incorrect procedures, have used correct procedures inappropriately, or, in some way, "did it wrong." (c) Part of (a) and (b) is knowing when to accept a client to work with, when and to whom to refer, and being clear with the client as to the nature of the therapeutic contract and our mutual responsibilities during the process.

The Process

When therapy is successful, clients learn something, making it more a cognitive process than an affective or behavioral one. Affective (emotional) expression and behavioral change are important sometimes in and of themselves; however, they are more important insofar as they "feedback" and modify those cognitive structures which have served to organize the clients' experience. The basic cognitive structures which underlie the interpretation of one's experience and guide behavior relate to perceptions and evaluations of oneself, others and the relationships between people. These are learned early and are reinforced by oneself and others in the manner of a continual, self-fulfilling prophecy.

Eric Berne (1972) suggested we try to "cure" patients in a single session. If we fail, we should spend the rest of the week figuring out why. I don't see people as patients to be cured; they're clients who hire us to help them solve human problems. We have the responsibility of working as quickly and as effectively as possible. If we don't do our jobs, clients should fire us. We should also work toward making therapy a science, rather than keeping it an art and polishing our intuitive skills. If we want therapy to be an art, perhaps we should tell clients to pay us after they've seen the finished product. We might all starve.

As I spell out elsewhere (Steinfeld, 1980), I have developed a model called TARET Systems, which integrates the clinical theories of transactional analysis, rational emotive therapy, social learning theory and Eastern philosophy. Assessment is holistic—from the potential contributions of biochemical (neurological, hormonal, nutritional, etc.) factors to the reinforcement of behavior in the context of the family. Whereas I once believed that a family systems model required working with the entire nuclear family every session, I now feel I can work with any part of the system and there will be ripple effects throughout. My approach is similar to the multi-modality therapy of Lazarus (1976), but in addition to employing the broad spectrum approach, along with the technical eclecticism of cognitive behavior therapy, a systems model and the interventions of marital and family therapists are also used. But before specific procedures can be introduced, the client—individual, couple, family—must develop a contract which specifies the goals toward which each person wants to work. The type of contract is related to the type of goals, an outline of which follows.

Contracts Related to the Levels of Therapy

Level 1. At this first level of therapy, there is the alleviation of distressing emotional and behavioral symptoms, while increasing desirable thoughts, feelings and behavior. After assessment, goal agreement and contract development, clients are helped to:

(a) *Go Inside*: Become aware of the labels used to identify emotional states—the physiological reactions and the mental component associated with them. At the first level the therapist teaches new ways of reacting so as to alter negative feelings and increase positive ones. Any number of cognitive-affective-behavioral strategies may be used here. If behavioral change is the focus, the goals relate to expanding the clients' behavioral repertoire.

(b) *Go Outside*: Here the focus is on helping the clients induce changes in others, but the reciprocity involved in family relations is brought into awareness, e.g., what can you do differently to help your wife respond differently to you?

In general, the therapist teaches new responses which are less likely to be self-defeating and more likely to get the clients what they want, both in the short and the long run. To help expand behavioral repertoires, the therapist may employ behavioral rehearsal, risk-taking exercises, communications training to break dysfunctional feedback loops, sculpturing, etc.

Level 2. After feelings are in awareness and the behavioral repertoire is expanded to allow for appropriate emotional expression or suppression (i.e., clients should be comfortable choosing their mode as a function of the anticipated consequences for themselves and others, with regard to their long- and short-term goals and values), clients can learn, if they so wish, to focus on the cognitions which preceded their affective and behavioral reactions. Here, they learn to increase awareness of the automatic thoughts and discriminate differences in their dysfunctional cognitions, such as arbitrary inference, selective abstraction, overgeneralization, magnification and minification, personalization (Beck, 1976), irrational cause-effect relations, mind-reading, etc. All these errors in thinking lead to distortions of reality, under- or over-reactions, and behavior which is often self-defeating. More personal irrational ideas are brought into awareness, disputed cognitively, or via other behavioral and emotive procedures, as discussed elsewhere (Bandler and Grinder, 1975; Ellis, 1973; Meichenbaum, 1977).

Essentially, clients learn to recognize and challenge basic assumptions and expectations about themselves, others and the world. More specifically, they learn to apply the criteria of rational thinking (adult ego state) to their basic belief systems, including the "self-talk" that internal and external events arouse. Thus, the second level is geared toward altering clients' cognitions (i.e., programmed "sets," cultural and family scripts, the "shoulds" and other "musterbatory" ideas which drive them in self-defeating directions). Focusing on this level provides for the more "elegant" solutions to problems in living (Ellis, 1973).

The purpose here is not necessarily to express negative emotions, but to reduce and even eliminate their occurrence (i.e., to let go or not hold on to them), while simultaneously learning to express appropriate reactions in the most appropriate ways, i.e., ways which will tend to get clients what they want, enhance their feelings about themselves, while respecting the rights and feelings of others.

Level 3. The third level of therapy addresses itself to the relative nature of reality. Basic to this process is the clients' conception of themselves, and learning not to take themselves, others, situations and the world too seriously. Involvement with detachment is one of the primary goals, as is the understanding of one's past as it relates to the present and the future. If desired, clients learn to explore how they may have learned to view themselves as they do, and how they continue to perpetuate certain myths about reality and the "games of life." Here, script analysis (Berne, 1972) is undertaken, so that clients can gain some historical perspective. At this level, questions of values and ethical principles are explored so that long- and short-range goals can become consistent with their guiding principles. The meaning of one's life is the issue, and how thoughts, feelings and behavior can facilitate the actualization of one's potential. Meta-questions are used extensively here, e.g., How do I think and feel about how you feel (think and do)? The purpose is to constantly penetrate to the basic beliefs about the nature of the self and to challenge its rigidity. Work at this level, in contrast to levels 1 and 2, is likely to take place individually, but its implication for the family is always kept in mind.

To summarize, contracts overcome obscure goals of traditional therapy and help us know whether clients are getting what they are paying for. In this regard, behaviorally oriented clinicians and transactional analysts are the only groups who consistently make systematic use of contractual psychotherapy. Not only should goals and procedures be clear, but potential dangers of change should be discussed. Contracts also help do away with the concept of resistance, or, at least, minimize it as an excuse for ineffective psychotherapy. For therapists who want to hold onto this notion, I suggest they also apply the concept of counterresistance to their work, e.g., slowing down the therapeutic process or iatrogenically creating more problems for economic or psychological reasons. As you can see, clear contracts can help do away with interminable psychotherapy and make clients and therapists accountable and responsible for their respective contributions to the process.

References

Bandler, R., and Grinder, J. *The Structure of Magic*. Vol 1. Palo Alto, CA: Science and Behavior Books, 1975.

Beck, A. *Cognitive Therapy and the Emotional Disorders*. New York: International Universities Press, 1976.

Berne, E. *What Do You Say After You Say Hello?* New York: Grove Press, 1972.

Ellis, A. *Humanistic Psychotherapy*. New York: Julian Press, 1973.

Haley, J. *Problem-Solving Therapy*. San Francisco: Jossey-Bass, 1976.

Lazarus, A. *Multi-modal Behavior Therapy*. New York: Springer, 1976.

Meichenbaum, D. *Cognitive Behavior Modification*. New York: Plenum, 1977.

Steinfeld, G. J. *TARET Systems: An Integrative Approach to Individual and Family Therapy*. Jonesboro, TN: Pilgrimage Press, 1980.

GEORGE J. STEINFELD, Ph.D.
Director, Adolescent Program
Division of Children and Youth
Greater Bridgeport Children Services
Bridgeport, CT

20. Multifamily Group Therapy for Outpatients

Question:

Most of what I have read and heard about multifamily group therapy (MFGT) suggests that it is most often used in psychiatric inpatient settings. I have done a fair amount of couples group therapy, but no multifamily group therapy with outpatients. Doing it with outpatients just seems administratively overwhelming. Can someone offer some practical tips on how to select families for outpatient MFGT, how to focus the early sessions, in general, how to get started in a way that's likely to succeed?

Discussion:

Two questions seem to be raised here, which I have struggled to separate in my response, one on a practical level, the other on a more theoretical plane. Beyond the question of the mechanics of starting multiple family group therapy (MFGT) lies the more fundamental question of how innovations are successfully introduced in clinical settings, or,"How do you teach old systems new tricks?"

To begin, MFGT therapists need enough administrative control over their work so they may define the appropriate place, time and patient referral process for their group. This allows them to develop systems boundaries around their work, so they may select the families, supervision and challenges they are prepared for. MFGT usually benefits from cotherapists and may involve other staff, too. If MFGT is seen as innovative and exciting, is given support by senior members and supervisors from the staff, and is not covertly designed to show how certain individuals, families or therapies are bound to fail, then the group is more likely to succeed. Initial enthusiasm can be generated through simulated workshops, as Peter Laqueur advocated in an article published just before his death (Raasoch and Laqueur, 1979), or through available teaching video cassettes (Lurie et al., 1978).

Therapist social support and territories must be respected. At one institution which had some 13 MFT outpatient groups running at one time, the cotherapists formed their own mutual support group, which met over dinner after the family meetings and was strictly limited to those leading MFT groups. The dinners were largely social but sustained each cotherapy team and made MFGT the "in" thing to be doing. Other methods of sharing one's work with colleagues are also important (e.g., videotapes, presentations, etc.). It is particularly difficult to begin with "graduates" of other treatments (e.g., hospitalization) as other therapists are reluctant to give up those families who are their most successful and gratifying. As an alternative, a therapist may bring several of his/her families already in conjoint treatment together in a group under that therapist's leadership.

To paraphrase our most family-conscious president, "Ask not what family will do for your treatment, but what your treatment will do for the family." For which families is MFGT the treatment of choice? MFGT provides something which conjoint family therapy cannot—relief from the social and emotional isolation that so often accompanies families with severe medical, social or emotional problems. Whether the social isolation is a cause or consequence of the presenting problem is of secondary importance. MFGT is designed to "help teach families to help themselves" and considerable esteem can be generated for families who can help others through emotional support or such concrete resources as job leads and baby-sitting. The list of psychiatric diagnoses that are complicated by social isolation are legion, but most would be helped by MFGT, especially enmeshed and stigmatized families. The major exception is families with sociopathic or psychopathic behavior in one or several members. Highly disorganized, "hopeless" families and those with members who are chronic schizophrenics respond surprisingly well to MFGT and are frequently able to maintain members in the community for long periods of time with only this support. One group, which was made up of such families whose members were often admitted to the state hospital, "survived" a Christmas recess without a hospitalization even with both cotherapists on vacation. To the therapists' pleasant surprise, the group had met regularly in their absence in various members' homes.

Fortunately, the literature is not barren of examples of successful MFGT efforts in a remarkably wide variety of outpatient settings, as recent reviews in several different journals attest (Benningfield, 1978; Frager, 1978; Strelnick, 1977). A brief catalogue of the published reports suggests that very few outpatient settings have not supported MFGT! Success has been reported in all of the following settings: community mental health centers, psychiatric day centers, child guidance clinics, voluntary family service agencies, alcohol and drug treatment programs, family therapy institutes, psychiatric outpatient departments, hemodialysis units, intensive workshops, schools, churches and community centers. I am also familiar with MFT groups in a private practice, in the families' homes and in a state hospital aftercare program.

MFGT may be viewed as intermediate between therapy and a self-help group. Different families, groups and therapists will require different balances between these two poles. Families which may benefit most from the self-help model can be organized around similar problems, such as school behavior problems, reconstituted (step) families, chronic illness or adolescent rebellion, without the illusion that any two families with similar problems are homogeneous. Particular success has been found with the last category, as the MFT group provides the adolescent with age-appropriate peer-group support, as well as alternative adult relationships and cross-parenting. The issues of individuation and family loyalty generated by the adolescents frequently resonate to similar struggles in their parents' marriages. It is helpful to have several of the group's children about the same age. On the other hand, Peggy Papp, who gave up trying to match families for her first MFGT and just called three families randomly from a waiting list, launched what proved to be a successful, if disparate group (Papp, 1974).

Heterogeneous groups, such as might be found naturally in a psychiatric day center or an aftercare program, can maintain common goals of preventing further hospitalizations and normalizing the family's affairs without institutional interventions. The importance and difficulty of transition to the community, the stigma attached to hospitalization or being "crazy," the issues of medication and heredity will all be shared, and family communication will be a recurring theme in all groups.

In launching a new group the cotherapists will presumably interview the several families to be involved and share with them the nature and purpose of MFGT. These families need to be "engaged" in treatment before entering the group, even if only by thorough joining in a preliminary interview. Following the rounds of introductions where families may begin to share their common problems, the cotherapists—who have chosen to focus on individual family and/or group dynamics—may move to the similarities and parallels between families, the diverse skills and coping mechanisms which they possess, their many social and personal resources which can be valuable to others in the group, and the importance of families learning from each other. Relabeling and reframing problems at this point can be useful both in directing the discussion and modeling new, positive approaches to problem solving. Some therapists (Bowen, Papp) may work with just one family at a time, as the others observe and wait to share their comments without free-for-all group interaction.

Unless the group is made up of "graduates" of previous family therapy, it is likely that the families will continue to try to contain their problems in a single patient or incident, and marital conflict will be minimized. Premature exposure of these difficult problems may be too threatening, resulting in dropouts. Adequate time must be given for each session, as it will usually require a half hour for most groups to settle down to more than social conversation. Therapists will find that, after getting the group going, its momentum will make it very difficult to end. Sculpting, role-playing or other psychodrama techniques are useful for groups which get stalled or monopolized. Physical movement and group formation around family roles (e.g., fathers in a central subgroup talking about fathering, etc.) are good opening exercises and keep children interested.

The value of MFGT does not end the moment the therapist declares the session over; frequently the most valuable work is done in time preceding or following the official sessions. Some groups have capitalized on this by formalizing pre- or postmeeting coffee or meals, prepared and shared by the participants. These "administrative" embellishments are important components of the group's social network building and should be facilitated.

There are at least two approaches to help families overcome their fears of what might seem overwhelming and unhelpful. ("Don't we already have enough problems of our own?") The first, for families already engaged in therapy, builds upon their relationship to the therapist and his/her agency. In this "graduate seminar" approach, emphasis may be on the self-help aspects of the group. The second approach, treatment of choice, refers appropriate families to MFGT after the initial evaluation of the therapists that MFGT is the best treatment for these family problems. With the strong recommendation for MFGT from the "experts," a family in crisis may venture into this potentially threatening type of therapy. Engaging the family through careful joining during the evaluation interview is almost always needed.

The more theoretical questions involved in discussing initiating outpatient MFGT are the problems and consequences of innovation in ongoing systems. Each agency has its own chemistry and ecology. Both psychological and administrative resistance to change will be at work whenever a new modality is introduced into an ongoing system. These homeostatic ideologies contribute to the sense that MFGT will be overwhelming. No genuine innovation and change in a system are likely to be psychologically "pure." The successful catalyst may be an individual's need for experimentation or personal growth when other clinical work has lost its challenge, or it may be the innovative response of an agency to demands for increasing productivity or shortening waiting lists economically. The major problem lies in the therapist and his/her supports and not the families. If the therapist is prepared to face the initial confusion, de-skilling and anxiety of having several families together, then s/he may help those families overcome their fears of exposure and shame and make the group thrive. MFGT can then be an adventure in modifying the therapist's role and in learning how to step back to teach families how to help themselves and each other.

References

Benningfield, A. B. Multiple family therapy systems. *Journal of Marriage and Family Counseling*, 1978, 40, 25-34.

Frager, S. Multiple family therapy: A literature review. *Family Therapy*, 1978, 5, 105-120.

Lurie, A., Schwartzberg, N., Young, P., and Kovacs, E. Family and Multi-Family Therapy. Video Cassette, Blue Hill Education Systems, 52 South Main Street, Spring Valley, New York 10977, 1978.

Papp, P. Multiple ways of multiple family therapists. *The Family*, 1974, 1, 20-25.

Raasoch, J. and Laqueur, H. P. Learning multiple family therapy through simulated workshops. *Family Process*, 1979, 18, 95-98.

Strelnick, A. H. Multiple family group therapy: A review of the literature. *Family Process*, 1977, 16, 307-325.

ALVIN H. STRELNICK, M.D.
Martin Luther King
Health Center
Bathgate Division
Bronx, NY

21. Selection of Couples for Group Therapy

Question:

I am a marital therapist in a family service agency with a very large and increasing service responsibility. Because our funding for staff positions is limited, we are considering the idea of seeing more couples in group therapy. Our staff is generally quite experienced in work in conjoint therapy, but has limited group experience. Therefore, one of our major concerns is the question of group composition. What couples should be (and not be) in a therapy group together? Our clients represent a rather wide range of people, so that many types of couples groups are possible. Should the couples be about the same age, at similar developmental levels, have the same sorts of presenting problems? What range of individual psychopathology is tolerable, e.g., should alcoholic couples be mixed with more garden variety difficulties? In group selection and composition, what would be ideal and what would be the worst combinations?

Discussion:

The problem of group composition presents an interesting dilemma. It is usually approached as though the central issue were the question we have been asked, namely, "What couples should be (and not be) in a therapy group together?" This presents the issues as though the decisions to be made were primarily diagnostic and were made by the therapist. In fact the issues are approached better if we formulate the question as follows, "What sort of negotiations between the couple and the therapist are necessary and appropriate for the couple to agree to participate in group therapy (with the concurrence of the therapist) and to in fact follow through?"

What this rephrasing of the questions emphasizes is that the referral of a couple to a group is the end result of a process which may in fact often begin with the negotiations that involve the presenting patient being seen alone instead of as a member of a couple. Let us focus our attention on a couple who are in marital distress and to some degree or other are both willing to participate in therapy. Clearly, to arrive at this point involves a considerable amount of work, which usually includes some evaluation, support, empathy for each member, and almost always some change. It is rare that couples seek help who are not in acute and painful distress, and the type of individualized understanding, support and focused interventions that can alleviate to some degree the immediate situation are not readily available in groups. Individual patients also tend to require some individual therapy before a referral to group can be made.

This view of the negotiating process emphasizes that, for a referral of a couple to group to be successful, the couple must have received some help with the immediate precipitating situation. They must have a therapeutic alliance with the therapist in whom they feel confident so that they feel understood. Many couples will be satisfied with brief and relatively focused therapy (again this is true for individuals), but others will desire to get to the "bottom of things," or will see or can be shown that their problems are longstanding and require further intervention (Grunebaum, Christ and Neiberg, 1969). It is these couples who are appropriately referred to couples groups. Referring couples in the absence of a therapeutic alliance may help lower the treatment load of the clinic but does not help the couple since the attrition between the referral and true involvement in the group will be quite high. In fact, many couples will require some degree of support from the initial evaluator-therapist in order to be able to join a group, since group psychotherapy is often experienced initially as stressful.

Thus far we have emphasized the more general, negotiated aspects of referral to couples groups; now let us turn to a consideration of the composition of the groups. There is no research on this subject, so we are left with clinical experience as a guide. Therapists generally agree that in individual group psychotherapy a certain degree of homogeneity is desirable. The individual who differs too greatly by virtue of degree of psychopathology, age, intellect, social class, work or other characteristics is likely either to leave or to be extruded. A group should be viewed as offering the opportunity and challenge of peer relationships and groups will not accept anyone who is too different.

This criterion applies to couples groups as well as to individuals. Couples who are dealing with similar issues in the life cycle often do well together if they are not too disparate in other ways. Certain differences can be tolerated if there are other similarities. For instance, a couple in their forties who are newly married might do well in a group of somewhat younger couples who are also recently married.

However, if this couple's issues involve the clash of character styles rather than the problems of early marriage, they may do better in a group of couples the same age but who have been married longer. In general, I have found that couples who have similar degrees of psychopathology do better than those with great differences in functioning. In particular, the ability of couples to function socially is critical. Are they able to welcome other members to the group and show them how to become members, or are they too egocentric and lacking in social skills to do this? The presence of social skills, the ability to relate as a peer, is probably more important than particular diagnoses, although here again certain common problems such as drugs or alcohol may draw a group together. It is my experience that couples reasonably well matched in regard to mental issues tend to do well together in groups.

It should be emphasized that a considerable number of couples, usually those with ego-syntonic characterological problems of long duration, are difficult to work with and to change. Finally, a certain number of couples will inevitably choose to get divorced during any couples therapy. The goal should be to help them reach this decision mutually and with minimal destructive impact on themselves or their children.

In summary, I have emphasized the negotiating process necessary for successful referral to couples group psychotherapy. Similarity of developmental issues in the marriage and ability to relate to peers have been suggested as the most useful criteria for the composition of well-functioning groups.

Reference

Grunebaum, H., Christ, J., and Neiberg, N. Diagnosis and treatment planning for couples, *International Journal of Group Psychotherapy 19*: 185-202, 1969.

HENRY GRUNEBAUM, M.D.
Associate Professor
Department of Psychiatry
The Cambridge Hospital-
Harvard Medical School
Cambridge, MA

22. Screening Couples for Marital Enrichment Programs

Question:

Most of the marriage enrichment programs I've heard about (e.g., Marriage Encounter, Couples Communication Program) say very little about what criteria should be used to screen out couples from these programs. My question has two parts: 1) What should an enrichment program leader look for in screening couples out of these programs before they start? and, 2) What are some common signs that show up after the program is underway that indicate that a couple needs more than enrichment (i.e., therapy)?

Discussion:

This is a very pertinent issue that comes up for anyone working in the area of social skills training, in groups, couples and families (L'Abate, 1977, 1981). Indeed, very little data can be found about this issue, so that this response will be based mostly on the experiences of this writer rather than on published, objective criteria.

Before admission to a program. To begin, L'Abate (1977) suggested very basic and obvious criteria for screening out: (a) uncooperative or extremely hostile or angry couples who indicate the existence of projective identification and excessive use of blaming ("you"), generalizations ("never," "always"); (b) chaotic or disorganized couples in crisis, who indicate that they do consider, or have considered, separation or divorce, and who, in the screening interview, show confusion of goals in their own lives or marriage, or who think that the structured experience will have magical results or be a substitute for therapy; (c) couples who have experienced a recent loss (death of close relatives, moving away of children, etc.) and attempt to reinstate this loss through the experience of enrichment, encounter, etc., (d) couples with entrenched psychosomatic or delusional systems that make them externalize most of their tensions outside themselves and their marriage.

In addition to the above considerations, enrichment leaders should consider the following expressions of excessive defensiveness as contraindications to admission to such structured programs: (a) excessively defensive statements, such as strong denial of any tension and/or conflict; (b) either a very digital (either-or) or extremely vague, amorphous and diffuse view of life and themselves; (c) superficial and shallow goals and views about the nature of life and human nature; (d) mixed or confused priorities about self, marriage and children, or work and family, where the woman typically puts the husband and children before the self and the husband puts wife, children and work before the self (L'Abate, 1976); (e) inappropriate or incongruent affect, with a minimum of congruent "I" statements and a maximum of blaming, placating, distracting and computing statements; (f) excessive polarization in the marriage as shown by overexpressivity in the woman and underexpressivity in the man (sometimes this pattern is reversed).

All of the above criteria are subjective and experiential. If or when a screening battery is administered, as we do routinely (L'Abate, 1977), extreme scores on any measure of marital or personal adjustment need to be considered, especially if such deviance is shown on more than one or two instruments.

After admission. No matter how careful a screening can be, some unusual or excessively troubled couple will inevitably slip through. When that happens, it is important to neutralize their impact on other couples and to minimize costs. It is usually important for the trainer to: (a) defuse the impact of extreme emotionality by making reflective statements on their felt conditions, and (b) set limits (L'Abate et al., 1975) on what the couple can say or do to avoid focusing on themselves and attracting more attention than the rest of the group combined.

These couples usually give themselves away by showing many of the patterns that should have been picked up in a screening interview and in a screening battery. In addition, these couples show a tendency to call attention to themselves by being unable to learn and to master whatever skills are being imparted. Their decision-making and negotiation skills become bogged down, and they are usually unable to reach a satisfactory level of solution or completion. Excessive emotionality or withdrawal may be present and the trainer needs to use all of his/her skills to be able to: (a) ignore, (b) confront, or (c) limit the presence of patterns that may disrupt or slow down the process of training. In extreme cases it may be necessary for the trainer to call the couple away from the group ("I would like to have a conference with you both if you don't mind") to avoid setting limits or confronting them in front of other couples. It is very important for a trainer to avoid other couples' setting limits for the troublesome couple or assuming a role that belongs to the trainer alone. When this happens, it may indicate that the trainer has lost control of the group and abdicated his/her responsibility as leader and conductor.

After the program. In follow-up interviews with individual couples, which should always follow a structured program, the trainer may have a better chance to confront various issues with the troublesome couple, deal with their original expectations ("We really thought it was going to be like a therapy group"), defuse the excessiveness of their emotionality, and help them deal more realistically with what they need for themselves (L'Abate and L'Abate, 1977) and consider the various options available to them. Typically in our training program, such follow-up interviews are divided into three stages: 1) "What did you get out of this program?" 2) "Let me tell you my reactions to you"—whereby assets are first asserted and reviewed, and then liabilities are raised—"You may need to work on . . ." and 3) "Where do you plan to go from here?", whereby various options are listed (nothing, more enrichment, therapy) and, depending on the degree of satisfaction, suggestions, recommendations and pertinent referrals are made.

References

L'Abate, L. *Understanding and Helping the Individual in the Family.* New York: Grune & Stratton, 1976.

L'Abate, L. *Enrichment: Structured Programs for Couples, Families, and Groups.* Washington, D.C.: University Press of America, 1977.

L'Abate, L. Skill training programs for couples and families: Clinical and nonclinical applications. In A. S. Gurman and D. Kniskern (Eds.), *Handbook of Family Therapy.* New York: Brunner/Mazel, 1981.

L'Abate, L., and L'Abate, B. *How to Avoid Divorce: Help for Troubled Marriages.* Atlanta: John Knox Press, 1977.

L'Abate, L. and collaborators. *Manual: Enrichment Manuals for the Family Life Cycle.* Atlanta: Social Research Laboratories, 1975.

LUCIANO L'ABATE, Ph.D.
Professor
Department of Psychology
Georgia State University
Atlanta, GA

23. Marital Therapy and Child Management Training

Question:

Child management training, teaching parents to correctly apply learning theory principles to increase their children's desired behaviors and decrease undesired behaviors, has obviously had a tremendous impact the last several years. But often the child's deviant behavior is a direct outgrowth of conflict between the parents, but not just conflict over their child's behavior. My question is, in clinical practice how does a behavioral family therapist make the important decision of whether to focus on the child's problem (as requested by the parents) or to focus on the marital relationship?

Discussion:

Any practicing family therapist knows that resolution of child behavior problems requires parents' cooperation, often their active involvement. Parents enmeshed in bitter conflict, or parents struggling to convince themselves and others of their compatibility, are no great allies either for their child or the therapist.

But the blanket assumption that where there is a child behavior problem there are also marital difficulties is groundless. There is no evidence that children's difficulties are universally symptomatic of marital troubles. Suspicions about the quality of the marital relationship are not doubly justified simply because conflict between parents is not apparent.

Parents, as consumers of therapeutic services, deserve to have their requests treated as legitimate. And children, as people rather than chattel, deserve to receive treatment than enhances their individual growth, that does not merely force them to conform to parental and societal rules. To bypass parents' statement of a presenting problem that focuses on their child demands evidence that such intervention would either fail or harm the child. Evidence that would lead me away from child intervention and toward marital intervention can be summarized by a series of questions.

Is the child-related presenting problem legitimate? To design an intervention focused on a child requires evidence of specific excessive or insufficient child behaviors. If systematic observations of the child revealed that the presenting problem was either unfounded or unsound, given knowledge of the range of normal child development, I would explore with the parents the connection between their worries about the child and their relationship with each other. Must parents be involved in intervention? Some child problems can be successfully treated with little or no parental involvement. School-based interventions can be designed for most academic and many social, emotional and symptomatic behavior problems. All that is needed is some manifestation of either the problem behavior or a desirable competing behavior in the school setting and a working relationship with the classroom teacher. Shyness, aggression, phobias, hyperactivity occur at school and often interfere enough with academic progress that teachers gladly cooperate with therapists in efforts to remediate these problems. When the presenting problem occurs principally away from home, when the presenting problem involves peers not adults, parents can do little to help or hinder, and so regardless of their relationship, attention to the child's problem is justified.

Will the nature of the parents' relationship prevent them from active involvement in their child's behalf? Some parents who are openly unhappy with one another, and some who valiantly struggle to seal over dissatisfactions, are willing and able to participate in a child-focused intervention. An intervention plan always foresees potential hazards and prepares for them. Quarrels about childrearing and lack of cooperation between parents, together with a legitimate child-presenting problem, call for active parental involvement and a simple intervention plan that foresees numerous hazards. In its early stages of implementation, this plan must train parents to coordinate their efforts.

Will a successful child management plan strengthen the couple's relationship? The most conflict-ridden couples are those with children (particularly teenagers) at home. Much of this conflict is a natural side-effect of frustrating childrearing responsibilities for which none of us are adequately prepared. Too often children's problems are mistakenly attributed to defects in the parents' relationship. But this is just a specific instance of a general cultural tendency to assume parents determine children's behavior. The reality of family life in which parents and children continually affect each other is more complex.

An intervention plan that carefully foresees hazards to remediation of the child's problem in the parents' relationship might plan periodic, simple objective measurements of the parents' relationship. This permits feedback to parents not only about their child's improvement but also about spontaneous improvement in their own solution of problems together. Such spontaneous improvement is often unnoticed or dismissed as superficial. But it can be a catalyst for change.

In short, I recommend that the clinician determine with the family whether the child presenting problem is legitimate, whether parents need to be involved in its remediation, whether the nature of the parents' relationship really will interfere with their contribution to a child-focused intervention and whether the marriage might benefit from the parents' active involvement in a child-focused intervention. Some of this information can be gathered in one or two family intake interviews. Some of it might be gathered during baseline observations of the child's behavior by directly sampling relevant parent interaction.

The acid test of the contributions that parents can make to child-focused intervention will come during the intervention itself. Any intervention plan, designed with limited information at hand, may prove unsuccessful in practice and need revision. One likely revision in any child-focused intervention is alteration of the parents' role. If the second stage of a child-focused intervention eliminates parent involvement and succeeds in remedying the child's problem, while the first stage in which parents collaborated did not, the therapist and the parents gain important information. Learning the skill that earlier prevented them from helping their child is an ideal objective for marital therapy.

ELAINE A. BLECHMAN, Ph.D.
Research Associate Professor
Department of Psychology
Wesleyan University
Middletown, CT

24. Contingency Contracting in Behavioral Marriage Therapy

Question:

From various workshops I've attended the last couple of years, I've gotten the impression that behavioral marital therapists are less likely than they used to be to emphasize the importance of explicit contingency contracting with couples, i.e., to specify various concrete quid quo pro exchanges of behavior. Instead, they seem to place more weight on communication training and problem-solving training without necessarily following up on these methods with explicit, contracted exchanges. My questions, then, are, Just when *is* explicit contracting called for in behavioral couples therapy? and When should such contracting be done in more eclectic, nonbehavioral therapy?

Discussion:

Those who have followed the relatively brief history of behavioral marital therapy (BMT) will have noticed a recent shift in objectives. BMT began as highly *content-oriented* treatment in which reinforcement principles were directed to the elimination of a couple's presenting complaints. As such, contingency contracting attracted a great deal of attention as the most distinctive and innovative feature of the behavioral technology. Unfortunately, contingency contracting was sometimes presented as a treatment procedure that stood alone rather than as part of a more comprehensive, but less clearly defined, process of negotiation and behavior change.

Currently, the focus of BMT has shifted to improving the *process* of a couple's interaction so that, ultimately, the couple themselves can evoke self-directed relationship change and can reverse relationship setbacks. To meet this overriding aim, BMT has become a multifaceted, programmatic approach that encompasses a variety of objectives, e.g., increasing spouses' attractiveness for one another, restructuring family rules, improving listening and supportiveness skills, and developing problem-solving skills. Contingency contracting is a procedure that can be used to promote one or more of these treatment objectives but is not, in its own right, an objective of treatment nor a necessary treatment component.

To understand how contingency contracting fits into an overall process of therapeutic change, it is important to differentiate between contracts in general and contingency contracts. A therapeutic contract is any written agreement in which the conditions are clearly specified and completely understood by all participants. Contracts are often written to foster behavior change but may also be used for other purposes, for example, to delineate family rules. A contingency contract is a written agreement which, in addition to specifying a relationship change, also specifies consequences for compliance or noncompliance with the desired change. These contracts can take a *quid pro quo* format in which each partner's behavior change serves as the reinforcement for the other's behavior change. Or, they may be *parallel* contracts in which the reward that each spouse receives for contractual compliance is totally independent from the other partner's targeted behavior change (Weiss, Birchler and Vincent, 1974). For example, for a husband and wife who have trouble with finances, a quid pro quo contract might read:

> Wife agrees that each Friday she will pay all bills that have accumulated during the previous week. Husband agrees that on two Saturdays a month he will review the budget and on alternate Saturdays he will personally deposit both partners' paychecks in the bank.

The same target behaviors in a parallel contract would read:

> Wife agrees that each Friday she will pay all bills that have accumulated during the previous week. Reward: Husband accompanies wife on a walk that evening.

> Husband agrees that on two Saturdays a month he will review the budget and on alternate Saturdays he will personally deposit both partners' paychecks in the bank. Reward: A back rub that evening from wife.

In a therapeutic endeavor to evoke behavior change, both formats of contingency contracting are best viewed as extensions of problem solving. Regardless of whether or not one is working within a behavioral framework, contracting must follow a process of thoughtful negotiation; otherwise it is likely that the terms of a contract will be determined unilaterally, and the contract itself will become an ultimatum rather than a negotiated agreement. Furthermore, in any problem-solving process it is recommended that the negotiated agreement be put in writing and stated in specific concrete terms. What is less clear is whether an agreement actually benefits from the additional structure provided by contingencies, or whether the contingencies are in fact superfluous to the successful implementation of the change agreement.

Unfortunately, since research offers us very little guidance on the utility of applying contingencies to written agreements,* we are left to clinical speculation. It has been hypothesized that the utility of this procedure lies in both its stimulus control and reinforcing control properties (Jacobson, 1978b; Weiss, 1978). Stimulus control properties refer to the contract's function as a cue: Simply having a written statement, with or without contingencies, serves as a reminder that an agreement was indeed reached and obviates "forgetfulness" about the specific terms of the agreement. Additionally it is possible that the rewards themselves in a contingency contract possess cue functions (Jacobson and Margolin, 1979). If, for example, a husband is to receive his favorite drink as a contingency for arriving home on time, that drink may serve to cue both spouses that desired changes have occurred. In essence, the reward draws attention to the fact that the desired behavior has been emitted and, as such, may facilitate tracking desired behaviors and may lead to positive cognitions.

The reinforcing properties of a contingency contract are determined by the impact of the contract. In quid pro quo contracts with the two target behaviors linked, the receipt of the partner's target behavior is the reward for emitting one's own target response. An additional and perhaps more potent reward comes with the recognition that the partner's willingness to engage in the contracted behavior signals that person's investment in the future of the relationship. Since parallel contracts include a positive contingency for compliance, regardless of whether or not the partner fulfills his/her side of the agreement, there is an additional level of reinforcing control. Yet, the positive contingencies are often viewed by couples as "frosting on the cake." Couples frequently report that fulfillment of the agreement is the meaningful reward and sometimes even fail to award themselves the predetermined contingency.

Careful consideration of reinforcing control has also led to the speculation that contingency contracting may offer some clinical hazards. One practical issue is the difficulty in identifying reinforcers for adults. While the rewards in most contingency contracts are pleasant to re-

---

*Jacobson (1978a) offers some data comparing quid pro quo and parallel contracts. No study has yet isolated contingency contracting from other behavior exchange and/or problem-solving procedures and studied its relative effectiveness.

ceive, it is highly unlikely that they are responsible for eliciting the target behavior. Thus, a contract that is actually predicated on the reinforcing qualities of the contingencies, rather than spouses' good intentions and readiness for change, is a risky venture. An even greater danger is that the specification of the reward actually reduces its reinforcing power (Jacobson and Margolin, 1979). If the motivation for the reward is attributed to the contract per se rather than the partner's good intentions, then the desirability of such a reward may be reduced. Through an extension of this reasoning, the import of the behavior change itself may be threatened if the recipient believes that the contract "forced" the desired behavior.

Faced with these potential advantages and disadvantages, the clinician must decide when contingency contracting is clinically indicated versus when it is ill-advised or simply redundant. Consider the situation of a wife who feels that her husband does not do his share of the household chores. Contingency contracting around this issue would be ill-advised if, upon careful exploration, it became evident that this complaint is merely a smoke-screen for a different issue, for example, the wife's desire to take a job outside the home. A contracted solution to the original issue may indeed lead to a temporary increase in the husband's activity around the home, but this premature effort to elicit behavior change would stymie understanding of the more general issue. For this couple, therapy should be directed toward exploring the overall impact of the proposed change in life style and restructuring relationship rules, rather than resolving one specific complaint.

Another possible scenario regarding the same presenting complaint is that the couple simply lack adequate problem-solving skills. Once the wife's request is clearly stated and the couple brainstorm a variety of possible solutions, the husband may be quite willing to comply with the new arrangements. In this case, since the requested changes are not at great cost to the husband, specific contingencies for his behavior change may be unnecessary. If, however, housekeeping represented a highly sensitive issue, so that the problem-solving agreement would be fulfilled only with great reluctance, then a contingency contract may be in order to insure that the husband receives something in exchange for his efforts. Furthermore, if the wife were not particularly skilled at spontaneously showing her appreciation for the husband's new activities, the contingency would guarantee her acknowledgement of the husband's change.

In sum, contingency contracts are seen as applicable for issues that have such a long and difficult history that there is a question about whether or not the change agreement will be enacted without the additional structure of the contingency. Since we lack data on what couples ultimately benefit from contingency contracting, the decision to introduce this procedure rests with the clinician. In making this decision, it is important to keep in mind that instructing a couple in how to write contingency contracts is a relatively cost-efficient process, requiring less than one hour. The time invested in this process has the added benefit of communicating to the couple the seriousness of their contractual agreements. For couples who reject the idea of prespecified consequences, there is no reason to force-feed this strategy—particularly if they fulfill their agreements without the contingencies. Yet, many couples are favorably disposed to the approach, appreciating its business-like quality or finding it a face-saving way to make changes that they have long resisted; for these couples, contingency contracting can become an integral part of their problem-solving process.

References

Jacobson, N. S. Specific and nonspecific factors in the effectiveness of a behavioral approach to the treatment of marital discord. *Journal of Consulting and Clinical Psychology*, 1978, *46*, 442-452.(a)

Jacobson, N. S. A stimulus control model of change in behavioral marital therapy: Implications for contingency contracting. *Journal of Marriage and Family Counseling*, 1978, *3*, 29-35.(b)

Jacobson, N. S., and Margolin, G. *Marital Therapy: Strategies Based on Social Learning and Behavioral Exchange Principles*. New York: Brunner/Mazel, 1979.

Weiss, R. L. The conceptualization of marriage from a behavioral perspective. In T. J. Paolino and B. S. McCrady (Eds.) *Marriage and Marital Therapy: Psychoanalytic, Behavioral and System Theory Perspectives*. New York: Brunner/Mazel, 1978.

Weiss, R. L., Birchler, G. R., and Vincent, J. P. Contractual models for negotiation training in marital dyads. *Journal of Marriage and the Family*, 1974, *36*, 321-331.

GAYLA MARGOLIN, Ph.D.
Assistant Professor
Department of Psychology
University of Southern California
Los Angeles, CA

25. Combining Behavioral and Structural Family Therapies

Question:

Structural family therapy seems to me to often include a good deal of straightforward behavior modification techniques, e.g., reinforcement for weight gain in anorexia. Since behavior therapists are so much more "instructive" than structural therapists (e.g., making explicit their treatment goals, intervention techniques and their rationale, etc.), how can these models be consistently integrated in practice? Aren't there a lot of assumptions in each model that are diametrically opposed to the assumptions in the other model?

Discussion:

Questions such as these have become increasingly frequent, since the description in *Psychomatic Families* (1978) of the work of the Minuchin group with anorexia. Their brief behavioral inpatient program was used with approximately half of the 53 cases treated, all of whom received structural family therapy (SFT) for an average of six months. *Psychosomatic Families* takes pains to differentiate the SFT approach to anorexia from a behavior modification approach. It is my own opinion (despite being a member of that project and a confirmed advocate of SFT) that the two approaches are fundamentally quite compatible, and that it is possible to integrate them consistently in practice. In order to achieve this integration, it is important to examine some of the considerable differences that currently exist in clinical practice, to see whether these differences are based upon fundamentally different assumptions or upon biases that can be corrected without doing violence to either model.

The similarities between the two approaches are probably obvious to anyone familiar with both. Both focus on observable behavior and look for patterns of interaction in the present which are maintaining symptomatic behavior. Change in present behavior is valued more than insight about past events. Compared to other forms of treatment,

SFT and behavior modification are both characterized by explicit goals and a focus on the presenting problem as a criterion of success.

On the other hand, there are many differences between the two approaches in current clinical practice. Most notable is the handling of the primary symptom, as exemplified in contrasting approaches to anorexia. Behavior modification approaches tend to place heavy emphasis on the target behavior and on achieving control over the contingencies maintaining that behavior. In the treatment of anorexia, this has led to the use of highly structured inpatient programs, with the nursing staff carefully instructed in the application of reinforcement contingencies to weight gain. Behavioral change while an inpatient is seen as primary, with return to the family environment "merely" a problem in generalization.

By contrast, SFT regards change in the family system as the primary goal. When inpatient treatment is used at all (in roughly half of the cases), the inpatient phase lasts approximately two weeks, compared to an average of three months for typical behavioral programs. Inpatient treatment is used to obtain a beginning shift in the eating behavior, but more importantly to change the family's view of the problem from an involuntary medical problem to a voluntary behavioral problem of power and independence.

Symptomatic improvement is not devalued within SFT, but it is seen in the larger family and social context. In the treatment of anorexia, for example, weight gain is obviously important, but it is considered crucial to get the primary focus off the anorectic and to find some arena other than weight for the necessary teenage struggles for independence. For these reasons, the therapist will usually contract separately with the anorectic about weight and keep the weight secret from the rest of the family, using the family therapy sessions to focus on other issues. It would usually be seen as a major technical error to have the parents weigh the patient and have weight the focus of therapy, since this maintains the family pattern of focusing on the anorectic and detouring other issues through their focus on eating.

A common technique within SFT is the enactment of symptomatic behavior in the session, such as having lunch with the family of an anorectic, or having a fire-setter light a little fire. Such direct observation is seen as crucial because it is considered virtually impossible for the family to report accurately the pattern of family interaction that led up to the symptom, responses to the symptom, responses to those responses, etc. Charting of behavior might be used, but only after crucial sequences had been identified through direct observation.

The author of the question is correct in observing that instructiveness is another characteristic that differentiates behavior therapy from SFT. I do not mean to imply that a structural family therapist would never be instructive, never make treatment goals explicit, etc. The crucial distinction is that such therapist behavior would be seen within SFT as an intervention, rather than as a given in therapy, and as such would be judged in terms of the effect. If instructiveness leads to greater compliance and more rapid learning, it should be used; if, however, it increases the resistance of the family and impedes progress, it is a therapeutic error.

Implicit in the above discussion is the "world view" underlying SFT. Symptoms are seen as occurring in the context of the family system and larger social systems. The behavior of all the individuals in the family is governed by feedback from the other family members; the system tends to remain balanced or homeostatic through the operation of these circular feedback loops. The therapist cannot avoid becoming part of the system, and all interventions and conditions of therapy become part of the overall context.

In *Psychosomatic Families*, this circular open systems model is contrasted to the linear model of causality seen as underlying behavior modification. It does seem that a good deal of behavioral thinking is of the "A causes B" variety, and that this simplified thinking has contributed positively to the early progress of behavior therapy. However, I see no real incompatibility between an open systems model and a behavioral approach, and in fact it seems that behavior therapy is gradually evolving in this direction. An example of the greater sensitivity to the overall context of treatment is a recent British study which reported the effects of behavioral treatment of agoraphobia in married women (Hafner, 1977). While the behavioral treatment was highly effective in removing the symptom, it had a major disruptive effect in a large percentage of the marriages, which in turn led to a variety of consequences—marital dissolution, resumption of the symptoms and, in one case, psychosis. Inclusion of the husband in treatment was therefore seen as quite important.

Behavior therapists need to consider the multiplicity of factors maintaining symptomatic behavior and the consequences throughout the family system of change in target behavior. This means careful consideration in the choice of target behaviors, who should be involved in treatment, and what role the therapist should play. Structural family therapists, in turn, have much to learn from behaviorists in terms of precise treatment goals and highly effective specific techniques. While resistance and family homeostasis are important, SFT may have paid too little attention to the conditions when behavioral change is straightforward, when behavioral education (particularly of parents) is sufficient to produce change, or when only one or two family members need to be included in therapy. Both SFT and behavior therapy can profit considerably from clinical collaboration and careful research addressing these issues.

References

Hafner, R. J. The husbands of agoraphobic women and their influence on treatment outcome. *British Journal of Psychiatry*, 1977, *131*, 289-294.
Minuchin, S. et al. *Psychosomatic Families: Anorexia Nervosa in Context*. Cambridge, MA: Harvard University Press, 1978.

THOMAS C. TODD, Ph.D.
Chief of Service
Putnam Community Services
Harlem Valley Psychiatric Center
Carmel, NY

26. Home Rehearsal of Tasks in Behavioral Family Therapy

Question:

Home rehearsal of tasks has been considered an integral part of the change process in behavioral marital and family therapy. Although the purpose and types of tasks rehearsed have been described, the actual steps in choosing and developing the task assignment have not been clearly defined. What benefits are there in task assignment and home rehearsal for both the therapist and the family? What are the responsibilities of the therapist who chooses behavioral homework as a technique? What are the specific steps in the task assignment sequence?

Discussion:

Change in dysfunctional behavioral patterns is thought to occur when families experiment with new and different interactions which are positively reinforced. The rewarding experience then leads to the reoccurence of the new transaction which, with repeated performance, becomes integrated into the family's behavioral repertoire.

Therapists may structure this learning experience in different ways. The therapist designs a task which can be rehearsed during the counseling session, at home or in both places. Some therapists believe that change is maximally facilitated if the task is rehearsed at home, generalizing the new behavior to the couple's own environment.

There are many purposes for home rehearsal in marital and family therapy. One purpose is diagnostic. The rehearsal experience provides data about the problem area by further clarifying how family members interact. These data are the basis for the strategies the therapist may use in continuing therapy with the family. A second purpose concerns the reinforcement when practiced at home of a new behavior which has been directed and supported during the in-session rehearsal by the therapist. The encouragement of the therapist decreases anxiety and makes home rehearsal of the task less threatening and more rewarding. A third purpose for home rehearsal is the generalization of the therapeutic experience to the home environment where the learning of the new behavioral interaction is to be applied. And, finally, the family members are working together, perhaps a new experience, to develop new ways for resolving interpersonal conflicts.

It is the responsibility of the therapist to identify and assign an experience which facilitates the acquisition of more positive behaviors by family members. The therapist develops and translates this interactional task to the family during the therapy session, persuading them to agree to carry out the task by emphasizing positive individual consequences. He or she directs family members in how to implement this interaction within the home environment, encouraging them to risk new behaviors while, at the same time, accepting and supporting their anxiety. The therapist then follows up on the home rehearsal experience in the subsequent therapy session, lending importance to the task assigned as well as establishing it as a part of the treatment's developmental change process.

Task Assignment Procedure

1) The therapist meets with the family and observes the interaction among the family members. The transactional pattern of the family is observed and areas of conflict are identified.

2) One, and only one, area of conflict is chosen as the therapist focuses on the family's most urgent need. This choice usually involves the presenting problem which the family brings to the therapy session.

3) The therapist develops a task for the family which forces them to alter old, negative behavior patterns and substitute new, positive ones.

4) The new behavior is rehearsed under the supervision of the therapist during the session. For example, in the family where the presenting problem is the acting-out behavior of the adolescent child, it may be clear to the therapist that the child is blocking communication between the parents. Therefore, the child is in a very powerful position. In order to help the parents regain their power, it may be necessary to have the parents, as their task, unite to develop rules and consequences for the behavior of their adolescent child. Therefore, the attempts of the child to interfere may have to be blocked when the parents discuss these child management issues during the course of the therapy session. The therapist directs the parents to speak to each other about the child's specific behaviors that they would like changed and specific consequences for the child's actions. When the child tries to interrupt the parent's discussion, it is the responsibility of the ther-

apist to help the parents block the interference of the child. The increased communication between parents and the more clearly defined boundaries between parents and child are the goals resulting from the supervised rehearsal experience.

5) It is of the utmost importance that, in assigning the family the practice of this new interaction in the home environment, the therapist work with them toward structuring the specific context of the rehearsal experience such as time of day, the length of time for rehearsal and the activity each person will be performing during this rehearsal period. The reason for this clarity in task assignment is to block anything or anyone which may sabotage rehearsal. Based on the homeostatic component underlying change, there is a tendency for family members to return to past interactional sequences when new sequences are being learned. In predicting this regressive pull, obstacles for implementing new behaviors are anticipated and methods developed to decrease their power.

For example, if the parents of the acting-out adolescent were to schedule a specific time to discuss their child's behavior, there might be a tendency for the parents or child to sabotage that experience. Consequently, the home rehearsal structure should be formulated by both therapist and family members so that they have a personal investment in its successful completion. The parents should decide together what time is convenient for them to talk privately, excluding their children. The therapist should help the parents arrange realistic guidelines in planning for their discussion. For example, the parents may enthusiastically say they will discuss their child's behavior daily for one hour five times a week. The length of time and frequency of rehearsal are considered and the therapist decides what is realistic in terms of change goals or steps. Tasks should be designed which are realistic and appropriate for the life style and changes needed for each family.

Since the home rehearsal experience is often different from past interactional experiences, difficulty with implementation should be predicted and considered acceptable. Consequently, when problems occur, neither family nor therapist experience failure, yet they collect further information on family interaction and steps which may be necessary to implement change.

The family should be told that they will be reporting the results of the home rehearsal experience to the therapist during the following session. By directing the family to implement an activity independent of therapy, the therapist is already beginning to transfer some responsibility for change to family members. However, this change occurs under the supervision and with the support of the therapist.

Tasks to be rehearsed at home are developed during the therapy session and time is necessary for planning and reviewing the specific roles of individual family members regarding their home rehearsal experience. Family members need to verbalize reservations regarding the planned experience so as to predict those obstacles which may prevent its successful completion.

Implicit within the process of change is a step-by-step sequence of slowly letting go of old negative patterns of interaction and experimenting with more positive ways of relating. The home rehearsal experience can provide a testing ground for family members to experiment with new behavioral interactions under the supervision of a trained clinician. Most important is that this new experience can be tested within the home environment where these behaviors are to ultimately occur.

WENDY JOFFE, Ph.D.
Family Life Center
Miami, FL

27. Using Behavioral Strategies in Family Therapy

Question:

> I've worked with numerous families and found, just as the theory of family therapy predicts, that the child's problems are often reflections of conflict between the two adults in the family. I am familiar with some of the strategic and structural therapy suggestions (Haley, 1976; Minuchin, 1974) for changing family structure and, thus, resolving family problems. However, I'm wondering if there are any behavior therapy approaches to resolving these issues in family therapy?

Discussion:

This question directly addresses behavior therapy's application to family therapy and raises a related question, namely, Are there any connections between behavioral approaches and strategic family approaches? I think both questions can be answered affirmatively and that behavior therapy approaches can greatly aid family therapists in the task of family restructuring.

Step one in this effort is a reasonably decent behavioral analysis of the situation. I have found that one can facilitate this process by first drawing a crude, inverted triangle diagram of the basic family members, e.g., mother, father and identified patient. Siblings and extended family can be added if needed. Then, the therapist can look at each dyadic pair in the basic and other triangle relationships and can write down all the behavioral excesses and deficits occurring between each pair in the system. This "diagnostic" phase helps pinpoint areas where behavioral strategies might be applied to family system problems.

Perhaps an example is in order. One family showed the following general pattern: Mrs. S takes an overprotective stance with J, a handicapped (partial expressive aphasia, language disorder), 12-year-old third son. She protects him from the overt hostility of her husband and of the second son, R, a favorite of Mr. S. Mr. S criticizes his wife for babying J, rejects J fairly overtly, and clearly identifies with R who is allowed to "get away with murder" in the family. The family is split down the middle, J with mother and R with father. As a marital subsystem, the spouses are angry and distant.

Step two involves studying the behavioral excesses and deficits and stating needed behavioral changes. This family's analysis went as follows:

Mother—J:
   (a) Increase Mrs. S's reinforcement of prosocial, age-appropriate behaviors, starting with those available in J's repertoire. Proceed in small steps.
   (b) Decrease Mrs. S's reinforcement of J's responses which require her to defend and protect him by giving her ways of managing sibling fights, etc.
   (c) Increase Mrs. S's ability to use punishment with J as needed.

Father—J:
   (a) Decrease the frequency of Mr. S's overtly critical verbal remarks directed towards J.
   (b) Increase Mr. S's positive behavior with J and Mr. S's reinforcement of J's prosocial behavior.
   (c) Decrease Mr. S's overt critical remarks comparing J and R.

Father—R:
   (a) Decrease Mr. S's protective behavior toward R in order to force R "to shape up" in the family.

Mother—Father:
   (a) Decrease Mr. and Mrs. S's tendency to fight when attempting to manage J's behavior.
   (b) Increase positive, reciprocal behavior, paying particular attention to Mrs. S's desire for a decrease in jealous accusations by her husband.

J—R:
   (a) Increase reciprocal, positive responses between J and R.
   (b) Punish effectively big violations of "peaceful coexistence."

Step three involves designing behavioral interventions based on the behavioral analysis and always with an eye to changes in family structure. In the case example, the behavioral analysis set the stage for intervention. Following Haley's (1976) recommendation, I started with an attempt to modify parent-child interactions. Often one can use a contingency contract approach (Stedman, 1977), which directly addresses the behavioral excesses and deficits of the parent-child interactions. Because of Mr. S's strong resistance and the general level of intrusive behavior in the family, it was necessary to take a *very* small step approach to the contingency contract. I decided that the contract should involve only one issue, on the surface apparently small and superficial, but nevertheless one involving both parent-child interactions and siblings' interaction. This issue had to do with J's long periods in the bathroom getting dressed each day. This daily event drew sibling and paternal aggression, leading Mrs. S to rush to J's defense. In essence, this scene, played out each morning, replicated the global problems of the family.

I approached the issue by having Mrs. S manage the contingency contract, using an egg timer to structure J's time in the bathroom getting dressed. If this time limit was achieved, he was reinforced with various privileges and money. The original plan called for reinforcement by Mr. S, a strategy designed to create a positive link between J and his father. Though this link failed, Mrs. S was able to successfully use the strategy to get J dressed and out of the bathroom quicker, thus providing him with a clear behavioral expectation, and decreasing sibling and paternal aggression over the issue. This example illustrates how family structure, at the parent-child level, can be unjammed utilizing behavioral strategies.

As to ties between behavior therapy and strategic/structural family therapy, I think there are some. Most strategic/structural family therapists seek to rearrange the family "field of force," after careful (sometimes almost operational) analysis of the family problems. Haley (1976) seems particularly oriented this way. Additionally, most family therapists of this bent want to deal with the total family (or with parts of the family with an eye to the total family), to negotiate family change using various sorts of programming, to be conscious of generation boundary lines, to disengage overinvolved parents who form collusions with the children, to reinforce positive accomplishment and ignore or redefine (reframe) negative occurrences, and finally, to reconstitute harmony in the marital relationship. It seems that behavioral interventions, considered as one form of strategy by which to accomplish these broad goals, are quite compatible with strategic/structural family approaches and can be used alongside more traditional strategic interventions, such as reframing, paradoxical injunction, etc.

References

Haley, J. *Problem-Solving Therapy*. San Francisco: Jossey-Bass, 1976.
Minuchin, S. *Families and Family Therapy*. Cambridge, Mass.: Harvard University Press, 1974.
Stedman, J. Behavior therapy strategies as applied to family therapy. *Family Therapy*, 1977, *4*, 217-223.

JAMES M. STEDMAN, Ph.D.
Associate Professor
University of Texas Health Science Center;
Chief Psychologist
Community Guidance Center of Bexar County
San Antonio, TX

28. Denial of Marital Conflict in Agoraphobia

Question:

A couple has been referred to me for marital therapy by their daughter's school counselor. The woman is agoraphobic. I am convinced, as was the school counselor, that the women's phobias are required by the family system. Though the couple agree that they are in conflict and the children are being negatively affected, they maintain that everything would be fine if it were not for the phobias. I am getting nowhere. How do I break out of this impasse?

Discussion:

This is a typical situation with such couples. Often the phobic person has sought psychiatric treatment repeatedly, only to find that verbal therapy is not useful. Consequently she (most agoraphobics are women) becomes discouraged about further treatment and settles into the patterns of the syndrome, with the family adjusting to it as well. In such cases problems with the children will bring her back into treatment. By this time husband and wife are convinced the woman has some illness and are highly resistant to focusing on marital problems which may seem obvious to others.

The strong use of denial which characterizes agoraphobics and their spouses is particularly frustrating for the marital therapist. While this denial is certainly reinforced by the avoidance of uncomfortable issues, the therapist needs to recognize that an additional factor is at play. The agoraphobic and her husband are legitimately focused on the very real effects of this crippling syndrome on their lives. The subtleties of interpersonal and intrapsychic conflict seem largely irrelevant in the face of such disability. To quote an oft heard comment, "So what's my being mad at my husband got to do with my being scared at the grocery store?" For this reason we find it more useful to begin by accepting that the phobias and panic are of primary importance at the moment*

---

*Of course this strategy might also be viewed as "joining the resistance."

and work in the reverse order of the appearance of the symptoms. This comment requires some explanation of the development of the syndrome.

It is helpful to understand that the agoraphobic symptoms are usually formed in the context of interpersonal conflict in which the preagoraphobic feels helpless and incapable of finding solutions. The usual course of development of agoraphobia is as follows. The preagoraphobic woman is likely to be highly sensitive to separation and loss, unassertive, and "hysterical" in her fashion of dealing with conflict and stress. By the last statement we mean that she does not make connections between how she feels and antecedent stressors such as a death or threatening conflict with a security figure. When she reaches a point in life where separation is threatened, for example, by finding herself in an unhappy marriage and having thoughts of leaving, then symptoms are likely to develop. The ongoing, poorly recognized conflict leads to chronic anxiety which reaches panic proportions at some point in time.

Her response to the panic, given the hysterical style discussed above, is *not* to say to herself, "Look what this situation is doing to me, I've got to make some changes!" Rather, she begins to obsess about the panic, believing it to be a sign of impending madness or of a potentially fatal disease. With the occurrence of several panic episodes she develops an autonomous conditioned fear to any sensations which may be interpreted as signaling the onset of another panic attack. Minor discomforts that we all have day to day become frightening and are avoided. Thus she begins to avoid not only places but also confrontations which might be upsetting. Now that she is "sick" and unable to leave the house alone comfortably, her conflict about leaving the marriage is reduced. It is impossible to leave. Instead of feeling trapped in her marriage, she feels trapped in myriad places.

It is understandable that the marital therapist's suggestion of difficulty in the marriage is very threatening and likely to be flatly denied because such thoughts will stir up the conflict. Increased panic and anxiety may result, and termination is likely. By helping the client cope with her symptoms first, we increase her ability to tolerate the anxiety caused by facing her marital conflict and indirectly flush out her husband's own fears and insecurities. In dealing with the "fear of fear" and resulting avoidance behavior, it is important for the therapist to recognize that whatever the secondary gain, a genuine and powerful conditioned fear has formed. Therefore, insight will not be sufficient.

We deal with the fear of fear symptoms by teaching the client ways to cope with anxiety and by exposing her to situations in which she believes she will panic. In programs especially designed to treat agoraphobia, this is usually done by taking people out in groups to department stores, grocery stores, expressways, etc., all the while helping them to learn ways of gaining control and reassuring them that they will not go crazy or die as a result of the anxiety. Usually within several weeks of work they are getting about more freely, their anxiety attacks have moderated, and they begin to be aware of the interpersonal difficulties that led to the development of agoraphobic symptoms in the first place. This comes about most often when the spouse becomes threatened by the increasing independence of his agoraphobic wife and starts to exert control over her behavior. Alternatively, as the agoraphobic becomes freer of anxiety about being alone, she will also become more assertive and expressive in the relationship. This change may lead to conflict. At this time there is usually high motivation from both partners to engage in marital or family therapy.

Once the client is no longer chronically anxious and panicky, it is easier for the couple to observe the spikes of discomfort associated with interpersonal events such as arguments, unexpressed anger and threat of separation or loss. Through this observation, facilitated persistently and patiently by the therapist, the couple learns to accept anxiety as a signal for unacknowledged psychological distress. The impasse is now broken, and "regular" therapy may proceed. The sensitivity to separation threat often continues and may require some individual work with the agoraphobic. When the spouse can react in an emotionally supportive fashion to the expression of these feelings, however, their intensity is greatly diminished.

The aspect that may prove most difficult for family therapists to deal with is the fear of fear which requires getting out on the street with the client and the application of some specialized behavioral methods. Descriptions of these methods are available in the literature (Chambless and Goldstein, 1980a, 1980b). However, it may be preferable to coordinate treatment with a program especially designed for treatment of agoraphobic avoidance behavior. There are a number of facilities throughout the country that have time-limited groups for effecting exposure treatment. Agoraphobics usually benefit from these programs but require the couples to work to stabilize or extend the benefit. Some programs, such as the Agoraphobia Treatment and Research Program at Temple University Medical School, have short-term intensive programs which include participants from other cities. These participants are encouraged to follow this treatment with psychotherapy once back in their hometowns. With coordination of therapists, this approach has often worked well.

128 QUESTIONS AND ANSWERS IN FAMILY THERAPY

References

Chambless, D. L., and Goldstein, A. J. Agoraphobia. In A. J. Goldstein and E. B. Foa (Eds.), *Handbook of Behavioral Interventions*. New York: Wiley, 1980a.
Chambless, D. L., and Goldstein, A. J. Clinical treatment of agoraphobia. In M. Mavissakalian and D. Barlow (Eds.), *Phobia: Psychological and Pharmacological Treatment*. New York: Guilford, 1980b.

ALAN J. GOLDSTEIN, Ph.D.
Associate Professor
Department of Psychiatry
Temple University Medical School
Philadelphia, PA

and

DIANNE L. CHAMBLESS, Ph.D.
Assistant Professor
Deptartment of Psychology
University of Georgia
Athens, GA

29. Family Therapy with Families of Mentally Retarded Children

Question:

I have just begun working with a family that has a mentally retarded child and am interested in doing family therapy with them. They are all willing to come meet with me, but I am uncertain about which approach would be most effective. Please give me some ideas for useful therapeutic interventions.

Discussion:

First, you should not assume that, because there is a mentally retarded child in the family, family therapy is the most appropriate intervention. A mentally retarded child is not necessarily an identified patient. In fact, I have found in 10 years of working with families of developmentally disabled children, that the most common problems they face can be best handled through other modalities, such as parent groups, referrals to specialty clinics and family counseling. Common problems include realistic confusion, encounters with societal stigma, social isolation, general stress and mourning. Let me give some specific examples of what I mean, and you can determine whether they fit the problems your family is presenting.

When parents are challenged with raising a developmentally delayed child, they usually must act without the support of role models. It would be the exception if their parents, relatives or friends had experiences in this area. They, then, often turn to professionals, distrusting their own parenting skills. Their questions are concrete and demand specific information, e.g., How do I toilet train my eight-year-old boy? They may receive vague responses and turn from one community resource to another. These parents are realistically confused about how best to provide for their handicapped child, yet could also be labelled as denying their feelings.

When parents with a mentally retarded child routinely experience curious stares and judgmental comments in public places, they are encountering social stigma. They themselves often shared the lay stereotypes about mentally handicapped people before their child was diagnosed, and these tense transactions can restimulate feelings of guilt and/or shame. In a society which prefers to isolate the deviant in rural institutions, the plight of parents who struggle to keep their child at home in a semblance of a normal living is difficult. This response can be exacerbated by professionals who themselves have often been underexposed in their training to the needs of the mentally retarded child.

Another kind of situation which families of mentally retarded children experience more often than families of normal children is social isolation. The causes of this, I think, are a combination of excessive burdens of child care resulting in exhaustion, and a decreased interest in pursuing social events, as well as the documented difficulty of obtaining ordinary baby-sitting services which would enable the parents to go out. As mental health professionals, however, we might easily interpret the isolation as pathological in origin.

Families with mentally retarded children whose delays are moderate, severe or profound come from all social strata and, prior to the diagnosis, are indistinguishable from normal families. After the diagnosis, they do *not* suffer from increased divorce rate, mental health problems, alcoholism, etc. They do, however, indicate mildly increased signs of stress. These may be related to the issues I've just mentioned. Appropriate interventions for these families, I feel strongly, lie in such interventions as linkages to specialty clinics, referrals to parent groups with an educational and sharing orientation, referral to organizations of parents for support, etc., rather than family therapy.

The most common problem which these parents experience is that of grief. All parents hope for a normal child during the pregnancy, and these parents are not exceptions. When a diagnosis of a permanent disability such as mental retardation is delivered, the parents not only confront an extensive number of unfamiliar and stigmatized demands (as I have mentioned) but they also mourn over the loss of the fantasized normal child. Although this is most intense in the year following the diagnosis, it is regularly restimulated over time. Normal developmental milestones which with a normal child would be cause for celebration can become periods of sadness for parents of the mentally retarded child. How can you be happy about the first menses of a severely retarded daughter? Transitional stages into school or out of school also activate these feelings described as chronic sorrow. These predictable periods can bring a family to a mental health professional and the treatment of choice here would be family counseling with a supportive attitude towards their chronic sorrow and an educational stance about the understandable nature of that sadness. I must add here that it would be a mistake to assume that because they are grieving several years after the diagnosis that they are having a pathological reaction.

On the other hand, there are times when family therapy is the most effective approach to use. These rare families would be characterized by their identification of the mentally retarded child as being *the* problem of the family. Rather than being confused about what to do with an atypical child, rather than wondering how to manage encounters with curious or judgmental neighbors, rather than finding child care so stressful that energy for social outings is minimal, and rather than mourning over time for the lost fantasized normal child, these families would focus their general malaise on the handicapped child. The child afflicted with a developmental delay would assume the additional role of being the problem in the family. Essentially, the mental retardation would take on a symbolic meaning for the various family members, and coalesce the family through that symbolism.

I have encountered three different ways in which this has taken place. In the first, the family members have very low self-esteem, and the mental retardation is evaluated as another example of their inadequacy. They treat the retardation as external proof of their own negative feelings about themselves. They respond to this by rejecting the child, never speaking to or holding the little one. Rather than attending to their own issues of poor self-confidence, they blame their own child and work to emotionally disengage the child from the family.

In the second, the family scapegoats the mentally retarded child. Here, the child is blamed for all of the family discontent: the deteriorating marital satisfaction of the parents and the lack of popularity of the adolescent. The child affords the family members the opportunity to avoid confronting their own problems. The child is a necessary member of the family because his/her presence maintain the family equilibrium.

In the third, the family members become involved in a joint enterprise actively to delude themselves about the mental capabilities of a severely retarded child. The family delusion serves the function of keeping the very stressed and very vulnerable family intact. They avoid sending the child to appropriate educational programs because they believe him/her to be normal. Although they observe that outsiders consistently perceive the child to be retarded, they explain this by saying that the child deliberately embarrasses the family through a "dumb act."

In each of these situations, the family role of the mentally retarded child extends beyond that of a disabled child. The retardation functions as a stabilizing factor for the pathological families. This role is destructive to the welfare of the child but benefits the family as a whole, as would be the case for any identified patient symptom.

If your family resembles one of these three types, I would recommend family therapy. The therapeutic goal in these situations would be to move the family focus from the mental retardation back to the felt inadequacies of the other family members. Since family therapy directs its energy away from the identified patient, the specific nature of any presenting complaint is minimized. Whether you chose to use structural, communication, existential or strategic family therapy would ultimately be less consequential than would be your initial assessment of the family's real need of family therapy.

LYNN WIKLER, Ph.D.
Assistant Professor
School of Social Work
University of Wisconsin
Madison, WI

30. Composition and Length of Treatment in Anorexia Nervosa

Question:

I work on the psychiatric unit of a community hospital doing family therapy. I have just encountered my first case of anorexia nervosa, and though I've done some reading, I'm still unsure about exactly how to approach certain issues. It seems like everyone has a different opinion. I have heard some claim that brief, strategic therapy is what works best; others say long-term work is needed. Some emphasize the need to have all family members in every session; others emphasize working with the motivated family member. How do I make the decision as to design of my treatment plan?

Discussion:

Among the many problems a therapist encounters when working with anorexia nervosa in a family context, you have focused on two, length of treatment and composition of the sessions. Decisions in both areas are going to significantly influence the overall effectiveness of the therapy. Decisions in both areas are difficult to make.

The issue of composition of the sessions in the treatment of anorexia nervosa calls to mind the debates regarding composition for family therapy in general. If we take family therapy to be an epistemological point of view rather than a technique, we don't necessarily need to confine ourselves to any stereotyped notion of who should be in a room to do family therapy. There are, then, a number of possible permutations for intervention, such as the nuclear family, all of the members of the household, or the parents only.

The choice of composition will reflect theoretical beliefs about change in families, thus the wide range of opinion regarding the unit of intervention. For example, Minuchin et al. (1978) castigate Bowen for selecting as his unit of intervention only part of the family system. They claim that Bowen's style of working with smaller units than the family "would certainly not be correct in treating anorectics" (p. 79).

Their position, however, is unclear. They state shortly after this that "The systems therapist's unit of intervention, however, is always a subsystem" (p. 80). They also describe differences in composition based on the age and developmental level of the identified patient.

My own thinking about composition in the sessions is based on my theoretical biases. I believe that all of the contemporary models of family therapy have certain strengths, yet the phenomena of the family are so complex that no one model is totally adequate. I am, therefore, in the process of developing an integrated model of family therapy which includes the strengths of several schools of thought. The model is composed of two main sections, with subsections in each area. The first broad area is called "self and the family," with the subsections being differentiation, structure, communication and behavior. The second broad area is called "time and the family," with the subsections being the nuclear family life cycle and genealogy. All of these areas can be seen as different dimensions of the family, all of which exist simultaneously.

All of the issues are not addressed simultaneously in family therapy, so the question in regard to composition becomes, "What particular combination of individuals from the family can be brought into a family session in order to most effectively address the issues which need to be addressed?" This is an ongoing decision which is pertinent for family work with anorexia nervosa as well as with other symptoms. There are two assumptions underlying this approach. First is the premise that there is no one right way of approaching the issue of composition, and second, the idea that composition of the sessions can change throughout the course of treatment.

There are potential pitfalls to this approach. One would be the potential for the therapist to be "triangled in" to some subset of the family; a second would be the possibility of the family manipulating the process so that crucial issues were avoided rather than addressed more effectively. A thorough assessment of the family helps to avoid these pitfalls. The therapist needs to have information about the general level of family functioning, coalitions and alliances in the family, patterns of communication, behavioral patterns, the family history, the family's connection or lack thereof to extended family, and some beginning idea about multigenerational patterns.

Gathering this information in the beginning stage of the therapy can be done best by including as many members of the household and the nuclear family as possible. There will occasionally be siblings who, due to distance, cannot take part in all of the sessions; however, some contact with them will broaden the assessment. Regular sessions with all available nuclear family members will be the most productive composition in the early stages. Oftentimes, siblings are especially helpful. I have noticed that the symptomatic member of the family is initially quite unable to verbalize thoughts, impressions and ideas about the family. The parents, though often articulate, are quite unable to see family process and describe it. But frequently there is a sibling who takes the role of family spokesperson, identifying conflicts and expressing feelings. Particularly in the early stages of family treatment of anorexia nervosa, this content can act as a catalyst in the therapy.

Later in the therapy I have found it advantageous to vary the composition of the sessions, using two guidelines. First, always see a minimum of two people in a session. This helps to minimize the potential for the therapist to be viewed as aligned with any one family member, and also helps to minimize the process of the therapist getting caught up in family secrets. Second, always restrict the content of these sessions to issues pertinent to the family members present. In other words, absent family members and issues related to them are not discussed. This type of contract establishes a climate of safety in that the absent family members need not be concerned about being able to give their perspective on issues discussed.

The theoretical thinking behind varying the composition of sessions has to do with the premise that person-to-person relationships between all the family members will enhance individual and family functioning. The sessions are then used as a way to help cultivate these relationships. They can symbolically emphasize a subsystem in the family merely by convening that group without the other family members. They can operationally emphasize a subsystem by providing an opportunity for issues to be worked on which would strengthen the relationships involved.

Looking specifically at anorexia nervosa, the issue of variable composition is influenced directly by thinking regarding length of treatment. If the treatment is short-term, there simply isn't going to be enough time to have several different sessions with several different combinations of family members. The question as to short- or long-term treatment, then, has to be considered early.

I would advocate long-term treatment. In my work with anorectics and their families, I have seen an initial period of symptomatic change in the identified patient accompanied by beginning changes in the family system. This can be seen in a relatively short period of time, possibly three to five months, and with relatively few family sessions, possibly 20 to 30. Termination of treatment at this point is misleading both to the family and the therapist. Either a plateau or a regression often follows, and continued contact with the therapist provides an opportunity to work through these periods. Beyond that, there is an even more subtle dynamic involved, having to do with separation. Generally, this issue permeates the anorectic family and is expressed by all of the family members in different ways. A unifying theme is often that a cut-off is the only way to separate from the family; the only perceived alternative is to be drawn into the family in a way which promotes loss of self.

Selvini-Palazzoli (1978) expresses a concern that if the family therapist continues with the family for longer than 20 sessions, there is a risk of his/her being incorporated into the family. On the other hand, I believe that it is at just this point that more in-depth work on differentiation in the family can begin. There is indeed a danger of the therapist being "triangled in," but this can be continually monitored. If the therapist in fact cuts him- or herself off from the family for fear of this, s/he is modeling the very fear that is central to the emotional process in the family.

How long is long-term? A distinction needs to be made between calendar time and therapy time. All of the cases I am familiar with have continued for one or two years or more. You will obviously not have the identified patient hospitalized that long. Probably s/he will be discharged after that initial period of symptomatic improvement. But it is important to plan on the family continuing in therapy after this, and in fact, having as one of the inpatient goals establishing a contract with the family regarding the continuation of treatment.

As far as therapy time is concerned, the sessions will be more frequent in the early stages and less frequent in the later stages. While the identified patient is hospitalized, sessions can be held weekly, and many families are capable of productively using twice weekly sessions. In the later stages, sessions at monthly intervals work well. The agenda for the follow-up treatment can include altering the composition of the sessions in a way which would symbolize the separation of the different generations in the family: in-depth work on the parents' relationship with their families of origin, and continued work on person-to-person relationships in the family. Occasional crisis-oriented work will probably be necessary. Anorectics have an uncanny ability to become more symptomatic in later stages of the therapy, at times when motivation to change in the family is waning.

In summary, the issues of composition and length of treatment in anorexia nervosa are difficult and debatable. I believe that a long-term treatment plan will offer the greatest potential for individual and family change. This can include sessions with the whole family as well as a carefully planned and carefully executed series of sessions in which the therapist is working with select subsystems from the family.

References

Minuchin, S., Rosman, B. L., and Baker, L. *Psychosomatic Families:Anorexia Nervosa in Context.* Cambridge, MA: Harvard University Press, 1978.
Selvini-Palazzoli, M. *Self Starvation: From the Individual to Family Therapy in the Treatment of Anorexia Nervosa.* New York: Jason Aronson, 1978.

DAVID MOULTRUP, M.S.W.
Clinical Instructor
Department of Psychiatry
University of North Carolina
Chapel Hill, NC

31. The Rejected Scapegoated Child

Question:

Reading the family therapy literature I realized that "scapegoating," or severe rejection of a child, must have been one of the prime motivations for seeing the family as a group rather than as individuals. I read plausible ideas, such as the detouring of marital conflicts through a shared rejection of a child. I also find the notion that the parents reject "unwanted" aspects of themselves, denying that they own them and seeing them in a child who then gets rejected. I can certainly see that such a move will lead to repercussions, and a rejecting system will be set in motion. Yet, when faced with a parent who is really virulently attacking a child, it is often extraordinarily difficult to stop it. Plausible explanations, confrontations or even structural moves can be rejected, interpretations scorned. One is left filled with distress oneself in identification with the scapegoated and often very unhappy child. I wonder what sort of approaches are really effective in practice.

Discussion:

This question involves one of the basic issues that a family approach has to be able to deal with if it is to see itself as a meaningful way of work. If scapegoating cannot be dealt with adequately, then what can! My own feeling is that there is probably no one technical approach that is going to be right for every case, but I do feel that there are a number of basic steps which have to be taken if one is to be successful.

The first step is to make a satisfactory formulation of how the scapegoating relates to the family system as a whole. In achieving this, the second step of firmly joining with all family members, and particularly the scapegoater, has to be achieved. The next step is to formulate a therapeutic strategy and approach.

Our approach, which we have developed over some years, we have called "focal family therapy" (Bentovim, 1979; Bentovim and Kinston, 1978, Kinston and Bentovim, 1978). In this approach we attempt to make our formulations of the family's current problem by combining salient factors from the family's current life and from their families of origin. We are currently trying to find a way of making such a formulation more systematic than the somewhat arbitrary way that we proceeded earlier. In arriving at a formulation we try to understand why the family requires a scapegoat. We would see scapegoating as an aspect of the family's "surface" system, which we see as the repetitious, circular, self-maintaining and compulsive pathological system which has a dominating, urgent quality, quite overriding apparently destructive consequences (Bentovim and Kinston, in press). We also see this surface system as having a "deep" structure of common meanings which maintain and "explain" the surface system. The family may be quite unconscious of this deep structure, which the therapist feels. Such "depth" structures are myths or shared beliefs which arise as reactions to events in the parents' own early childhood and families of origin, or events which have occurred in the life of the current family. These have been integrated into a meaningful pattern by the family, which has resulted in a characteristic surface system which requires that a family member must be rejected or scapegoated.

For example, in a family I saw recently, the surface system was a mother continuously rejecting her five-year-old daughter, who, of course, responded with stubborn silence or defiance. Each triggered, reinforced and activated the other to ever-increasing emotional heights until somehow defused. Emotionally traumatic events had happened to the little girl, including physical abuse and emotional abuse, such as the removal of her "transitional" object—her teddy bear—as a punishment for lying!

At the same time, as a manifestation of the surface system, I noted, when the mother and daughter were asked to enact their conflict, that the two younger children played at the far end of the room, and the father sat near his wife yet looked away from the conflict. When asked what he was doing and how he felt he was helping, the father indicated that he knew that if he joined his daughter he would find himself in a fight with his wife, and that if he joined his wife his daughter would be even more rejected. So the father's silence acted to maintain the mother/daughter relationship. His silence supported mother against daughter and, of course, allowed the daughter to feel that she had his shoulders to climb on in this symmetrical battle with her mother—a battle which she, of course, had to lose. The two younger children were quite outside this dysfunctional triad.

When we got to know this family better, we came to realize that this surface system was being maintained by a deep, avoided but shared, sense of failure that both parents experienced. This had originated from extremely critical, demanding and undermining parents, which both parents had in rather different ways. Such factors had played an important part in their mutual choice of each other as marital partners and yet ensured a repetition of the pattern in the next generation. Although the parents complained vigorously about the grandparental generation, they were quite unaware of their own identification with such highly punitive parental figures themselves.

The question is, then, "What practical effects result from this particular formulation?" We feel that this way of looking at families can direct one's therapeutic strategy. Whatever one's approach, however, the first task is to join with the family. The single most important act is for the therapist to join with the *rejecting* parent in the first instance. Rejecting parents need sympathy for finding themselves saying such bitter, angry, painful and hateful things towards members of their own family, their own flesh and blood, part of themselves that they helped to bring into the world, have parental care of and yet who are the cause of so much pain, anger, shame and humiliation. It is also important to sympathize with the parents having to come to a professional and say such bitter, cruel and hard things about their own children. This major statement of joining is an absolute prerequisite for any sort of therapeutic move, particularly before joining with the rest of the family, the other parents who have to experience their partner in such pain, the children who experience it, and the other children who have to be party to the pain. I have used the word "pain" prominently since I believe that this is the most helpful reframing of anger and the most useful way of linking the therapist and the family.

Once initial joining and adaptation enable the therapist to arrive at an understanding of surface and depth manifestations in the family, s/he is then in a position to follow a particular strategy. If a structural model of work is chosen (Minuchin et al., 1978), the strategy is to persuade the family to adopt a new set of rules—that is, to work with the surface system. In the case example, a whole array of moves may be necessary to persuade the peripheral parent to be far more central, to decenter the child, to help parent and child to persist in face-to-face negotiation with each other until they find a new way of relating. This might include attempts to be warm at the therapist's urging. From there the therapist would need to pick up silent cues between the parents which are maintaining the triangular system and which need to be made explicit. They, too, have to negotiate and find a new way of parenting, of control without attack. Through intense, regular and persistent work using the therapist's expertise and power, the new rules have to be reinforced and made to stick.

Such a structural method does not work directly with the depth structures concerned with failure, although it may well affect them. If the aim is to work with the deep system of powerful parental images, then one's approach would be more dynamic (Pincus and Dare, 1978). Interpretation and confrontation of such identifications and repetitions in the current family of patterns from the family of origin would be needed. If a painful sense of failure structures the meaning that family members give to interaction, one would need to confront the mother for behaving like her own father in being so intensely critical of her daughter. Alternately, of course, the daughter might be seen to be like the mother's own critical father, causing the mother to feel like the helpless child. The father is then seen as belittled and dominated, as his father was in his family of origin. The therapist would inevitably be drawn into the pattern and would need to deal with the repetition that will inevitably occur with him- or herself and the multiple layers of meanings that focus on the conflict.

Alternatively, if the therapist takes a systemic view and tries to take in both surface and depth systems, as Selvini-Palazzoli and her group (1978) describe, then the family may well need to be told paradoxically that the system they are living in, although painful, may be preserving them from something worse. In the case example, the therapist would need to point out that, because of their loyalty to their families of origin and the need to avoid the absolute rage and murderousness felt towards their parents, one of their own children must be sacrificed and must continue to sacrifice him- or herself so that such anger can find a place. The family might be told that they should continue to scapegoat one of the children and that the father should hold the balance between mother and child in their battles, because something far worse might happen if anybody does anything different, at least until more therapeutic work is done. It might even be necessary to prescribe a ritual which would involve all members of the family scapegoating someone outside the family rather than inside. Hopefully, such an approach would make the family system that felt "spontaneous" appear more purposeful, so the only way of getting back to spontaneity would be a leap to a new and healthier system.

Clearly the way in which therapists deal with problems such as scapegoating depends on what they feel comfortable with and what they feel competent to practice. Making the sort of formulation I have described can help give a sense of direction, whether along familiar channels or new ones. It also helps the therapist make some sort of prediction as to what to expect if successful, so that both surface systems and depth systems would be modified in a predictable direction.

References

Bentovim, A. Towards creating a focal hypothesis for brief focal family therapy. *Journal of Family Therapy*, 1979, *1*, 125-136.

Bentovim, A. and Kinston, W. Brief focal family therapy when the child is the referred patient. I. Clinical. *Journal of Child Psychology and Psychiatry*, 1978, *19*, 1-12.

Bentovim, A. and Kinston, W. Brief focal marital and family therapy. In S. Budman (Ed.), *Forms of Brief Psychotherapy*. New York: Guilford, in press.

Kinston, W. and Bentovim, A. Brief focal family therapy when the child is the referred patient. II. Methodology and results. *Journal of Child Psychology and Psychiatry*, 1978, *19*, 119-143.

Minuchin, S., Rosman, B. L., and Baker, L. *Psychosomatic Families: Anorexia Nervosa in Context*. Cambridge, MA: Harvard University Press, 1978.

Pincus, L. and Dare, C. *Secrets in the Family*. London: Faber and Faber, 1978.

Selvini-Palazzoli, M., Boscolo, L., Cecchin, G. F. and Prata, G. *Paradox and Counterparadox*. New York: Aronson, 1978.

ARNON BENTOVIM, F.R.C.Psych.
*Consultant Psychiatrist to
the Hospitals for Sick Children
and the Tavistock Clinic, London*

32. Therapeutic Confusion Produced by Too Close/Too Far Family Systems

Question:

Working with enmeshed families towards greater distance and autonomy, I have become more and more convinced that intimacy poses them with even greater problems than does autonomy. Am I working in the wrong direction? I have also noticed the converse: When helping family members who are very disengaged to get closer, contrary to first impressions, what emerges is that they have enormous problems in handling autonomy. Much of the literature on family therapy techniques makes it sound as if the direction in which to work is clear. Is the theory too simple or are my impressions misleading?

Discussion:

I find that attachment theory helps me to make sense of the apparent paradox that you have spotted (Bowlby, 1977). Visualize a boy of two with his parents: He will play for a while, come back to make contact with one or another parent and, when he feels secure in the knowledge that his parents are available, physically and emotionally, he will trot off to play again. Thus, real autonomy is founded on the availability of good intimate contact with others. If this trust is not achieved through intimacy, family members can be reduced to continually monitoring each other (leading to enmeshment), or when despairing of making meaningful contact, they may disengage. Thus, enmeshment and detachment *are not opposites* but different styles of dealing with the same problem: a failure to establish secure bonds through intimacy. Both styles often exist in the same family. An example would be the classical triangle of an overinvolved mother/child dyad with a distant father.

Another way of conceptualizing this is to see it as a too close/too far system (Byng-Hall, in press). In the disengaged marital system, the husband feels too close and pulls away, his wife feels too distant and pursues, he backs off further and so on. The two boundaries have

143

converged and then crossed over so that the marital partners are simultaneously too close for comfort but too separated to feel safe. The
resulting mutual positive feedback system could (and sometimes does)
lead to a break up of the relationship, but, if the wife disengages, the
husband often feels left out and comes in closer. This reversal of roles
reveals the shared nature of their problem. In families it is more complex. For example, a girl who is also fearful of abandonment and intimacy can, if her parents threaten to break up, do something to bring
them together, or if they become too close, insinuate herself between
them. Her ambivalence then becomes their distance homeostat. The
family system stabilizes, but the price is that the go-between may
become delinquent or symptomatic. Every member of the family, it
will be noticed, is fearful of both loss and intimacy, so the proximity
in one dyad and the distance in the other are both still uncomfortable.

Let us return to the basic problem, a failure of intimacy. The enmeshment solution includes ignoring the boundaries between people,
giving the illusion of knowing exactly what the other is thinking, thus
gaining some relief from the fear of abandonment. If you think you
know exactly what is going on in someone else's mind you can predict
his or her every move. In order to maintain a shared illusion that all
is under control, hostility or wishes to escape may be excluded from
overt communication (conflict avoidance) but, of course, the deception
provokes even more diligent "mind reading" plus monitoring of every
move. The detached system within the marriage also involves loss of
boundary, in that frequently both spouses imagine that they know the
intentions of the other. The remote quality of the relationship comes
from not bothering to monitor the other, either because the one is
doing the monitoring for both, or because of the defense, "I don't care
if you go because I'm longing to go anyway." Real intimacy involves
honest exchange of personal information. If this is merely a reflection
of what the other wants to hear, or is forcibly extracted, it will not be
trusted. To enable a freer exchange, the therapist has to remove the
overlap of the distance boundaries so that the point at which there is
a wish for more space is not also experienced as being so separated
that relationships are threatened. Only then can both autonomy and
closeness be freely shared and enjoyed.

One technique for changing boundaries taken from structural family
therapy (Minuchin, 1974) is to escalate the tension between the
mother/child dyad, for example, by letting a girl cling to her mother,
then having the parents join together in making a decision about the
child, such as how to get her off the mother's lap, or out of the parental
bed, or how to get her to school. Although this draws the parents
together, it also differentiates them because they have to make their

communications explicit and specific. If they do not the child will not respond, and the therapist can point out the contradictory or blurred messages.

If the therapist can tolerate ensuring that the intensity rises beyond usual thresholds, parents are forced to allow their fury to emerge unmonitored. At last, a genuine communication; the child will usually label it as such by obeying. The fear of catastrophic consequences of anger is broken. The open expression of previously covert hostility in the context of parental decision making is, I often find, the first and sometimes the crucial step towards intimacy. If the couple can discover that anger can both be tolerated and used creatively, and the child (or children) observe this, then the "too close" boundary can be drawn in closer, and sexuality can on occasions suddenly flood back into the marriage.

This answer is of course oversimplified. In other families open hostility may be used to avoid depression. In this case the spontaneity of intimacy is experienced as threatening because the pain of loss would flow out. The therapeutic task is similar to the previous one; that is, the parents have to be able to experience the hidden feelings without the child being used to block them. It will probably still be necessary to start by using structured family therapy techniques to reestablish parental authority, which has been undermined by the mother/child alliance. With particularly resistant families one can use a paradoxical approach, telling them not to change their fighting for the time being (so long as it is not dangerous). Once the family is secure enough (say the third to sixth session), historical material is brought in. A genogram may be used to identify the important unmourned losses. The aim is to experience the memories of loss at a higher intensity than is normally tolerated, allowing mourning to be completed, so clinging to the "replacement" figure can be reduced. To facilitate this, the therapist can use photos, homemade movies or videotapes, sessions at home in the dead person's bedroom, visits to the grave, etc., but above all he can invoke vivid memories through recollections. With these techniques the "too far" boundary can be moved outward.

Family sculpting can be used to recalibrate both boundaries. Often in the first sculpture of the family "as it is," members of the family are placed either very distant—or very close. For instance, father might be put halfway out of the door, with son sitting on mother's lap. The sculpture should be held long enough for this to become uncomfortable, allowing the family to experience father as too far and son as too close. Intensity can be added, if need be, by pushing the son further onto mother's lap, tipping him over on top of her, and then half closing the door on father. This provides the impetus for a rebound in the subsequent "as you would like it to be" sculpture, in which they might bring father in very close to mother, and son might be separated somewhat from mother. One mistake is to leave it at that. It is important to let them then experience the discomfort of the converse: father too close, son too far from mother but too close to father. This is done by letting them "stew" for a bit in the new position. The approach/avoidance conflict can then be understood. After exploring their ideas and feelings about both experiences, the boundaries can be actively moved back. The family is asked to move repeatedly from the "as it is" position to the "as you would like it" one. This is repeated perhaps 10 times until it is tedious, then they are invited to "try whatever comes." As the family is beginning to be bored with both positions, they often find a completely new solution. Father may go up to the boy, hold him by the hand and put his arm round his wife's shoulders. She may then snuggle up to him, not her son.

Once the "too far" boundary has been moved out beyond the "too close" boundary, the fundamental distance conflict is removed. Both autonomy and intimacy can be explored without transgressing boundaries. Many families choose to finish therapy at this point. Some, however, want to improve the quality of their intimacy. Other fears associated with intimacy, such as catastrophic loss of identity and sexual anxieties, can then be tackled, often in a marital or sexual dysfunction contract.

You will notice that I use techniques from many schools, e.g., structural, strategic, experiential, insight, etc. To use this wide repertoire you need a clear conceptual framework, or as you noted, confusion will follow. A fuller exposition of my particular conceptual framework and its therapeutic implications can be found in Byng-Hall (in press).

References

Bowlby, J. The making and breaking of affectional bonds. I. Aetiology and psychopathology in the light of attachment theory. *British Journal of Psychiatry*, 1977, *130*, 201.

Byng-Hall, J. J. Freeing the index patient from the role of marital distance regulator. *Family Process* (in press).

Minuchin, S. *Families and Family Therapy*. Cambridge, MA: Harvard University Press, 1974.

JOHN BYNG-HALL, M.R.C.Psych.
Consultant Child Psychiatrist
Co-Chairman Family Therapy Programme
Tavistock Clinic, London;
Chairman, Institute of Family Therapy
London

33. Integrating Redecision Therapy and Family Therapy

Question:

> How can I integrate individual and family systems work? If, for example, I think in terms of reasons for individual behavior, I may be admonished by a systems person for involving linear causality. If, on the other hand, I use paradoxical techniques or am a therapeutic activist, I worry about being manipulative. I know that individuals have a past history that must be somehow relevant to their current systemic problems, but I don't know how to put these two together. What do you know about successful ways of resolving this dilemma?

Discussion:

The several schools of family therapy differ in the extent to which they rely on theory developed from a general systems approach, an individual approach or from small group behavior. Proponents of each mode imply that their approach considers the other. For example, Minuchin (1974), utilizing his structural approach, states that he works with individuals as well as the "structure," and Bowen (1978), while working with an individual, aims his intervention at the family system in absentia.

Our three-stage family therapy model actively integrates family system theory and individual theory. This is done so that the individual "personal" work makes sense to the family, and the family work both gives birth to and develops from the individual work. We will first describe the model that we have developed and then focus on the details of the individual work. It may be helpful to know at the outset that our overall approach makes use of an integration of the principles of family systems theory, transactional analysis (with particular emphasis on redecision therapy) and gestalt therapy.

The Three-Stage Model

Stage 1 is a "here and now," process-oriented stage in which we

147

utilize, as they apply, principles of general systems theory together with small group theory. We emphasize the here-and-now process orientation. This is significant because it represents one essential difference between our work and more traditional family systems work. We observe, clarify, vivify and exaggerate the ongoing process that occurs in the office rather than rely on inferences from the family history. We use historical data to support our observations. We conceptualize ongoing process as repetitive patterns of behavior and believe that people behave in a current situation based on information, assessment and decisions which they made in the past. The importance of systems dynamics is that rigid systems, for example, make it exceedingly difficult for people to change behavior even when the situation calls for such a change. In Stage 1, we identify these repetitive patterns which occur in the here-and-now process and intervene in such a way as to interrupt a typical pattern at a "nodal point" (Selvini-Palazzoli et al., 1978). Following a successful interruption of the pattern, one or more individuals become available to move from the first stage of our model to the second stage, allowing them to change their own behavior with less likelihood of restoration of the old homeostasis than if Stage 1 work had not been done.

Having identified the nodal point, we move to Stage 2, from the "here and now" to the "there and then." We mentioned earlier, and it is useful to reemphasize, our belief that individuals operate in the here and now based on decisions made in the past. These early decisions, often not made in awareness, were made on the basis of a person's perceptions of events, and with the goal of surviving or getting needs met in the family of origin. These decisions were made with the psychic impact of the magical fantasies of a child and are carried into present life situations as if these past factors were still relevant. Psychoanalytic thinking suggests that repeated working through will lead to resolution of the early impasses. We believe that if we can facilitate temporary regression so that the individual is at one moment in time back in the there and then, redecisions can be made that carry the same psychic impact as the earlier decisions. We combine the tools of gestalt therapy, bioenergetics, psychodrama and many others to facilitate this regression, following which we utilize the techniques of redecision therapy to facilitate the actual resolution of the impasse.

Once the redecision has been accomplished an individual usually looks, acts, sounds and feels different. We next move into integration, Stage 3 of our model, in order to solidify second stage changes. We recognize the systems and individual tendency toward reestablishing the old homeostasis, so in this stage we help people practice behaving in ways that are consistent with their new perceptions of self and other. Thus, our third stage is both here and now and future oriented. Certainly the techniques of the third stage are markedly different from those of first and second. There is more cognitive work, more focus on actual behavior, more focus on learning, and less affective work. The therapist is more at a distance than in either the first or second stages, more of a guide than an intervener or transference figure. Similarly, the time frame between sessions is different. The first stage is often crisis oriented, so we use frequent and long (two to four hour) sessions; the second stage is intrapsychic and we use a once or twice weekly schedule; the third stage requires the occurrence of real life events for actual planning and follow through. Thus, two to three weeks and sometimes even four to six weeks between sessions may be common. Stage 3 then leads naturally into the termination phase. This may be less well defined for us than in individual work because the family members are relating again to each other rather than to the therapist, and they will have reformed their external boundary with less sense of loss than if we had stopped at the end of the first or second stage.

A case example will now focus on three separate issues: recognition of the important here and now events or nodal point; transition from the here and now to the there and then, and finally what to do when you get back to the there and then.

Case Example

In one family session, preadolescent boys were drawing pictures on large papers in the center of the room, mother was talking, while the two-year-old girl was climbing all over her. The little girl then moved down and tromped all over her brothers' papers. One brother kept on working as if nothing was happening, the other made his drawing smaller and enclosed his drawing by a dark heavy border. As this was occurring, father sat back looking more and more distant.

The here and now issue that we chose to address at this time was not the presenting problem, one brother's learning disability, or the marital issue that mother was currently talking about, but the little girl's invasion of everybody's space, while neither parent set limits for her. This was not the only here and now issue that we could have chosen but clearly one that was important to the family. The boys had previously complained bitterly that their rooms at home were inadequate, that no one had his or her own closet space and that they each resented their young sister's intrusion onto the family scene. Mother and father frequently fought about finishing their incomplete shell of a house. Thus, all members of the family were at some level concerned about space.

We reasoned that if either parent changed in the dimension of limit setting, profound changes in the family would follow. Furthermore, we intuitively felt that mother was less defensive than father, so we elected to intervene with her. When we asked mother to set limits, she was reluctant to do so and we pursued. She then began to talk about how, when her daughter was born, she let this little girl become her central focus. We then helped mother into a description of her own childhood, and she related how she had felt unimportant. As she talked, her eyes became glazed and she began to look like a sad little girl. She was, at that moment in time, being that little girl from her past, so we used a two-chair gestalt technique to resolve the impasse between her and her mother. As a little girl, she had decided that she didn't count, and she was acting that early decision out in her present life with her daughter by parentifying her daughter and making her more important than herself. As she made sure that her daughter counted more than anyone, she also acted this decision out with her husband and sons, as she felt she had no significant impact on them and was not heard by them. Of course, they cooperated and didn't listen.

In the gestalt work, mother reexperienced the power of that early decision and its inappropriateness to the present, since she was no longer that little girl but a grown woman (a role she thoroughly enjoyed). She redecided that the sad little girl did count, her wants and needs were important, and that she would be willing to express those needs now even though she didn't express them then. As she heard her own words, experienced her affect and energy, she sat up straight, voiced relief and subsequently succeeded in the early stages of effectively parenting and setting limits for her daughter.

Obviously, there was much more to this work because, as we said, the whole family was involved in this pattern. Father, in fact, permitted and somewhat enjoyed his daughter's rampant behavior. By focusing on her he could most effectively hide. This hiding was an important piece of here and now behavior stemming from an early decision to never openly express hostile feelings for fear that he would seriously hurt someone. This, too, was worked with in the family setting. He made a redecision that ultimately led to the direct expression of his feelings.

The child with the learning disability was acting as if he had no abilities whatsoever. He had, in fact, figured out that the parents did not want him around anyway and had been thinking that if things went bad enough he would eventually kill himself. Watching his parents do their work stimulated him to ask lots of unasked questions about his birth and his reading disability, and to talk about his anger at himself. Ultimately, in a new drawing in which he used all of the space on the paper, he expressed his own redecision to stay alive and, with some additional help from the therapist, his decisions to take care of himself and to think for himself.

Finally, after all this work had been done (over several sessions) we were ready to begin the reintegration phase. The family now had at least one active parent, mother, and was considerably more open about hostile feelings. Father had barely touched the surface of his work and mother carefully planned how she would carry through on her redecisions even if father did not maintain his. She had separated herself from her mother, could separate from her daughter, and was more available to her sons. This was not to be the end of therapy for this family, but is a good place to stop and summarize our view of individual (redecision) work in the context of family therapy.

The essence of redecision work with families is that we start from the here and now behavior in the system, behavior that represents the old decision, interrupt the systemic pattern, move back at an affective level to the there and then, help persons resolve the impasses with the self and parents of old, and then return to the here and now (but in a future-oriented sense) to reintegrate the family unit, to establish a new homeostasis based on new decisions and new ways of behaving.

References

Bowen, M. *Family Therapy in Clinical Practice*. New York: Jason Aronson, 1978.
Minuchin, S. *Families and Family Therapy*. Cambridge, MA: Harvard University Press, 1974.
Selvini-Palazzoli, M. Cecchin, G., Prata, G., and Boscolo, L. *Paradox and Counterparadox*. New York: Jason Aronson, 1978.

LESLIE B. KADIS, M.D.

and

RUTH McCLENDON, M.S.W.
Project: Family
Aptos, CA

SECTION III

Resistance and Countertransference

34. Resistance in Behavioral
Marriage Therapy

Question:

I recently read a debate in family therapy journal about behavioral marriage therapy. One issue in that debate really caught my eye because it's something I've run into rather often when I do marital therapy, most of which I do along behavioral lines. Specifically, what behavioral strategies have been found to be helpful for dealing with resistance?

Also, are different approaches to a couple's (or one partner's) resistance called for when there is resistance about different issues? For example, I've seen several couples who seemed to buy the ideas of a behavioral approach, but repeatedly failed to bring in their homework sheets (or even failed to record faithfully). I've tried such things as making the length of sessions contingent on their compliance with these tasks, using a response cost such as the potential loss of money to an organization that is distasteful to the couple, shaping their compliance by going back and starting over with simpler homework assignments and gradually expecting more homework, etc., but none of these efforts have paid off very reliably. Also sometimes one or both partners just wouldn't go for the reciprocity idea, since they felt that, as one husband said, "If you have to ask for it, it isn't worth getting." Any suggestions about how to deal with resistance in behavioral marriage therapy in general, or in particular kinds of resistance situations, will be very appreciated.

Discussion:

It is most exasperating when couples reject carefully thought out behavioral interventions which, according to the last behavioral marital therapy (BMT) workshop attended, should work flawlessly. Problems of resistance in BMT are one of the most important yet least well described aspects of such approaches to intimate relationships.

A crude typology of resistance forms helps focus either external or

155

internal explanations for not completing homework assignments, failing to implement newly learned skills, etc. Reasons which are external to the dyad are: (a) dislike of the therapist; (b) behaviorism is unacceptable, runs counter to previous therapy experiences, is nonhumanistic, etc.; (c) requirements of BMT exceed basic skill level of couple, e.g., some persons would never track daily events, appointments, etc.; and (d) one or both partners do not subscribe to the therapeutic contract as defined by the therapist, e.g., "I'll go through with all this only as long as my implicit goals are being met."

Those forms of resistance which are best described as internal to the relationship are more difficult to define and even more difficult to alter. In the first instance they reflect the "politics" of the relationship and can be understood only through deciphering the plan of the relationship. They are more difficult to alter because the therapist must become a master manipulator, an impression manager and an expert in metaphor. The step by step application of this or that behavioral technique does not seem to increase compliance. BMT seems to be the culprit, but it more often merely provides a net for catching these relationship difficulties. Consider three forms of internal resistance: (a) Frozen Spontaneity—The best example is that provided by our correspondent, viz., "If you have to ask for it, it isn't worth getting." Other variants include, "She is only doing it because you told her to," or, "If you *really* loved me you wouldn't need to be asked." (b) We Don't Dare Change—The central theme is that something horrible would happen if either person or the relationship were to change. Couples can go to extremes to make this point, and may even use therapist assignments to "prove" the malevolence of the other, i.e., the failure of one partner to complete an assignment now becomes the basis for last night's fight! A spouse may assure the therapist that the partner will not comply, whereas the predictor most assuredly will comply. (c) Devitalized Relationships—these may be the dull, low activity level or aversiveness-driven type of relationship, the super-uptight "nothing-ever-happens" couple, or the quiet battlers. For each of these prototypes, resistance to BMT is part and parcel of the relationship itself and will require the helper to adopt an unfamiliar helper role vis-à-vis the couple.

The message in the first example of internal resistance (Frozen Spontaneity) is that someone does not feel appreciated. Appreciation is the product of two differentially weighted factors: Commodity value *times* sincerity of intention. The latter communicates the personal worth of a partner. (We teach our children that it is the thought that counts when presented with a ceramic ashtray the size of a meteorite.) Since intention is weighted more heavily than commodity value, a sumptuous dinner arranged for questionnable intentions loses on all counts. Merely showering a spouse with relationship "pleases" on an assigned "love day" is likely to misfire if the therapist has not carefully prepared the intentionality of the act.

The partners in this same example are also acknowledging to the therapist that each still has the power to proffer worthwhile commodities. Running the other person down ("It isn't *worth* asking for!") helps them lose sight of their resentment over not getting a worthwhile commodity from the other. The therapist's task is to effect an exchange of commodities without anyone losing face. I once suggested to a husband that he paraphrase his wife's statements about the difficulty they were having with their child. This otherwise mild mannered man became flushed and tensed with inner rage since for him "paraphrasing" meant agreeing with his wife's position, and he was not about to give in.

What the We-Don't-Dare-Change couple cannot tell the therapist is that they would be unable to relate to one another should they give up their ritualized patterns of interacting. Some writers (Haley, 1976) stress the importance of recognizing that partners protect one another with their symptoms. "He won't do it no matter what you say, Doctor," is an example of wife protecting husband from failing. Although she is labeled as a nagging wife (and worse), we note that somehow Ol' Dad never has to risk being more responsible. The teeter-totter effect is familiar to marriage therapists: As soon as one person's depression abates the other become symptomatic.

For the third type of couple (Devitalized) some threat to the status quo prompts their seeking "help," although the outcome they seek is a return to the status quo. Many relationship enhancing techniques (emphasizing positive exchanges) for these couples would be analogous to telling a depressed patient to go out and make friends, have fun, be active, i.e., all those behaviors which the patient now sees as impossible.

If the remedies are not to be found among specific behavioral techniques, where are they to be found? The BMT practitioner might become a strategist distinguishing between skill deficits on the one hand and programmatic relationship dysfunction on the other. Ideas expressed by the communications writers (Haley, 1976; Watzlawick et al., 1974) are quite applicable to BMT. Here then are some specific strategic applications to BMT:

1) The BMT practitioner must command the couple's attention. This

is done best by being consistently brilliant! Make truly empathic responses, remember important details of the couple's lives together, and be predictively correct by suggesting future events which actually do happen. We must relate idiomatically to each couple, using metaphor and images which convey a familiarity with the content of the couple's life. Notice a shared "naughtiness" and comment how much the couple actually enjoys it. For example, husband may secretly enjoy his wife's walking across his desk top to get his attention, yet still complain bitterly about her being a spend-thrift. It is essential that the therapist be seen as a real live person who understands the texture of their lives. It is even more essential that the couple be understandable to the therapist.

2) Use of Reframes. A reframe is a plausible explanation which has an exceedingly low probability of being thought of by the couple. A nagging spouse's behavior can be reframed as showing the concern of an altruistic person for the wellbeing of the spouse; that by showing such concern the one is shouldering too much responsibility for the relationship, etc., etc. Reframes can be used to deal directly with resistance: "It is a good idea that you are not completing all your assigned tasks. Obviously I am moving you people too fast for your own good. I'll follow your lead and slow down so that we don't threaten your relationship."

3) Creating a Different Problem. A couple will always beat the therapist when it comes to yes-butting on their own territory. Rather than trying to deal with their ritualized solutions to their problem, the therapist creates a new problem which now defines him or her as the expert. After listening to each partner harangue the other's traits the therapist may ask: "All marriages impose an obligation on the partners to be attractive to one another. How do you two make yourselves attractive to one another?" The "problem" is how they will solve this ex cathedra pronouncement about marriage. (We have now implicated the relationship, not the traits of each person.) Or the therapist may inquire, somewhat absentmindedly: "Marriage relationships exist for mutual support. I wonder how you two have decided to support one another?" For high rate, acting out couples (overtalking, mindreading) it is often helpful to ask: "I wonder if you have ever thought that it's possible for you both to make your relationship look bad? Do you make each other look worse than you really are?" It is impossible to deal with this therapist-created problem unilaterally, e.g., "Well, *she* makes me look bad, but *I* don't make her look bad." If he agrees that she makes him look bad he is also agreeing that he knowingly complies with what she is doing! Q.E.D. They are both partners in crime.

4) Changing the Ground Rules. If partners engage in high rate chaos, or one dominates the sessions, it is helpful to change the rules by saying that the therapist understands their problem, and that he/she will be doing things from time to time which they are not yet able to understand, but which are designed nevertheless to help them. This creates a new problem in the sense of their having to track the therapist rather than acting out ritualized distractions. They must now join forces to figure out what this mad (albeit plausible) therapist is about!

The strategic moves being suggested here are based upon the therapist's understanding of the politics of the relationship. They are designed to decenter the relationship so that BMT techniques become acceptable. Refocusing requirements onto the relationship, or onto the therapist rather than the individuals, is always helpful. With less distressed couples the idea that the relationship (they jointly) must attain some therapist-set production goal is helpful. The strategy throughout is to make noncompliance with assignments evidence that one does not wish relationship benefits, i.e., that one has *no* self-interest! Once the natural reinforcing contingencies take hold (couple actually enjoys small segments of togetherness), the resistance issues shift, and in our experience, the couple now faces new challenges which highlight their skill deficits. But the therapist predicts these: "Of course you're feeling awkward. That is exactly how you should feel, and that tells us you are now ready for the next exercises."

The issue of resistance in BMT is truly complex and probably now involves more artifice than many of us would like to admit. Yet it is well to remind ourselves that performance is still largely a function of its consequences; couples develop ritualized exchanges which must be altered by the BMT practitioner. The therapist must become an effective source of reinforcement for the couple in order to compete from their own stabilized system of exchanges.

References

Haley, J. *Problem-Solving Therapy.* San Francisco: Jossey-Bass, 1976.
Watzlawick, P., Weakland, J., and Fisch, R. *Change.* New York: Norton, 1974.

ROBERT L. WEISS, Ph.D.
Professor
Department of Psychology
University of Oregon
Eugene, OR

35. Management of Resistance in Early Phases of Marital Therapy

Question:

As a marital and family therapist in a large community service agency, I see a great variety of cases. However, over the past year my case load has shifted to a predominance of marital cases. Approximately two-thirds of these are young and/or recently married couples with adjustment and attachment issues depicted in communication, sexual and child-rearing problems. My problem is with the other third who appear to be basically neurotic individuals. They have been married as long as 10 to 20 years, but their relationships display chronic periods of intense conflict and dissatisfaction. While their needs appear so great, I have been unable to keep them in treatment very long. I see them conjointly and, after a couple of sessions of getting acquainted and history-taking, they typically cancel their next appointment and then drop out of treatment. I believe I am missing something in understanding and recognizing some early resistance. I would appreciate your suggestions.

Discussion:

You are correct in differentiating the early adjustment and attachment issues from the more chronic patterns of neurotic marital interaction. The former group are generally somewhat healthier in their own personal development and patterns of relationships. The latter group tend to reflect earlier developmental deficits demonstrated in problems with object attachments, immaturity and dependency in relationships, and an inability to separate present adult interactions from (often unconscious) family-of-origin issues. The most common stumbling block in working with this latter clinical population is the failure to recognize the powerful *reciprocal processes* which are apparent in neurotic marital interaction.

You have identified the traditional neurotic traits in these spouses. Generally these individuals have a tendency to select as mates other

160

individuals who share similar levels of personality development and maturity. Dicks (1967) has termed this process a "mutual signalling system" by which each prospective partner senses in the other both similar developmental needs and complementary personal resources that may potentially fill in lost parts of one's own development. Complementary neurotic patterns have been identified elsewhere in the literature: Mittelman (1944) has identified five patterns, ranging from dominate-passive to emotionally detached-craving affection; Martin and Bird (1959) identified the lovesick wife and cold, sick husband; Barnett (1971) explicated the obsessional-hysteric marriage.

In these marriages the relationship becomes essentially a "projection screen" (Dicks, 1967) onto which unresolved intrapsychic and family-of-origin tensions become displaced. The two traits typical of these marriages which reveal the reciprocal processes are *projective identification* and *collusive resistance*. In the former, each spouse projects onto the other unacceptable or disavowed aspects of the self (e.g., aggression or passivity) so that the actual perception of the other in the relationship is altered. Zinner (1976) has suggested that this is the point at which intrapsychic conflict is transposed to the interpersonal sphere. Thus, in effect, each spouse begins to react to the specific complementary traits which originally attracted them to one another. For this process to be maintained, each partner enters into a basically unconscious collusive bond which allows the projection to be accepted and serves to employ the relationship as a protective mechanism against the identification of internal personal deficits. Generally, the more severe the personal deficits, the greater will be the collusive bonding.

As you suggest in your question, the chronic levels of conflict in these marriages may not surface for five to 10 years when the early idealization has subsided and/or when one partner begins to move away from the collusive defense. The early resistance of these couples is subtle but apparent in their reluctance to remain in treatment. If you look at the conjoint intake process you describe for history taking, you will probably find that it is the third or fourth session before you begin to move in on substantial personal and/or interactional issues. This is, of course, when the resistance of cancelled appointments appears. Basically, you are hitting head-on the collusive bond of the couple. Looking back over an early interview, you might recall a period where the couple was expressing a lot of anger at one another. As you probed the relationship or focused on one of the spouses, a dramatic shift occurred where the anger was gone, the couple seemed closer and aligned with one another. They were either withdrawn, defending one another, or expressing some anger toward you. Your movement toward the relationship triggered the mechanism of collusive resistance where the marital conflict became secondary to the need to employ the relationship to ward off your potential threat of discovering their hidden internal deficits. Once you stumble upon this it is very hard to back up and retain the spouses' involvement in therapy.

In the early phases of marital treatment, the establishment of clinical control by the therapist is crucial. It is gained by communicating from the onset a supportive and yet objective milieu, and moving toward developing a rapport with the couple and a sense of attachment with each individual spouse. The structure of the early phase of treatment has been useful in managing the aspects of collusive resistance. I have employed a form of combined conjoint and concurrent treatment over the initial four to six weeks. I will see the couple together the initial session and then see each spouse in individual sessions the second, third and occasionally the fourth week. I will then see them conjointly again to review my assessment and to make recommendations—normally for ongoing conjoint or family treatment, as indicated.

The initial conjoint session allows clarification of the "identified problem," the management of early anxiety, and the development of early rapport with the couple. The only particular history I will look at here will be an excursion into their courtship and mate selection experiences. This is usually accessible to both conflicted and devitalized couples because it triggers their early idealized fantasies of one another and the relationship. Utilizing this material bypasses an early confrontation with the collusive resistance; at the same time it utilizes their recall to momentarily bridge some of their distance and ambivalence and allows the present situation to feel somewhat more manageable. The following concurrent sessions allow the development of rapport and attachment with each spouse separately, as well as the gathering in some depth of individual, family-of-origin, and relationship histories. The therapist will learn a great deal about the quality of the marital relationship from the manner in which each spouse handles the relationship with the therapist in these individual sessions.

This suggested approach allows the therapist to establish a relationship with both the couple and the individual spouses. This approach avoids the trap of an early confrontation with the collusive resistance and allows a more natural flow of therapeutic control. When the sessions return to a conjoint format, and presumably for ongoing treatment, the therapist must then rely on additional skills in blending historical material with relationship issues and gradually identifying the projective identification and collusive dynamics.

References

Barnett, J. Narcissism and dependency in the obsessional-hysteric marriage. *Family Process*, 1971, *10*, 75-83.

Martin, P. A. and Bird, H. W. The "love-sick" wife and the "cold-sick" husband. *Psychiatry*, 1959, *22*, 246-253.

Dicks, H. *Marital Tensions*. New York: Basic Books, 1967.

Mittelman, B. Complementary neurotic reactions in intimate relationships. *Psychoanalytic Quarterly*, 1944, *13*, 479-491.

Zinner, J. The implications of projective identification for marital interaction. In H. Grunebaum and J. Christ (Eds.), *Contemporary Marriage: Structure, Dynamics, and Therapy*. Boston: Little, Brown, 1976.

CRAIG A. EVERETT, Ph.D.
Director, Graduate Program in
Marital and Family Therapy
Department of Family and Child
Development
Auburn University
Auburn, AL

36. Couple Therapy Resistance Based on Early Developmental Patterns

Question:

I am a marital and family therapist and I work with couples primarily in conjoint sessions. Recently I have been identifying a type of impasse that is related to the early developmental patterns of the couple. For example, a couple well-versed in communication skills can listen and respond to each other, but then, for no apparent "reasonable" reason, one spouse is triggered into an angry, irrational response. On questioning, the spouse can identify the origin of the unreasonable response as a remembered similar incident in the family of origin. I can label the behavior as transference or "projection," but what I am requesting are procedural suggestions. How do you help the spouse to consider a behavioral change, and how do you use the combined approach of individual and conjoint sessions in that process?

Discussion:

The problem of the marital therapy impasse that is related to early developmental patterns recurs frequently and can be difficult to integrate into the ongoing process of therapy. Also, as you have indicated, selection of a treatment plan relates directly to the issue of the combined use of individual and conjoint sessions in marital therapy.

An important consideration in formulating a marital therapy treatment plan is an evaluation of the level of ego functioning of the individuals concerned. In a discussion of the psychoanalytic perspective in marital therapy, Meissner (1978) points out that the tendency to repeat the pattern of relationships from one's family of origin depends on "a poorly developed and relatively undifferentiated self." I concur that the issue is one of lack of differentiation, and that most persons who seek marital therapy do have the tendency to repeat dysfunctional patterns of relationship. However, I think that Meissner's concept has a somewhat more universal application, and that most couples under stress have such tendencies. How, then, do you determine the ability

164

of persons in therapy to tolerate stress? In general, in my experience, couples who are able to commit themselves to the possibilities of change in their relationship can also tolerate the anxiety of modifying the dysfunctional patterns of behavior. If one or both partners are relatively uncommitted to continuing the relationship, then the procedure that I am about to describe may not be helpful.

Given the required level of ego development, a model that has been useful to couples in coping with the defined problem is one in which together, in the conjoint session, the couple and the therapist identify and label the "unreasonable" response, and then contract that the spouse involved work toward resolution in an individual session. Perhaps a description of the process with a particular couple will illustrate the method.

Susie and Bill came for help because of their violent arguments during which, at times, they fought physically with each other. The arguments were initiated by either spouse over what seemed to be trivial matters, e.g., whom to invite to dinner, what to serve for dessert, etc. The recommended structure for therapy, which they accepted, included alternate weekly conjoint and individual sessions. In the beginning phase, therapy in the conjoint sessions was focused on clarifying their contracts with each other and learning communication skills. Although both partners expressed more satisfaction with the relationship, the bitter fights continued to occur from time to time, and they seemed triggered by unimportant details of their life together.

Fortunately, early in the therapeutic process, the problem presented itself, live, in a conjoint session. During a discussion of the budget, Susie said that she thought they could not afford to spend money on a planned vacation weekend that month. Bill suddenly became very angry and said that he was no longer interested in discussing anything with Susie and that he was ready to terminate therapy. My therapeutic procedure was to intervene and question Bill about his feelings of the moment. He explained that he felt panicked, helpless and angry. The next step was to assist him in identifying the anger of the moment as similar to his feelings during an upsetting event that occurred in his family of origin when he was seven. At that time his uncle gave him some money, part of which he spent on a much-wanted harmonica that he had been unable to get because his family income was sufficient to cover only essentials. Bill's father was outraged. He said that Bill had wasted the money, and he took away the remainder of the gift. Bill felt helpless and angry at what he perceived as a gross injustice and act of control on the part of his father. Out of this and similar experiences he developed an assumption that, if anyone made a demand on him regarding money and other issues, he was facing a threat of control of his entire being.

I explained that having identified the "out-of-awareness" trigger of his anger, Bill could spend time in his individual therapy exploring the issue in greater depth. Bill agreed with the suggested procedure. Usually, it is helpful at this point to explain to couples that when they encounter sudden, overwhelming feelings that are also "unreasonable," they can assume that the feelings are related to an earlier developmental problem that is unresolved; it is not particularly related to their ability to be rational persons. Couples are reassured by this explanation and helped to understand their own seemingly inexplicable behavior. The explanation also helps lessen their embarrassment over the temporary loss of emotional control.

In the conjoint session, we returned to a discussion of what was happening with Susie in the interactional process and explored with her how she understood Bill's sudden, strong feelings. In addition, it was helpful to clarify Bill's perception by discussing what Bill had heard Susie saying and to emphasize that Susie was referring specifically to the budget without the intent of controlling Bill. Usually, as in this instance, the couple can then proceed with the issues of the conjoint session.

In Bill's individual sessions during the following weeks, therapy was directed to three phases of the resolution of the identified problem. The phases necessarily overlap and do not proceed smoothly or within any prescribed time frame. The first phase was to help him to bring to his cognitive awareness the times when his assumption or belief that any perceived demand on his money, time, etc., was threatening to control his life.

The second phase was his reconnecting with affect to specific incidents in his early history with his family of origin in which the pain and the hurt had been hidden from himself, and to reexperience and reexamine what had happened at that time. The use of the Gestalt "empty chair" technique was useful to him in working through family scenarios. Also, his dreams provided for him meanings that had previously been unconscious. As his attachment to the early painful feelings diminished, he was open to looking at alternative perceptions of the meanings of the events.

The third phase involved behavioral change in which, as the new alternatives were assimilated and/or integrated, they could be put into practice. As his world view became less egocentric he was able to consider new possibilities of behavior.

In conjoint sessions, we continued to identify the trigger issues as they arose, and gradually over the months their power diminished. Bill was able to hear suggestions, even about the use of his money, without the old feelings of panic and anger.

Susie, similarly, reached impasse points in the conjoint sessions. As a child she had developed an assumption that if a person of significance in her life expressed criticism of her, it meant that she, Susie, was an unworthy person and she became depressed and withdrawn. She also contracted to utilize time in her individual sessions to move forward to a resolution of the early beliefs, feelings and behavior.

I have described one method of helping couples work with the impasse that hinges on beliefs and behavior that were learned in the developmental process with families of origin. The method described is only one of the methods of working therapeutically with such impasses and of helping couples to come to terms with the "irrational" feelings and behaviors that result in a dysfunctional marital interaction.

Reference

Meissner, W. W. The conceptualization of marriage and family dynamics from a psychoanalytic perspective. In T. J. Paolino and B. S. McCrady (Eds.), *Marriage and Marital Therapy*. New York: Brunner/Mazel, 1978.

THELMA DIXON-MURPHY, Ed.D.
*Chairperson, Marriage and Family
Therapy Program
Blanton Peale Graduate Institute
Institutes of Religion & Health
New York, NY*

37. Resistance to Role Playing in Marital Group Therapy

Question:

About six months ago, my agency began offering group therapy services to couples. Attempting to capitalize on the unique opportunities groups offer for peer feedback and multiple models, I usually request couples to engage in a fair amount of role playing. Periodically, a couple will be very resistant to this procedure. I have tried to deal with these couples by techniques such as: describing the value of role playing, letting other couples role play first, and suggesting they try practicing at home. Although occasionally successful, I have not achieved any consistent positive results. Any suggestions you can offer regarding additional ways of overcoming couples' resistance to role playing will be appreciated.

Discussion:

Role playing is an important procedure in group marital therapy. Consequently, clients who refuse to participate in role playing deprive themselves of a potentially valuable therapeutic technique as well as affect the group functioning in a negative way. In order to understand couples' resistance to role playing and what to do about it, a brief enumeration of some of the sources for such resistance may prove helpful.

In my experience, six sources of resistance to role playing in couples groups are seen most frequently. 1) Some couples simply experience "stage fright," that is, anxiety about performing in front of others. This fear seems to derive from "evaluation apprehension" over how well they can perform their assigned roles or their unfamiliarity with this form of expression. In most cases of this type, resistance is usually easily dispelled. 2) Some couples believe role playing is not "real" and, therefore, of marginal value to improving their relationship. These couples are often in a hurry to get to the "heart of the matter," seemingly eager immediately to tackle their most severe relationship problems. 3) Some couples resist role playing because they fear that exposure of some personal aspect of their relationship to the group will result in ridicule or criticism. Unlike couples in the stage fright category, these couples do not fear performing *per se*, but rather group reaction to some idiosyncratic aspect of their relationship. 4) Occasionally a couple or spouse will fear the exposure of an implicit interpersonal contract or interactive pattern which, although appearing exploitive or destructive, serves some maintenance function in their relationship. Since the viability of this arrangement is dependent upon its remaining covert, role playing is viewed as highly threatening. A cue to this type of resistance is the spouse who repeatedly sabotages role playing by refusing to be serious or "forgetting" what to do. 5) A related type of resistance occurs when a spouse is unwilling to interact positively with his/her partner. Frequently, this person is not highly committed to the relationship and is using therapy to "prove" to his/her spouse the futility of any attempt to salvage the marriage. A tip-off to this type of resistance is the individual who can easily role play with other group members or with his/her spouse if the role play's content is neutral or negative (for example, "Role play how your spouse makes you feel bad"). 6) Some resistance may be caused by group-level factors. Development of antitherapeutic norms, lack of group cohesiveness and ambiguous group goals may contribute to couples' unwillingness to role play. This type of resistance may be relatively independent of the dynamics of a particular couple's relationship, but depend on understanding of the group purpose, their relationship to the group leader(s) as well as to each other. The unwillingness of more than one couple in the group to role play may be a sign of this source of resistance.

Understanding the source of a couple's resistance aids the therapist in choosing a procedure with a high likelihood of success. Since different forms of resistance may have certain determinants in common (e.g., anxiety, anger), more general procedures can often be used in a first attempt to deal with the problem. For instance, when the major stumbling block to role playing is anxiety, any procedure which will result in anxiety reduction is likely to be of some value. In this situation, I have found the following procedures useful: relaxation training, giving group members control over termination of the role play, reading or describing (rather than acting) one's part, observing the group leader role play the resistant group member's part, performing only a small segment of the role (e.g., one sentence) and cognitively rehearsing one's role play. These procedures have two advantages: They are relatively easy to implement and they permit—through observing the group's response—further assessment of the sources of resistance.

A pregroup orientation meeting with each couple is valuable as a general method of *preventing* resistance. During this meeting, the therapist should be very explicit about what he/she means by role playing, how it will be used in the group and why it is important. Any signs of unease or confusion on the couple's part can be dealt with immediately and with less difficulty than in the group. In most cases, I would recommend that a trial role play be performed during the interview. This assures clear communication of what is expected and also gives the therapist a chance to detect misunderstandings or skill deficits that might interfere with successful role playing.

For more specific sources of resistance, I have found a number of procedures useful, of which the following are a sample. The "exaggerated role play" involves the therapist or group member burlesquing their role (a good example can be found in LoPiccolo and Lobitz, 1973). This serves two functions for couples: reducing concern that the idiosyncratic nature of some aspect of their relationship (e.g., the way they express affection) will be denigrated by the therapist or group, and helping couples to imbue their role playing with greater affect and, hence, more realism. This latter function is particularly important since the effectiveness of role playing seems related to the degree it approximates all relevant dimensions of the actual situation.

Role reversal—having each spouse assume the role of his/her partner—can facilitate participation of couples who avoid traditional role playing around certain issues associated with past communication breakdowns and aversiveness. Essentially the role reversal restructures the interaction, reducing anticipated unpleasant consequences associated with the spouse's usual role. Further, it provides a novel framework for communication, offering each partner the opportunity to present his/her perception of the other. For best results, role reversals should be carefully structured. Spouses should speak in the first person, no interruptions, and opportunities for feedback. One caution: While the insights gained through role reversal are often enlightening for the couple, a strong emotional reaction may also result from observing one's "self" through the eyes of another. Therapists must, therefore, carefully plan the timing of this procedure so as to minimize possible negative consequences.

Spouses weakly committed to relationship change may still continue to resist these procedures. In these instances, defining the role play as "just for fun" may be helpful. Paradoxically, this metamessage—"Your behavior in this situation is not real"—is also useful for clients who resist on the grounds that role plays are "not real." Rather than defending the use of role plays, the therapist empathetically agrees with the client but asks him/her to just go along with the game. Such qualifications rarely obviate the potential benefits of the procedure.

Spouses who are content with the present structure of their relationship (i.e., how each partner's role is defined) may be particularly resistant, since the cost of any relationship change is perceived as outweighing any expected benefits. Thus, resistance is likely to persist unless the possibility of relationship gains worth the effort can be demonstrated. The procedure I have found most useful here is the "shaping role play." In this procedure nonthreatening role plays (and other procedures) are used to develop a context in which later role plays, dealing with specific relationship issues, can be successful. For example, teaching spouses communication and sexual enhancement skills and "programming" mutually enjoyable extragroup activities may demonstrate to the resistant spouse the potential benefits of increased cooperation. Essential to this strategy is to temporarily steer around highly threatening topics, concentrating on teaching relationship skills which stress *mutual* positive outcomes.

All of the aforementioned recommendations assume the presence of a positive group environment. As was the case with the pregroup orientation, many problems of resistance can be avoided or more easily overcome by sufficient attention to group-level variables. For example, carefully choosing the topic and participants for role plays in the first few sessions of the group will facilitate development of group norms which support role playing as an important expression of group membership. Pressure to conform to these norms will be related to the degree of cohesiveness among group members and how attracted they are to the treatment program. Two methods for achieving these objectives are creating a highly reinforcing atmosphere among group members and therapist, and providing couples with "promising" information (for example, presenting a novel conceptual framework to view their relationship or using an exercise which is likely to produce some new insights) as a sample of the program's effectiveness. The therapist must never forget that he/she is dealing with a group as well as couples. If this happens, *individual* resistance will seem a small problem.

In this discussion, I have tried to highlight some of the salient sources of resistance to role playing and procedures for overcoming them. This is certainly not an exhaustive account and the group marital therapist should expand these procedures based on his/her assessment of group, individual and relationship needs.

Reference

LoPiccolo, J. and Lobitz, W. C. Behavior therapy of sexual dysfunction. In L. A. Hamerlynck, L. C. Handy, and E. J. Mash (eds.), *Behavior Change: Methodology, Concepts and Practice*. Research Press: Champaign, Illinois, 1973.

STANLEY L. WITKIN, Ph.D.
Assistant Professor
School of Social Work
Florida State University
Tallahassee, FL

38. The Symbolic Meaning of Behavioral Exchanges in Marital Therapy

Question:

I am a practicing family therapist whose interest in behavior modification has grown considerably over the years. Recently, I have become interested in using contingency contracts in my work with couples. Some couples with whom I work, however, become quite resistant when I introduce contingency contracts into their treatment program. These couples typically say that they cannot understand how a simple agreement to exchange specific behaviors, increase their rates of pleasing responses or decrease the incidences of punishing responses will improve their marriage, because they believe the causes of the partner's problem behaviors to be "deeply rooted and unconscious." Behavior modification is meaningless for these couples, because it goes against their belief that insight into the causes of problem behavior is necessary if "true" behavior change is to be achieved. Can you suggest some techniques that I might use to help couples overcome their initial resistance? Can clients retain their beliefs about the nature of the behavior change process and still learn to use behavioral procedures, or is conversion to a behavioral viewpoint necessary before behavioral procedures can be used effectively?

Discussion:

In such a situation, it is important for the therapist to recognize that he/she is confronting a belief system about human behavior and behavior change which is tied inextricably to a model of personality formation and motivation which differs drastically from the basic philosophy which underlies behavior modification practices. Changing this belief system, however, probably will prove to be difficult and time consuming. Nevertheless, little therapeutic progress can be expected to occur unless the therapist can persuade antagonistic spouses to collaborate for the ultimate goal of improving their marriage. In such cases, it often is necessary for the therapist to devise strategies which do not require alterations in the belief systems of clients but which will allow spouses to work cooperatively and utilize behavior modification procedures in spite of their negative feelings toward each other and their mistrust of behavior modification.

One means of fostering collaboration between spouses is to ask the spouses to treat the presenting problem as if it were external to the relationship, a problem that can be solved only through the concerted efforts of both spouses. For example, if a wife complains that her husband does not spend enough time with her, or if a husband complains that his wife does not show him enough affection, the complaint can be reframed as a problem that both must solve. The therapist might recast the complaint as one of the spouses "having a problem finding a common time when they can enjoy each other's company because of their busy and often conflicting schedules," or "having to learn additional communication skills that will enable them to communicate their needs more effectively." The problem's resolution becomes a superordinate goal to be attained by both spouses. Once the couple agrees to focus on solving the problem at hand, the therapist gradually can introduce behavioral procedures such as modeling the skills to be learned, having the couple practice at home the problem-solving and communication skills learned in the therapist's office, having the couple implement a procedure where they gain a joint reward for the successful completion of a task together, etc. In essence, the therapist begins to shape the couple's behavior in such a way that they begin to incorporate behavioral practices into their own behavior patterns. If these new behavioral skills are satisfying for the couple, the probability that they will become an integral part of their way of interacting is increased. Contingency contracting then can be introduced into the treatment regimen.

If the therapist is unsuccessful in getting the couple to accept this procedure, another technique might be employed which also does not require the clients to alter their cognitions, but will allow them to assimilate behavioral technology into their already existing belief system. I have found the procedure which I will outline below to be effective in helping couples increase the rates of pleasing behaviors exhibited toward their spouses and accept the use of contingency contracting as part of the treatment process.

When spouses express doubts about the relevance or applicability of behavioral procedures for their particular relationship difficulties, or when they insist that the only way to produce lasting behavior change is by gaining insight into the deep-seated psychological causes of the problem at hand, the therapist should avoid debating these issues with the clients or trying to change their belief system. As is true of all psychotherapeutic approaches, the therapist's first task is to establish a trusting relationship with the clients. Questioning the clients' belief system at the outset of therapy, therefore, may be counterproductive. Once a trusting relationship has been established, however, the therapist can begin to help couples assimilate behavioral practices into their already existing set of beliefs about the nature of human behavior and behavior change.

Having gained the clients' trust and acceptance, the therapist can begin to direct the couple to a specific problem area that they would like to tackle. Once the couple has identified this area, both spouses are asked to pinpoint the specific behavior exhibited by their mate that they consider to be problematic and would like to see changed. The spouses are given the opportunity to:

1) Explain to their mate how they feel when the problem behavior is exhibited or fails to be exhibited. By doing this the offended spouses have the opportunity to express feelings which might have been suppressed for some time.

2) Discuss their personal interpretation of the problem behavior and the intentions that they attribute to their spouse whenever he/she performs or fails to perform the behavior in question. This process helps the offending spouses begin to understand how their behavior is being interpreted by their mate. This procedure also helps spouses role play and enables them to begin to understand how their mates perceive them. The spouses begin to experience their impact on their mates.

3) Disclose what they say to themselves covertly before, during and after their spouse behaves in a particular fashion or fails to behave in the desired manner. This aspect of the process is extremely important because these covert statements often serve as antecedent cues for affective and behavioral responses. If spouses interpret their mate's intentions as malicious, there is a good chance that their self-statements will be inflammatory and the affective responses which accompany these statements most probably will be those of anger, shame, anxiety or guilt. The offended spouses, therefore, will be likely to respond to their mate in a hostile or coercive manner.

At this time, the offending spouses are given the opportunity to discuss their actual intentions. As is often the case with distressed couples, one finds that the behavior exhibited by the offending spouses is not mal-intentioned but has been perceived as malevolent by the offended spouse. In such cases, intervention at the cognitive level is called for. The offended spouses can be taught to relabel and reinterpret their mate's behaviors in more accurate and less malevolent terms. Inflammatory self-statements can be replaced by statements which serve as cues for verifying the partner's actual intentions, open communication and constructive problem solving.

The three step process outlined above may provide enough insight for a given couple to allow them to increase their performance of rewarding behaviors for their spouses, because now they understand the meaning that these behaviors have for their mates. At this time, contingency contracts might be introduced into the treatment process.

The final step in this process is reserved for those individuals who believe that insight into unconscious dynamics is a prerequisite to lasting behavior change. In such cases, the following procedure may be used.

Spouses are asked to discuss the symbolic significance that the problem behaviors exhibited by their mates have for them as these behaviors relate to past childhood experiences. For instance, I recently treated a couple where the wife became enraged because her husband did not share his work day experiences with her in the evening. She interpreted his characteristic introverted behavior as "withholding" and "punishing." When asked what this experience brought to mind from her childhood years, this woman recounted that her older sister would never share her toys with her and her mother always gave her the silent treatment when she was bad. When this client was asked to identify what specific behaviors she would like her husband to exhibit, she indicated that she would like him to "talk with me in the evening after dinner" and "spend some time alone with me after the children have gone to bed." When asked to discuss the significance of these behaviors as they might relate to childhood experiences, this woman related how as a child she rarely spent any time alone with her parents, especially her father. The only time that she could remember getting her parents' undivided attention was when her older sister spent time away from home visiting relatives.

Obviously, the husband had been unaware of the importance that talking to his wife about mundane events and spending time with her in the evening had for her. This insight served as an incentive for the husband's behavior change. This couple then was able to contract for specific times when they could talk about the day's events and spend some time together.

When contingency contracts are introduced, it is important for spouses to discuss the symbolic significance that particular rewarding behaviors have for them. This is done so that the spouse who is being asked to perform the behavior can appreciate its importance to his/her mate. For example, a contingency contract for a dinner of roast duck may take on a different meaning when the cook sees the meal as symbolic of shared love and commitment, commemorating a meal that the couple enjoyed together on their honeymoon. Similarly, a quiet walk alone with a spouse may take on a deeper importance if this walk is understood as a display of silent affection which recreates a childhood experience that the recipient once shared with a beloved parent or sibling.

In our work with families, it is important for us to remember that some treatment approaches may be appropriate for some families and inappropriate for others. While some individuals might feel comfortable learning to use behavioral techniques to change undesirable interaction patterns, others might find a behavioral approach to be "superficial," "mechanistic" or contrary to "humanistic" and "dynamic" psychology. Such individuals may better be served by a referral to a therapist who shares their theoretical orientation. This, however, is an empirical question. From my perspective, the ultimate goal of family therapy is the modification of dysfunctional interaction patterns which impede the growth and development of the family members and the family system as a whole. It should not matter whether family members change their belief systems about the nature of human behavior or whether a family subscribes to a particular viewpoint. What does matter is whether family members can be taught to use functional problem-solving strategies and positive behavior change techniques in their dealings with each other.

DENNIS A. BAGAROZZI, Ph.D.
Assistant Professor
School of Social Work
University of Georgia
Athens,GA

39. Management of the Treatment-Destructive Resistance in Family Therapy

Question:

Many practitioners are aware that there has been a change in the type of family who enters treatment. More recently, families are coming for help who are not self-referred and who often might be thought of as character disordered. Naturally, since they are not self-referred, and since their pathology is perceived by them as ego-syntonic, they pose a challenge for the practitioner insofar as it is very difficult to sustain them in treatment. What should the practitioner bear in mind in working with this type of family?

Discussion:

Before answering this question, it probably would be helpful to look at the problem somewhat broadly. Such an understanding may enable the clinician to view the problems of these sometimes disturbing family members from a more benign point of view.

The negative thrust of the treatment destructive family stems from the basic biological processes which are common to all organisms. These are anabolism and catabolism, or the building up and breaking down of the cells. When a correct proportion of mental energy is devoted to each of these functions, then the organism is well-balanced and can exist in a harmonious manner in its environment. In some families, this is not the case.

This disproportionate emphasis on the negative results stem from a child-rearing experience in which the parent wishes the child dead and communicates this message to the child. If the child cooperates with this injunction, as an adult, he will be prone to reject people who seek to help him and behave in a generally self-destructive manner (Bloch, 1965).

A case in point is the Z family. Mr. and Mrs. Z consulted me about their 10-year-old son who had been observed behaving in a peculiar manner in school. Mrs. Z told me that her son's problems were entirely the fault of the school, and she could see no good reason why he should need any treatment. I told her that, indeed, there were many school practices which were not in the best interest of the child and that perhaps this was the case here. She said to me that if, in fact, the school was to blame, why should she bring her child in for treatment. I told her that the child did not have the problem that the school thought he had, but rather he was not able to convince the school to treat him in the way that he wanted to be treated. I also told her that I was in a position to teach him to do that, if they were interested in availing themselves of my service. They said they were, and we concluded with arrangements as to fee, time frequency, etc. (cf: Strean, 1978).

I want to point out here that even though a family may be initially won over and appear to be positively disposed toward the therapist, it must be clear to the reader that their negative feelings will naturally emerge in the course of time. Assuming that this will happen, I tell the family that they are not going to like me no matter what happens. If the child does not appear to be progressing as rapidly as they would like, they are not going to like me because they will feel dissatisfied. On the other hand, if the child makes a lot of progress, they are not going to like me because they will feel that I did a better job than they did. The parents generally "pooh-pooh" these statements, but forewarned is forearmed. I want to point out that both of the interventions described, so far, communicated to the family, and the parents specifically, that the therapist understands them. All of which adds thrust to an effort to bring the family into the mainstream of the shared positive values of the culture, rather than the destructive path upon which they are embarked.

As treatment progresses and the family becomes more involved with the therapist, they will demonstrate their destructive patterns in other ways. Specifically, they will fight in the therapist's office. Generally, these fights are, again, attempts to place the responsibility for the difficulty on someone other than the principals. It is this unfortunate tendency to deal with problems in this manner that makes them insoluble. If the family perceives the therapist as doing nothing about this situation, they will remove themselves from the treatment situation. Such an atmosphere of recrimination and animosity is not good for the therapist either, and his/her personal interests are well served by bringing an abrupt halt to this kind of misbehavior. A common-sense explanation of the inadvisability of this behavior, as well as a suggestion for some alternative approaches, will serve this situation well.

References

Bloch, D. Feelings that kill; The effect of the wish for infanticide in neurotic depression, *Psychoanalytical Review* 52:51-66, 1965.
Strean, H. Paradigmatic interventions in seemingly difficult therapeutic situations. In Marie C. Nelson (Ed.), *Roles and Paradigms in Psychotherapy*. New York: Grune & Stratton, 1978.

MICHAEL J. BECK, Ph.D.
*Dean, Long Island (N.Y.) Institute
for Psychotherapeutic Studies
Babylon, NY*

40. Impasses in Negotiating Solutions in Behavioral Family Therapy

Question:

Imagine that you are conducting a behavioral family therapy session with a mother and father and their 15-year-old daughter, June, who argue repeatedly about a variety of issues. You are trying to teach them effective problem-solving communication skills. They are discussing June's curfew. They define the problem clearly, generate a list of solutions, and evaluate each solution. You are excited because they are finally learning to use the techniques that you have been teaching them for several sessions. Suddenly, at the final stage, when you least expect trouble, they get bogged down. They are unable to negotiate a compromise. Each family member rigidifies his/her position, flatly refusing to consider the others' perspectives. The atmosphere is emotionally charged. You feel a sinking sensation in the pit of your stomach. What do you do?

Discussion:

This discussion will describe three social psychological and cognitive-attributional techniques which I've found useful for helping families overcome such disagreements. These techniques are 1) fractionation of the conflict, 2) appeal to a higher authority figure, followed by graduated reciprocal initiatives in tension reduction, and 3) cognitive restructuring. I have found these techniques particularly helpful during discussions of heavily value-laden issues such as premarital sex, religious beliefs, and marijuana smoking.

Fractionation of the conflict (Fogg, 1974). This technique entails breaking a dispute into several elements that might each be settled separately. The more easily managed elements are dealt with first to build up a reciprocity of positive interactions. If such reciprocity is not forthcoming, a partial solution may at least be salvaged. As an example, consider the case of the Janis family. Mrs. Janis found several marijuana cigarettes in her son Tom's dresser. She had suspected that Tom was smoking marijuana and had surreptitiously searched his room. Tom was incensed by his mother's invasion of his privacy and refused to give up smoking marijuana. His mother was unalterably opposed to Tom's use of marijuana, at home or outside the home, and had responded to her discovery by grounding him indefinitely. They were unable to resolve this dispute.

The therapist fractionated the issue into three elements and addressed each individually: 1) Tom's use of marijuana outside the home; 2) Tom's use of marijuana at home; and 3) Mrs. Janis' invasion of Tom's privacy. Even though Mrs. Janis could not condone marijuana smoking anyplace, she did recognize that it would be difficult to prevent her son from smoking outside the home. After an extended discussion, she "agreed to disagree," i.e., to cease making an issue of marijuana smoking outside the home, although she made clear her continued opposition to his smoking. Tom was able to provide convincing evidence that he was discrete in selecting the locations where he smoked. Given the positive climate created by his mother's compromise, Tom agreed to refrain from smoking and storing marijuana in the home. The resolution of the first two issues set the stage for a discussion of Mrs. Janis' invasion of Tom's privacy. Mother and son agreed to communicate future suspicions directly rather than obtain information surreptitiously.

Appeal to a higher authority, followed by graduated reciprocal initiatives in tension reduction (Fogg, 1974). This technique entails locating a higher authority whom the parents, the adolescent, or both respect, and arranging for the authority to sanction a compromise by one or more family members. Such authorities may be friends of the family, clergymen, physicians, political or media personalities, or even psychics. The therapist prepares one family member to announce a "spontaneous" deescalation of the conflict, taking the others by surprise. As a consequence, the other family members feel obligated to follow suit with a second deescalation step, reciprocated by further compromises, and the conflict is rapidly resolved.

This strategy was inadvertently used in the case of a disagreement concerning religion. Sixteen-year-old Joey was a passive adolescent who was unable to verbalize this opinions and feelings to his parents; instead, he would "save up" his affect until he exploded, "acting out" in an aggressive manner. During the first two therapy sessions, I taught Joey to define problems assertively to his parents, and the family appeared to be benefiting from treatment. Then, we held a

discussion of church attendance. Displaying his newly acquired assertive repertoire, Joey stated for the first time that he was agnostic and
therefore considered it hypocritical to continue attending church services. Father turned livid; Mother began sobbing uncontrollably; Father
stated that his son would be damned for the remainder of his life if he
ceased attending mass every week. Enraged, Joey threatened to run
away if his parents forced him to continue attending mass. Tempers
were running so hot that I adjourned the session after instructing each
family member to consider the issue very carefully during the week
but not to discuss it without my help.

The parents consulted their priest, who advised them that a flexible
attitude was appropriate with teenagers who were going through the
stage of doubting religious beliefs. With permission from the priest,
a credible higher authority figure, the parents were willing to announce a "deescalation" of the conflict at the beginning of the next
session: They suggested that Joey attend church twice a month and
read a passage from the bible on the Sundays when he did not attend
mass. Aware of his parents' orthodox religious beliefs, Joey was genuinely surprised that they would even consider a compromise. He indicated that, since he recognized how much religion meant to them
and what a great sacrifice they were making, the least he could do was
attend church twice a month "to please them," even though he would
continue to maintain his agnosticism. Impressed by the power of the
priest's permission-giving, I decided that when I open my next family
clinic, I will hire a liberal clergyman as a consultant.

Cognitive restructuring. This technique, a step-child of rational
emotive therapy (Goldfried, 1979), is designed to teach a family to
identify the illogical beliefs preventing the resolution of a dispute,
challenge the validity of these beliefs, substitute more reasonable cognitions, and increase family members' receptivity to each other's solutions to the dispute. The therapist formulates a hypothesis concerning
the illogical cognitions presumed to mediate the family's argumen-
tative behavior and expresses the hypothesis to the family at an op-
portune moment during the discussion. Such a hypothesis is best
expressed Socratically by "catching" a family member committing a
logical inconsistency and then humorously introducing a challenging
statement, perhaps in an exaggerated, catastrophic fashion. During
the ensuing moments of surprise and embarrassment, the therapist
firmly but graciously challenges the credibility of the illogical cognitions. The family is asked to marshal evidence illustrating the unrea-
sonableness of the faulty belief, and alternative, more flexible beliefs

are modeled. Finally, the therapist requests that the family try a brief experiment: Assume that the more reasonable beliefs may be appropriate, negotiate a solution to the dispute, implement the solution for one week, and evaluate its effectiveness. If the solution is effective, then the more flexible belief system is supported. If the solution is ineffective, the therapist notes that the family member can always retain the previous beliefs. Most families find that they cannot refuse the offer of the experiment, when presented in a balanced manner by an empathetic therapist. The experience of success in trying a new approach to a touchy problem then helps to solidify the new belief system.

Conflicts concerning adolescent sexuality have proven fertile ground for the use of cognitive restructuring. For instance, Mr. and Mrs. Jones refused to let their 15-year-old daughter, Betsy, stay out past 10:30 p.m., but could not present a satisfactory reason for their position; they simply asserted that she was "too immature." Betsy angrily denounced the curfew and accused her parents of ruining her social life. I suspected that her parents believed that if Betsy stayed out past 10:30 p.m., she would become precociously involved in heterosexual activities, possibly becoming pregnant, and that only by restricting her curfew could they avoid a catastrophe. When the family reached an impasse during the discussion, I personalized their dilemma:

> You know, Mr. and Mrs. Jones, if I had a 15-year-old daughter who wanted to stay out late with her friends, I'd be very worried. Even more worried than you are. I'd worry that she might get involved with boys sexually; that she might get hurt physically and emotionally; that she might have sexual intercourse; and even worse, that she might get pregnant and ruin her future. Sure, she would regret it afterwards, but teenagers act without thinking so often. So I'd really be worried. As a parent I'd want to protect my daughter. I'd do anything, including keeping her in the house. Do you feel at all this way?

Mr. Jones writhed; Mrs. Jones cried. They proceeded to tell their daughter how frightened they were about her budding sexuality and how unsure they were about her ability to handle herself with boys.

Betsy was surprised by her parents' anxieties and hurt by their lack of trust in her judgment. I pointed out to the parents that if Betsy were determined to engage in sexual relations, she would find the opportunity despite a 10:30 curfew, and therefore the more basic fears concerning her sexuality should be discussed directly. Betsy indicated to her parents that she enjoyed kissing, petting and other noncoital sexual activities, but that she had no intention of surrendering her virginity to the first boy who asked; in fact, she vehemently insisted that the last thing she wished to do was become pregnant, and that when she did have sexual intercourse, she would use contraception. Mr. and Mrs. Jones were reassured by their daughter's sincere, common-sense attitude towards sexual matters, and were able to adopt more realistic beliefs. I proposed a trial period with a later curfew and the family agreed.

Conclusion. When parents and adolescents become bogged down during the negotiation stage of problem solving, my goal is to interrupt their perseverative interactions, prevent an escalation of the disagreement, and redirect their discussion in a more productive direction. The three strategies reviewed here accomplish these goals by permitting family members to distance themselves from the ongoing interaction and take another's perspective concerning the issue under discussion. It is hypothesized that the strategies are effective because of the tendency of individuals in intense, long-term relationships to be willing to meet each other's needs when they can do so gracefully, "saving face" and preserving their individual dignity and personal values.

References

Fogg, R. Some effects of teaching adolescents some creative, peaceful conflict resolution approaches to international conflict. *Theory and Research in Social Education*, Fall, 1974, 51-67.

Goldfried, M. R. Anxiety reduction through cognitive-behavioral intervention. In P. C. Kendall and S. D. Hollon (Eds.), *Cognitive-Behavioral Interventions: Theory, Research, and Procedures*. New York: Academic Press, 1979.

ARTHUR L. ROBIN, Ph.D.
Assistant Professor of Clinical
Child Psychology
Department of Pediatrics
Wayne State University School of Medicine
Detroit, MI

41. Managing Resistance to
   Behavioral Family Therapy

Question:

What guidelines can you offer to deal with resistance to behavioral family therapy in general, and to behavioral rehearsal in particular?

Discussion:

The best "cure" for resistance to behavioral or other therapies is to prevent its occurrence in the first place. Preventing or minimizing resistance entails developing rapport and a working therapeutic alliance from the very start of treatment. While most therapists are selected and trained for listening skills, empathy, genuine human concern and warmth, few consciously employ specific behaviors which can cumulatively promote a favorable therapeutic relationship. A partial listing of these relevant therapist's behaviors follow, derived from suggestions made by Fisher (1974):

1) Give careful directions for finding the way to the therapist's office before first visit.
2) Provide equitable physical distance between therapist and patient:
   (a) Possibly avoid having desk as a barrier;
   (b) Possibly allow patient to sit near the door;
   (c) Shake hands *after* initial visit instead of at opening introduction;
   (d) Greet patient at the door or in waiting room and walk with patient to the door at end of session. Say "goodbye" and remind patient of next appointment;
   (e) Use touching and "pats-on-the-back" with discretion and discrimination of the patient's comfort and values.
3) Ask permission before using patient's first name—give patient the option of how he/she wants to be called and addressed.
4) Apologize if you are late for an appointment.

5) Show patient where toilet is located and give permission to use it whenever needed—even in midst of session.
6) Avoid looking at clock or watch when *patient is talking*.
7) Let occasional sessions go overtime—don't end every session strictly "on-the-60-minute-hour."
8) Acknowledge patient's birthday and anniversary verbally and possibly with a card.
9) With discretion, greet patient when crossing paths in the community.
10) Use good "personal effectiveness" nonverbal style–eye contact, resonant voice, fluent and slow speech, gesture; leaning toward client, smiling and appropriate, reflective facial expressions.

Building Favorable Expectations

It is well-accepted and empirically documented that adequate orientation to the particular treatment being offered will promote favorable expectations and better outcome for the patient. In behavior therapy, orientation is made easier by the concrete, down-to-earth, and direct nature of the therapeutic approaches. In fact, the Association for the Advancement of Behavior Therapy has published a brochure that explains, in layman's terms, what behavior therapy involves (AABT, 1979). Rationales are particularly important for patients with chronic problems as confusion about the disorder has often been fed by multiple and frustrating experiences with therapists of differing persuasions. Behavioral practitioners are well versed in rationales that can help to clear up confusion in patients suffering from agoraphobia—for example, explaining how environmental overstimulation of a vulnerable autonomic nervous system can produce recognizable symptoms and how escape from or avoidance of feared situations reinforces the phobia.

As another example of offering the starting patient a rationale for a particular therapy, the following excerpt is given from a client's introductory brochure for social skills or personal effectiveness training (Liberman et al., 1975):

The purpose of this Introduction is to give you an idea of what social skills training is all about so that you will know what to expect. Social skills training helps people to improve the way they communicate their feelings, their emotions, their requests, and their wishes to others. It also provides better ways of responding to the communications of others. It is a form of "assertive training," which is a way of teaching people to deal directly, positively, and effectively with other people. In the training we concentrate on some elements of communication that are often overlooked. The words we use are important, but more important than the specific words is how we put our message across.

What's different about how we use our words? Simple things, and so obvious that you might easily miss them. The way you hold your body, how you use your eyes, your hand gestures, your tone of voice, the volume of your voice, and your facial expressions are the elements that make or break a message. Smiling when you're angry, mumbling when you want to be "perfectly clear," looking away when you should be steadfast in your irresistible gaze, all these are extremely important. But they don't come naturally; they are learned. If they can be learned, then they can be taught—efficiently and directly. Two elements are necessary in the training. The first is rehearsal. Practice in lifelike situations is very important. Actors memorize their lines and their moves, but before they can become comfortable in their roles, they have to practice and rehearse. The famous psychologist William James once said that the soul of learning is repetition, and he was very nearly correct. Practicing your new skills, trying them out on a variety of different people, watching others show how they would handle the same situation are all part of what we call "behavioral rehearsal" in social skills training.

Some people are a little nervous at first about this part of social skills training, but it passes very quickly. One reason is that the individual practice sessions or "scenes" are very short, and seldom last more than two minutes. Things happen so fast and you are so busy that there is practically no time to get nervous. And soon, as you begin to pick up new skills, this will become the most enjoyable part of your training. Also, a little nervousness can even be a good thing. Even the best clergymen, actors, salesmen, and lawyers admit to feeling a bit nervous before a big event. The observer doesn't see it, however. He sees the confident, capable, effective person convincing others to see things the way he sees them. Last, but of equal importance to feedback and rehearsal, are real-life assignments. As each new skill is learned, you will receive assignments to be completed at home, in stores, restaurants, or on the job. What should you expect when you attend your first session? Getting into a new social situation, especially one that may involve some of your personal problems, is a little like going swimming. Once you're in the water, its comfortable; getting there is half the agony.

From the excerpt, it can be seen how the patient's expectations for a positive experience and outcome are raised, even while predicting some of the discomforts that require adaptation. The patient is informed about the role of the therapist as well as the patient, including modeling and homework assignments. The patient is told what will happen, why and when. Preparing the patient for specific elements of the therapy procedure cannot be done only once at the start of treatment, but rather, must be presented repeatedly as therapy proceeds. In undercutting resistance that might otherwise develop, an astute behavior therapist will also spend time on catharsis and determining the patient's reasons for coming for help. Sufficient opportunity for ventilating feelings and concerns—even at the risk of temporarily reinforcing maladaptive tendencies—is important to provide *before* engaging the patient in goal-setting and structured therapy. If the patient feels he or she has not been "heard" before therapy commences, counterproductive complaining and foot-dragging will often occur during the therapy. It is also incumbent upon the therapist to assist the patient in formulating the reasons for coming to a mental health professional *now*. Future resistance to inappropriately chosen goals and techniques can be obviated by employing a "customer" approach with the patient. In doing this, the therapist helps the patient articulate poorly understood needs and wishes and actively pursues the patient's hopes, fears and desires for change and for the treatment experience itself.

Overcoming Resistance to Behavioral Rehearsal

One of the key techniques in behavioral family therapy is behavioral rehearsal. In behavioral rehearsal, the therapist sets up a clinically relevant interpersonal scene and has the couple or family practice the interaction. Going through a "dry run"—as the family members have interacted in the past—provides the therapist with direct evidence of the kinds of deficits in communication and problem-solving that are contributing to the family's distress. Thus, the initial "dry run" is an extension of behavioral assessment and serves as a point of departure for therapeutic interventions. Interventions, built around behavioral rehearsal, include instructions, cognitive restructuring, prompting, cueing, modeling, coaching, positive feedback and homework assignments. Usually, a therapist will have the family members repeatedly rehearse a problematic scene until they have demonstrated some clear improvement in their communication style and problem-solving ability. The sequence of steps in the behavioral rehearsal process is shown in Table 1.

TABLE 1

Training Procedure for Behavioral Rehearsal in Family Therapy

1. Specify the interpersonal problem by asking:
   —What affects or communications are lacking or not being appropriately expressed?
   —Where, when, and with whom does the problem occur?

2. Formulate a scene which simulates or recapitulates the features of the problem situation
3. Observe while the family members rehearse the scene ("dry run"), and position yourself close to the action
4. Identify the assets, deficits and excesses in the patient's performance during the "dry run" and give constructive feedback
5. Give instructions and prompts to initiate changes in behavior
6. Use models to demonstrate more adaptive expressive skills
7. Focus on all dimensions of social competence:
   —Topical content and semantic choice of words and phrases
   —Nonverbal components
   —Timing and reciprocity
   —Perceptual and discrimination skills
8. Give positive feedback to reinforce progress or even effort as the patients again rehearse the scene in a "re-run"
9. Shape behavioral changes in small increments. Start where the patients are and don't expect too much improvement at any one time
10. Generalize the changes over settings, responses and time by:
    —Repeated practice and overlearning
    —Specific, attainable, and functional "homework assignments"
    —Positive feedback for successful transfer of skills to real life
    —Training in self-instructions and self-reinforcement
    —Fading the structure and frequency of the training

Since behavioral rehearsal is such a key element in behavioral family therapy, overcoming resistance to practicing expressive and communication patterns is important. It would be very nice, indeed, if all our families behaved as mature adults and cooperated with our efforts to engage them in behavioral rehearsal. Unfortunately, our patients come to us because they are not mature adults and their resistance to behavioral rehearsal may be symptomatic of a wide range of affective, cognitive and social problems. Effective methods of coping with resistance, then, depend upon identifying the sources of the resistance. With a family member suffering from schizophrenia or severe depression where biologically mediated symptoms are interfering with attentional, cognitive and motivational skills required by the behavioral rehearsal, it may be necessary judiciously to use medication for overcoming resistance induced by symptoms. With a spouse who is paying "lip service" to marital therapy but who lacks any interest in improving the marriage, a direct exploration may be required of the person's ambivalence and possibly greater desire for separation. The following suggestions for surmounting resistance to behavioral rehearsal are offered with the assumption that the experienced clinician will use them in the context of a proper evaluation of the types and sources of resistance.

Acknowledging sources of resistance. Many times, resistance can be quickly dissolved by the therapist simply reflecting back the emotions, inhibitions and anxieties that are behind the negativism. This is particularly effective when mild anxiety or embarrassment are at the root of the resistance. Straightforward performance anxiety can often get in the way of direct practice of family scenes; acknowledgment dilutes the anxiety, gives "permission" for experiencing discomfort, and promotes confidence and rapport with the therapist. It is important not to overreact to resistance by offering elaborate psychological interpretations which may only serve to reinforce the resistance. Simple and direct acknowledgment should be quickly followed by prompts for engaging in the desired behavioral rehearsal. For example, a therapist might say, "I can understand your anxiety going through this difficult scene, but let's give it a try even though you may be a little uncomfortable."

Modeling for the resistant patient. Borrowing from psychodramatic techniques, the clinician can "double" for the family member who is reluctant to rehearse a scene. By doubling or providing an auxiliary ego, some of the pressure for initiating or processing a family problem can be taken off the resistant patient who can repeat, word-for-word, the phrases spoken by the "double." Another use of modeling is to have the patient observe the therapist taking the patient's role and then asking the patient to criticize, revise or elaborate on the therapist's performance. This gives the patient a chance to learn vicariously through observing the therapist and to become involved in the task. With very anxious and inhibited patients it may be necessary to allow the patient to watch others engage in behavioral rehearsal for a session or two before prompting action on the patient's part.

Shaping participation in small steps. A sensitive therapist can subtly slip the resistant patient into rehearsing by asking the patient to describe in concrete, graphic details what generally happens in the actual problem situations. The patient will usually volunteer descriptions of who did what to whom, after which the therapist can prompt, "When he said that to you, you said . . . (pause)?" Even getting a patient to take the first person position during a single interaction is a step toward full participation in rehearsing a scene. Other ways of breaking down the rehearsal into smaller responses include setting up a brief, and emotionally nonthreatening scene that has no "heavy" personal loading for the patient. Therefore, in trying to gain the participation of a resistant adolescent, it would be counterproductive to invite a rehearsal of a scene dealing with parental confrontation of marijuana use; instead, it would be wise to start with a mundane scene such as how family members greet each other or say goodbye to each other. Another use of shaping through approximations is to ask the resistant family member to take the role of a different person inside or outside of the family circle and play that person's part in a behavioral rehearsal. Once some practice in another person's role has been carried out, anxiety has usually diminished to the point where the patient can then rehearse his or her own role.

Using group process. One of the many advantages in conducting marital or family therapy in groups is the opportunity to overcome resistance to behavioral rehearsal. In a group, the therapist has the option of beginning the rehearsals with the most enthusiastic and cooperative patients or with those who are "veterans" of behavioral rehearsal. This capitalizes on their modeling impact on resistant and shy group members. Group process also promotes cohesion which has an anxiolytic effect on inhibited group members. In a group, the therapist can allow new or resistant members to simply observe the more active members. As they watch the others getting involved and gaining the therapist's interest and feedback, the more reluctant patients will be motivated to participate. Asking the more resistant patients to give verbal suggestions and feedback to other participating members serves as an approximation to their subsequent, more active involvement in the treatment process.

Strategic ploys. The use of paradoxical and other subtle methods can be useful in gaining the compliance of patients to therapeutic instructions for behavioral rehearsal and homework assignments. It should be emphasized, however, that therapists require some finesse and experience to effectively use these interventions. Some of the strategic interventions, useful in eliciting the cooperation of a patient, are:

1) Establish a "response set" for compliance and cooperation by initially making small requests that can be easily agreed to. Thus, after agreeing to pass an ashtray, use a different chair, and write a list of complaints, the patient has already begun to cooperate and may be more likely to respond favorably to larger requests in the future.

2) "Join" with the patient's resistance—identify with patient's concerns and thereby avoid a power struggle.

3) Emphasize positive behavior and downplay resistance in talking

with patient (e.g., "Despite your reluctance to being involved in family therapy, you *are* here today and have made an effort to get help.")
4) Establish *this therapy* as distinct and different from the other therapies which have failed in the past.
5) Give permission to engage in noncooperation and noncompliance:
   (a) Instruct patient to actually PRACTICE being resistant;
   (b) Schedule symptomatic behavior;
   (c) Introduce an "ordeal" as an accompaniment to resistant behavior.
6) Predict resistance.
7) Provide a choice or option for the patient to decide on, either of which is therapeutic.
8) Emphasize a worse alternative to behavioral rehearsal.

Summary

Resistance to the directive methods of behavioral family therapy is a common occurrence and should not surprise the experienced therapist. Many families will show little or no resistance if the therapist observes some basic procedures at the start of therapy which provide a rationale and orientation, enable catharsis, and build a positive therapeutic alliance.

Some patients will evidence noncompliance with behavioral methods such as homework assignments and role playing. Noncompliance and resistance are behaviors in their own right and require analysis of antecedents and consequences. It is helpful for the therapist to develop plans of action to manage specific types of resistance based upon social learning principles. Shaping approximations to the therapeutically desirable behaviors, modeling, use of a multiple family group, and strategic interventions all are useful tactics in overcoming resistance. Paradoxical techniques work by undercutting the social reinforcement that the patient expects to get by "defeating" the therapist. Dealing constructively with resistance requires the same careful behavior analysis and therapy that clinical symptoms demand. The types of families not suited for behavioral family therapy become very small indeed if the therapist develops and maintains a solid and positive relationship with all members of the family.

References

Association for the Advancement of Behavior Therapy (AABT). *Guidelines for Choosing a Behavior Therapist.* Available from the AABT, 420 Lexington Avenue, New York, NY 10017, 1979.

Fisher, D. *How to make a bad therapist good and a good therapist better.* Presentation at Oxnard Community Mental Health Center, Oxnard, California, February 10, 1974.
Liberman, R. P., King, L. W., DeRisi, W. J., and McCann, M. *Personal Effectiveness: Guiding People to Assert Themselves and Improve Their Social Skills. Client's Introduction* (brochure). Champaign, IL: Research Press, 1975.

ROBERT PAUL LIBERMAN, M.D.
*Professor of Psychiatry
UCLA School of Medicine;
Director, Mental Health Clinical Research Center for the
Study of Schizophrenia
Camarillo State Hospital
Camarillo, CA*

42. Countertransference Reactions
in Family Therapy

Question:

Time and again I experience intense feelings towards a family, or towards one or more specific members of a family. Sometimes these are positive feelings that seem nevertheless exaggerated, but more often they are negative feelings that have made sessions uncomfortable and difficult. These reactions seem different and more complicated than the countertransference reactions that I experience in working with individuals or groups. How best can I avoid or overcome these feelings in order to establish good rapport with families? Also, is it ever advisable to reveal my feelings to the family?

Discussion:

Countertransference is a psychoanalytic term for the repressed feelings and infantile wishes evoked in therapists by their patients. These feelings are viewed as detrimental to the treatment process. The analyst is encouraged to detect and consequently control or restrain countertransference tendencies (Eidelberg, 1968; Greenson, 1968). Countertransference is not confined to psychoanalysis; it is a phenomenon common to all forms of therapy. The experience of countertransference is familiar to anyone involved with treating whole families. It is evident when we sense that something feels wrong in our relationship with a family member or with the family as a whole. In individual therapy one attempts to locate the repressed feelings of the therapist in relation to the patient. In family therapy the process is much more complex since the therapist not only has reactions to each individual family member, but also to the family as a whole. Furthermore, there are reactions to the relationships between people in the family. When the therapist's reactions are obstructing the process of treatment, he/she is alerted to the problem by feelings of discomfort, defensiveness, or actual distress during and/or following a session. The therapist usually feels blocked, ineffective and bewildered. What is necessary at this juncture is to go beyond an understanding of the family's dynamics, and explore the therapist's affective reactions to the family and its members. Unlocking the countertransference reactions can lead to a renewed and more effective freedom of functioning for both the therapist and family.

Countertransference reactions in family treatment are not only more complex, but they are often more intense than in other forms of therapy. This poses a unique challenge in treating families. Unlike the individual therapist, the family therapist is generally more active and involved in interacting with family members. Consequently, his/her reactions are more difficult to conceal. A family member sensing dislike or antagonism from the therapist may react by forcing or contriving a premature termination of treatment. Losing one member invariably means losing the whole family. While negative feelings are clearly obstructive to a therapeutic working alliance, even positive feelings, if inappropriate, may disrupt treatment by creating an imbalance in the therapist's relationship with various family members. Stierlin (1977) points out that the therapist should be involved but impartial, so that he/she remains basically fair towards each family member. Thus, he defines countertransference in the family therapist as a deviation from this therapeutic position of involved impartiality.

Why is it that families arouse such powerful feelings in therapists? The key lies in some unique characteristics of the family as a social system. It is a group, not reducible to a collection of separate individuals. The complex history that binds members of a family is a chronicle of the development of deep-seated attitudes and feelings. Each family that contacts a therapist represents a reservoir of intense feelings. The therapist experiences an intensity of feelings because the family members are intensely experiencing their relationships with each other. The client in individual or group therapy can much more readily maintain a social facade. Family members know each other intimately; they do not long permit social disguises. Close confinement with those who have had the greatest effect on one's life is unavoidably impactful. It is one thing to confide feelings about one's mother to a sympathetic therapist. It is quite another to actually face one's mother and express feelings that have long been held back.

The arousal of strong feelings in the therapist may be a normative experience in successfully engaging with a family. It is to the therapist's advantage to regard his/her reactions to the family as valuable data that can help the progress of treatment. The task for the therapist is to distinguish what is being conveyed by the family or individual members, from feelings that he/she may be inappropriately attributing to the family. An example may make this clear.

A trainee complained of feeling impotent whenever he had a session with a particular family. With some exploration in supervision, he became aware of experiencing marked fear of the father in the family. It was known that the father had, in the past, become physically violent towards his wife and children. He resolved to never lose his temper again, and there had been no such incidents for over a year. In family sessions he appeared restrained and polite but stiff and awkward. Family members seemed reluctant to engage with the father on an affective level, and they either avoided him or engaged only superficially. In effect, he was isolated in the family, both in the sessions and at home. The therapy had bogged down because issues involving the father were not broached, and the therapist unwittingly colluded with the family in avoiding the father. During supervision the therapist realized that he was sharing the family's sense of impotence. His fear of the father could be partially attributed to events in his personal family history. More to the point, however, his feelings also accurately reflected the feelings of most members of the family.

The therapist's countertransference became important as a source of information for changing the situation and promoting movement. The supervisor suggested that he make a statement in the next family meeting to indicate that people in the family seemed afraid to say or do anything that might make father angry. This intervention had the effect of a safety valve. The mother and children admitted their fear of the father, and in doing so became less fearful. They became aware of the extent to which they had avoided him, and how much they wished for closeness with him. On his part, the father expressed his own sense of impotence. He was so afraid that he would lose control if he gave way to his anger that he created extreme distance to minimize the impact of any possible provocation from other family members. He felt lonely and depressed, aware of keeping his family at arm's length, but seemed unable to bridge the gap.

This session resulted in a dramatic decrease in tension. Family members felt free to interact and the therapist was given (and had unwittingly assumed) a position of power. The fact of addressing the father's anger made the therapist seem unafraid. By sympathetically understanding the anger as a problem rather than as a threat, he removed a serious obstacle to therapy. The father and the other family members felt freer to interact knowing that the therapist was vigilant and strong enough to tolerate and monitor whatever anger may be generated.

In the preceding example, the therapist's feelings of impotence reflected the emotional climate of the whole family. Frequently though, a therapist may be encumbered by an overwhelming feeling towards only one member of a family. This type of reaction may be attributable to personal history, but once again it may pinpoint an important interpersonal problem in the family. How does the therapist cope with intense feelings of anger towards a particular family member? These feelings cannot be willed away, nor can they easily be disguised (as noted earlier). Confronting that family member with the reaction, by way of offering "insight," is inevitably counterproductive. The more effective strategy in this instance is to first determine to what extent the therapist's feelings reflect feelings of other family members. This is best done by facilitating the expression of such feelings. Thus, after the family member has said or done something particularly annoying, the therapist should turn to another family member (preferably the most likely to be annoyed) and innocently inquire, "How do you feel about what X just said?" When the second family member hints about feelings of irritation or anger, the therapist can supportively encourage the further expression of such feelings. The next step is for the therapist to turn back to X and say, "Were you aware that Y feels this way?" This may now lead to a direct interaction between the two family members. Once the ice is broken other members of the family generally chime in. This therapeutic maneuver can only succeed if the therapist is viewed as nonjudgmental and impartial. Invariably a gratifying consequence of this strategy is that the offensive behavior of the first family member becomes understandable to the therapist as he/she learns more about the interpersonal context in which it is occurring.

Caution is necessary in utilizing countertransference as a therapeutic aid. A number of excellent clinicians have demonstrated the skillful use of personal reactions in order to change the defensive style of families, and this has led to the popularization of the "use of self" in family therapy. Unfortunately, there is a thin line between the use of self to facilitate therapeutic process and the use of self to meet the needs of the therapist. Practitioners of the order of Carl Whitaker are dazzling to behold, frequently misunderstood, and difficult to emulate. Many therapists vent their countertransference reactions in the misguided belief that they are employing personal honesty to improve treatment. In fact, they burden the family with the inappropriate task of having to cope with the therapist's problems. The place for revelations of personal feelings is in supervision or in personal therapy. Unless there is some valid strategic goal (and honesty is required in order to determine this) there is no point in saddling the family with one's personal problems. The criterion for what is said by the therapist should be the therapeutic needs of the family and not the personal needs of the therapist. This distinction can be readily demonstrated by two brief examples.

A therapist was working with a couple who persisted in a characteristic mode of interaction. The wife spent much of her energy in vain attempts to please her husband and earn his approval. No matter what she tried to do, he remained critical and dissatisfied. During one session the wife described at length the preparations she had made to surprise her husband with a gourmet dinner the previous evening. The husband's sole reaction had been that it took too long for her to cook the dinner. The husband attempted to justify his reaction. At this point the therapist sighed and suggested with a half smile that he was thinking of having his own wife call this woman in order to find out how to make what sounded like an excellent meal so that he could enjoy such a rare treat. The husband was caught off guard by this comment and grudgingly admitted that perhaps he did take his wife for granted at times. Here, the therapist interjected a personal reaction, which was an effective therapeutic strategy.

Another therapist was working with a couple who were going through a difficult period of atempting a separation. He decided to share his own difficulties when he had gone through a similar experience. He explained to his supervisor (and to himself) that he was sharing his personal experiences in order to support the couple and show them that he could understand what they were experiencing. In fact, the therapy stalled after this intervention. The couple seemed most uncomfortable and were unsure how to react. After much inquiring on the part of the therapist in a subsequent session, the couple admitted feeling dismayed by what they had been told. The wife felt resentful that the therapist had gratuitously introduced his own personal difficulties. It made her feel that she may be burdening an already troubled therapist with her problems. The husband felt threatened that the therapist might be biased in favor of divorce (he was hoping to prevent a divorce), and that the therapist and wife would form an alliance against him. In this example, it seems that the therapist's self-disclosures were motivated by personal needs rather than by a clear sense of correct therapeutic strategy.

To conclude, then, countertransference reactions in family therapy pose unique and complex challenges. The arousal of intense feelings in the therapist should not be reduced simply to his/her unresolved problems. A more productive approach is to explore the possibility that such reactions reflect the feelings of the family. This can result in viewing countertransference as a possible source of significant data about difficulties in the family system. Personal reactions of the therapist should not be freely shared with families, unless it is clear that such expression has therapeutic justification.

References

Eidelberg, L. *Encyclopedia of Psychoanalysis.* New York: The Free Press, 1968.
Greenson, R. R. *The Technique and Practice of Psychoanalysis.* Volume I. New York: International Universities Press, 1968.
Stierlin, H. *Psychoanalysis and Family Therapy.* New York: Jason Aronson, 1977.

RODNEY J. SHAPIRO, Ph.D.
Associate Professor
Director, Family and Marriage Clinic
Department of Psychiatry
University of Rochester Medical School
Rochester, NY

43. Paradoxical Strategies and Countertransference

Question:

The clinical practicum in family therapy that I teach in a graduate school program is eclectic with an action-oriented, psychodynamic flavor. Over the last couple of years, as paradoxical techniques (e.g., prescribing the symptom) have become more popularized, I find a number of our trainees using them. I have no objection in principle to these approaches, but I find that trainees often use them when they feel cornered, locked out, frustrated or angry at families. How can I help my trainees use these paradoxical interventions *for* the family instead of *against* it? A related question is: When, aside from moments of the therapist's own anxiety, are paradoxical approaches *not* indicated?

Discussion:

Quite naturally, along with the increased interest in the use of paradox in family therapy comes increased confusion, as it is a complicated technique that requires skill and practice in its application.

In the Brief Therapy Project of the Ackerman Institute for Family Therapy we have been experimenting with paradoxical interventions over the past five years and have developed a certain criterion for their use. This criterion is based on our evaluation of family flexibility and motivation. If motivation is high enough and resistance low enough for a family to respond to direct interventions, such as logical explanations, suggestions or tasks, there is no need to resort to a paradox. Also there are certain crisis situations, such as violence, sudden grief, attempted suicide, incest or child abuse, in which a paradox would be inappropriate, as the therapist needs to move in quickly to provide structure and control. We reserve paradoxical interventions for interrupting long-standing, rigid, repetitious patterns of interaction which do not respond to a logical approach. A paradox can then be used as a weapon against resistance and to change the relationship between the family and the therapist. It should not be used unless the therapist understands the meaning of the symptom in the family and prescribes it in a way which *changes the functioning of the system.*

One prevalent mistaken notion is that simply prescribing the symptom is therapeutic. The symptom must be prescribed in a particular way and under particular circumstances to have any benefit. If it is scheduled, it should be scheduled at a designated time and place, with a designated member of the family. For example, in a case in which the presenting problem was persistent headaches in a nine-year-old daughter, the therapist, Olga Silverstein, defined the headaches as "worry headaches" and decided they were brought on by the child's need to help her mother worry about all the family problems, because her father refused to worry. The child's worry was spilling over into school time and interfering with her studying. She was instructed by the therapist to worry for half an hour every morning before school, so she wouldn't need to take time from her school work to do this. Her father was instructed to help her worry so she wouldn't feel alone. They were not to tell mother what they had worried about. This served the purpose of realigning the family and diffusing the relationship between mother and daughter, forming a closer relationship between father and daughter, and involving father in the family concerns without pressure from mother, to which he had become allergic. Merely prescribing the headaches without connecting them with the family system would have been of dubious value.

Another common misconception arises around the use of what we in the Brief Therapy Project refer to as a "systemic paradox." This is one in which the symptom is connoted positively, defined as serving an essential function in the family system, and prescribed along with the system. Beginning therapists often prescribe the behavior of various family members without connecting them. This *connection* between the symptom and the system is crucial. For example, in a family in which the son, Billy, was failing in school, the therapist connected his failure with a subverted conflict between mother and father over father's lack of ambition and failure in business. Turning to Billy, this therapist told him that for the time being it was important for him to protect father from mother's disappointment by keeping her disappointment focused on him. Otherwise, mother might begin to nag father and he might become depressed and withdraw. Since Billy was younger and more resilient, he could take mother's disappointment better than father and should continue to do so. The therapist thus defined the system which maintained the symptom, defined the *connection* between the two, and prescribed both. The formulation of a systemic paradox must be both accurate and at the same time unacceptable to the family. It was accurate to say that mother nagged Billy when she was disappointed in father, but defined and prescribed in this way it was also unacceptable to the family. The therapist had confronted them with the demands of their own emotional system.

A common error made by beginners in attempting this kind of paradoxical intervention is in simply prescribing the symptomatic behavior of the identified patient, such as "Billy, you should continue to keep mother's disappointment focused on you." This is meaningless and confusing. Another frequent error is in prescribing each individual family member's behavior separately, such as, "Billy, you should continue to keep mother's disappointment focused on you; mother, you should continue to nag Billy; and father, you should continue to withdraw." This lacks therapeutic impact, as here again the symptom is not connected with the system in a circular definition. The power of this type of paradox lies in the reason *why* each person should continue his/her behavior, as the reason why contains a definition of the symptom-producing cycle. Once this cycle has been exposed, the family finds it difficult to continue it in the same way.

PEGGY PAPP, M.S.W.
Co-Director, Brief Therapy Project
Ackerman Institute for
Family Therapy
New York, NY

44. Sexism in Family Therapy

Question:

Most family therapists seem to publicly endorse values (e.g., about marriage and family life) that are quite consistent with feminist ideas. Still, we're all human, and all products of the same culture. So, I wonder if someone could suggest some concrete "signs" for family therapists to look for in themselves to help make them aware of ways in which they may be communicating sexist values without intending to do so.

Discussion:

While family and marital therapists may publicly avow support for feminist ideals, such as equality for women and men, at the same time they may hold beliefs about the rightness (desirability) of traditional family roles and behave in ways that communicate sexism to clients and colleagues. As in other areas, therapists can become aware of and sensitive to signs in themselves of these pervasive biases by examining their knowledge, behavior and attitudes toward women. Here are a few questions therapists can ask themselves.

Knowledge. It is now recognized that much of the data that inform our theories of behavior and of therapy is based on past psychological studies which used only men as subjects or used subjects with sex unspecified. Therapists who are biased against women have been found to be misinformed or uninformed. Out-of-date or biased findings persist with the tenacity of myth. For example, recent controlled studies have found no evidence that depression in women is associated with menopause more than any other period in the life span. Yet textbooks as well as therapists continue to talk about menopausal depression and use it to explain behavior.

As a family and marital therapist, are you aware that a higher proportion of married women are depressed than single women or married men? Do you question why marriage is associated with depression in women? Have you read a book reviewing recent research on the psychology of women in the last couple of years? Do you believe that therapists working with women should have knowledge of the psychology of women?

Behavior. One sign of whether a therapist treats members of both sexes in the same way is the use of language. The English language may not be inherently sexist, but the speaker who does not make use of nonsexist options is. If you think you are using "man" or "he" to refer to all human beings, consider the following familiar logical examples:

All men are mortal.
Socrates is a man.
Therefore, Socrates is mortal.

If your assumption about the universal use of "man" is correct, then the following should also be appropriate:

All men are mortal.
Sylvia is a man.
Therefore, Sylvia is mortal.

The absurdity makes apparent that "man" is not a neutral term but refers to males, as is often the case. Similarly, those arguing that "he" refers to both males and females are not persuasive in claiming that "the secretary, he . . ." "the nurse, he . . ." imply both male or female persons.

Use of first names or diminutives with a woman when a man is not similarly addressed is a sign of sex bias. Do you use pejorative labels like "frigid" for a woman rather than inquiring about how much and what kind of sexual stimulation she receives?

Nonverbal beaviors also can reveal differential treatment of men and women. We tend to look at people we consider more important. Who do you look at most when talking? Research on nonverbal behavior shows that women are treated and behave as inferiors. Do you interrupt women more than men? Do you show more impatience when a woman is talking than a man?

Do you ask both women and men what they do? It is not unusual for the man to be asked what he does and for the woman to be asked what her husband does. Her work is often regarded as less important. Do you regard housework as fulfilling when you do not regard yardwork as fulfilling? Do you talk in a rational mode to the man and about feelings to the woman?

Do you comment on her appearance but not on his, reinforcing the idea that she, but not he, should make herself attractive for others? Do you suggest it would help if she made herself more attractive, but not he? Ageism and sexism are closely associated because in our society middle-age women are regarded as less attractive and interesting than middle-age men. If you describe a woman as "the sprightly grandmother of three" would you also describe a man as "the balding grandfather of three"?

Therapists may have to deal from time to time with criticism and questions from clients. Do you treat her challenges as more unreasonable, emotional or a consequence of limited ability to understand, but not his? Which do you answer more fully? The therapist's response can suggest who is entitled to ask questions and who is regarded as an equal of the therapist.

If you do cotherapy, do you model traditional forms of inequality based on the male therapist's having more experience, training, status or advanced degrees than the female therapist? This is a powerful message despite what may happen in the interaction. Who is the "co" in cotherapy?

Attitudes. Attitudes that communicate sexist values may be less obvious than behavior or lack of up-to-date knowledge and, therefore, be harder to identify and confront honestly. Do you typically regard either the woman or the man as the victim? Do you find yourself thinking, "What has this woman done to this man?" Therapists have been found to consider the woman in the family more at fault in causing problems.

What are your attitudes toward appropriate behavior for children in the family? Do you catch yourself thinking, "Boys will be boys?" Do you think it's nice for girls to help around the kitchen, but not for boys? Do you think boys should have more freedom than girls, be allowed out later, be less accountable?

Do you take a protective stance toward the woman, encouraging her dependency, but not the man's? Do you regard her as having too much power in the family or marriage, but not him? Since men typically have power and status in the society at large, therapists should be cautious about rushing to "restore" the power to the man, thus lowering the woman's self-esteem and limited authority. Do you believe that if he supports her, he has a right to tell her what to do, to have sex when he wants, to expect her to run the house to meet his needs?

A common assumption shared by many therapists is that, if they are persons of good will who have had conventional training, they are capable of treating women in an unbiased way. However, since sexism is so pervasive in our society, such bias usually goes unrecognized and unacknowledged. The questions suggested here are just a sample of those that a therapist who is concerned with changing might want to ask him- or herself. They provide a one-way mirror for self-analysis for those willing to look.

RACHEL T. HARE-MUSTIN, Ph.D.
Director
Community Counseling Program
Villanova University
Villanova, PA

SECTION IV

Treatment of
Severe Disorders

45. Family Therapy Goals in Short-Term Inpatient Hospitals

Question:

Most family therapy literature has been written by therapists who work with outpatients. However, family therapy is increasingly becoming a standard part of inpatient hospital treatment. In such a setting, the context in which the family therapy is conducted has a major impact in defining the nature of the therapy. How is family therapy in an inpatient setting different from family therapy in an outpatient setting? What goals are appropriate for family therapy on an inpatient unit? How must these goals be further modified if the therapy takes place on a short-term (less than 30 days) inpatient unit?

Discussion:

Table 1 shows many of the ways in which inpatient family therapy is different, because of the constraints produced by the context of hospitalization. These differences require that inpatient family therapy be viewed as a specialty in its own right (Anderson, 1977; Boyd, 1979; Fleck et al., 1957; Harbin, 1978; Tangari, 1974).

The fact that the patient has been admitted to a hospital must be considered the fundamental issue around which family therapy must be organized. The therapist must keep foremost in his or her mind the questions, Why is this person in the hospital? How can family therapy illuminate or alter the conditions that led to hospitalization? What is the impact of hospitalization on the family? How is the family relating to the hospital staff, and vice versa? And how can we arrange for the patient to leave the hospital, to rejoin, or to live apart from the family?

The reason any patient is admitted to a hospital is unique; however, in general people end up in a psychiatric hospital for one of the following reasons: 1) the risk of suicide or homicide; 2) a destructive interaction between the patient and family or other people; 3) the need

TABLE 1

Differences Between Inpatient and Outpatient Family Therapy

Inpatient	Outpatient
Treatment is usually time-limited, often between 2 and 12 weeks.	Treatment is not necessarily time-limited. This allows more extensive therapeutic goals to be realistically pursued.
The hospital has officially labeled one person as the "identified patient." This makes it harder to relabel the whole family as the problem.	If the therapist disagrees with the family's assignment of one person as the "identified patient," he/she may relabel the whole family as the problem.
The patient must still be treated even if some family members refuse to come in for family therapy sessions. The therapist must decide whether or not to work with those family members who are available.	The family therapist may coerce all members of the household into attending family therapy sessions by threatening to refuse to see the patient or anyone else unless the entire family participates.
The identified patient is usually psychotic or a severely disturbed borderline patient. The family is often extremely pathological, functioning at a low level of differentiation. Often the family is fragmented—either there is no family at all, a one-parent family, etc.	The identified patient is often healthier, and the family is often more differentiated and intact than is true of inpatient therapy families.
Since the patient is removed from the family, the family can temporarily ignore the conflict that the patient stirs up. They can claim that things are tranquil now.	The patient remains in the family as a potential irritant and focus of conflict.
Family therapy is one of a multitude of different forms of treatment. The different therapists must be in communication with one another. Family therapy must be coordinated with group therapy, individual therapy, medication, milieu, etc.	Family therapy is usually the sole modality of treatment.

for evaluation and diagnosis; or 4) the need for treatment. For each of these reasons, family therapy can significantly contribute to understanding the situation and producing therapeutic change.

1) *Risk of suicide or homicide.* To understand this problem, the family therapist must assess the extent of family collusion to encourage or provoke the patient to commit suicide or homicide. It is also important to help the family deal with the anxiety, fear, anger and guilt stirred up by these acts.

2) *A destructive interaction between the patient and family.* The fact that the patient has been removed from the family and placed in a hospital automatically places some limits and restraints on the patient's destructive influence on the family, and vice versa. Hospitalization represents a psychosocial moratorium. However, the therapist must be very sensitive to some common dangers: The family may feel guilty or stigmatized by the hospitalization, or they may feel that the patient and/or the hospital staff is seeking to blame the family for the crisis that led up to hospitalization. These problems can easily lead to the family's withdrawing and becoming unavailable for family therapy. The therapist must address these problems gingerly and adroitly. The family therapist also may need to confront other staff members about the way in which they mistreat the families of patients (Anderson, 1977; Appleton, 1974; Fleck et al., 1957).

3) *The need for evaluation and diagnosis.* The family is an invaluable source of information about a patient's present illness and developmental history. Assessment of the family structure also reveals the way in which the family might be affecting the patient, and in which the patient's illness has been affecting the family. Much of the assessment of families in an inpatient setting is the same as the assessment in an outpatient setting and involves issues such as generational boundaries, triangular alliances, bizarre communication patterns, etc. But since a psychiatric inpatient is usually significantly impaired, the therapist must assess how realistic the family is about that impairment. For example, a young schizophrenic may be admitted to the hospital floridly psychotic, yet the parents believe that they have a normal child.

4) *The need for treatment.* The therapeutic approach to families is much the same for inpatient family therapy as for outpatient family therapy. It involves restructuring, detriangulating, clarifying boundaries, etc.—the types of maneuvers which are well known from the family therapy literature.

Short-term Hospitals

So far, we have been addressing the special qualities of family therapy on any inpatient floor. However, family therapy on a short-term (less than 30 days) hospital unit is somewhat different from family therapy on longer term units. This difference is important to emphasize because there are more and more short-term hospital units. Furthermore, there are reasons to anticipate that the trend toward brief hospitalization will continue, both because of financial reasons (hospital cost containment) and because the best available research has shown that hospitalization of less than 30 days is as effective as three-month hospitalization (Glick et al., 1976 and 1977; Herz et al., 1977 and 1979). There have been more than 18 studies comparing short-term hospitalization to longer hospitalization, and they have all reached the conclusion that longer hospitalization offers no advantages (President's Commission on Mental Health, 1978). Patients in a short-term hospital get better faster than do patients in a hospital for two to four months.

On a short-term unit family therapy must accommodate to an extremely time-limited framework. On some hospital units the average length of stay is seven to 10 days. This sort of time-limited treatment is less personally satisfying for the therapist, who often feels that he or she hardly has time to get to know the family before the patient is discharged, and certainly does not have time to alter the structure of the family. What is clear with these short-term units is that definitive treatment is not going to be provided inside the hospital, because there simply isn't time. A corollary is that outpatient therapy assumes much more significance. Indeed, the primary task of inpatient family therapy in a short-term hospital unit should be to assess the need for outpatient family therapy and make an appropriate referral to an outpatient family therapist, recognizing that definitive treatment will occur in the outpatient setting.

While this sounds very logical and straightforward, it is very difficult in actual clinical practice. The author's experience is that there is a wide gulf separating inpatient units from outpatient clinics. Usually inpatient therapists do not facilitate a smooth or rapid transition to outpatient therapy; and in outpatient departments it is often a month or two before a patient discharged from the hospital is picked up for treatment. Although there is usually poor communication and poor coordination between inpatient and outpatient services, the needs of families dictate a much closer working alliance. This is especially true when a patient is discharged after a brief hospital stay, but the crisis in the family is still volatile.

One of the main tasks for a family therapist on a short-term inpatient unit is to decide, in collaboration with the rest of the staff, what form of outpatient therapy is most appropriate for a given patient and family. One particular group of patients for whom family therapy is always the outpatient treatment of choice are those schizophrenics who have families that express a lot of intense negative feelings about the patient. Research in Britain has shown that schizophrenics who return to live among relatives who are highly emotionally involved with them are much more likely to suffer a relapse of florid psychotic symptoms than are schizophrenics who return to live among families with less expressed emotion (Brown et al., 1972).

If the decision is that family therapy is the outpatient treatment of choice, the therapist must cultivate and prepare the family for this referral. The outpatient family therapist should meet with the family one or two times *before* the patient is discharged. Without such preparatory work, there is a strong likelihood that the family will drop out of sight as soon as the patient has been discharged, and will never come to the first outpatient therapy meeting. It is also imperative that the inpatient family therapist communicate with the outpatient family therapist about the nature of the patient's illness and the family's problems.

References

Anderson, C. M. Family intervention with severely disturbed inpatients. *Arch. Gen. Psychiatry*, 1977, 34, 697-702.

Appleton, W. S. Mistreatment of patients' families by psychiatrists. *Amer. J. Psychiatry*, 1974, 131: 655-657.

Boyd, J. H. The interaction of family therapy and psychodynamic individual therapy in an inpatient setting. *Psychiatry*, 1979, 42: 99-111.

Brown, G. W., Birley, J. L. T., and Wing, J. K. Influence of family life on the course of schizophrenic disorders: A replication. *Brit. J. Psychiat.*, 1972, 121: 241-258.

Fleck, S., Cornelison, A. R., Norton, N. and Lidz, T. Interaction between hospital staff and families. *Psychiatry*, 1957, 20: 343-350.

Glick, I. D., Hargreaves, W. A., Drues, J., and Showstack, J. A. Short versus long hospitalization: A prospective controlled study. IV. One-year follow-up results for schizophrenic patients. *Amer. J. Psychiatry*, 1976, 133: 509-514.

Glick, I. D., Hargreaves, W. A., Drues, J., Showstack, J. A., and Katzow, J. J. Short vs. long hospitalization: A prospective controlled study: VII. Two-year follow-up results for nonschizophrenics. *Arch. Gen. Psychiatry*, 1977, 34: 314-317.

Harbin, H. T. Families and hospitals: Collusion or cooperation? *Amer. J. Psychiatry*, 1978, 135: 1496-1499.

Herz, M. I., Endicott, J., and Gibbon, M. Brief hospitalization. *Arch. Gen. Psychiatry*, 1979, 36: 701-712.

Herz, M. I., Endicott, J. and Spitzer, R. L. Brief hospitalization. *Amer. J. Psychiatry*, 1977, 134: 502-507.

President's Commission on Mental Health. Research panel report. Volume IV, *Task*

Panel Reports Submitted to the President's Commission on Mental Health Washington, D.C.: Government Printing Office, 1978, p. 1765.
Tangari, A. Family involvement in the treatment of a psychiatric inpatient. *Hosp. and Community Psychiatry*, 1974, 25: 792-794.

JEFFREY H. BOYD, M.D.
Department of Psychiatry
Yale University-
Connecticut Mental Health Center
New Haven, CT

46. Using Family Therapy to Plan for Discharge of a Hospitalized Family Member

Question:

I work on an inpatient unit and think it important to do therapy with the families of the patients that are hospitalized. Whenever I attempt family therapy, however, I inevitably experience a great deal of difficulty in a variety of forms. In particular, the problems being presented by the family often become diffuse and are hard to focus on, or the family continues to stay organized around the identified patient. Would you please describe some of the ways I might become more effective in working with families who have a member hospitalized?

Discussion:

The problem you describe is frequently encountered by those who attempt to treat families with a hospitalized member. It is complex because these families are complex and, perhaps more importantly, because inpatient units are also complex.

The reaction of the family to the hospitalization itself is almost always one of relief, particularly if the identified patient has been disruptive. In terms of theory, we might say that the identified patient's behavior is related to the distress in the family itself. As the distress increases, the patient acts, causing the family to focus on that disruption. This shift, in consequence, lowers the level of distress among other family members. Hospitalization can thus be regarded as the ritualization of distress relieving maneuvres, resulting in the family stabilizing around the disturbance of the identified patient. One way of maintaining this stability is, of course, by avoiding other issues, making them diffuse or focusing on the identified patient. The idea of stabilization seems viable, particularly when the identified patient occupies a position which is either psychologically or functionally critical to the stability of the family over time.

In some families, however, the hospitalized patient is not critical to stability, but is being extruded as a peripheral part. The family organizes around the disturbance and the hospitalization in a way that enforces the extrusion. You may see this happening with some families with an elderly member, particularly when the patient is the mother or father of the peripheral parent in an over-involved parent-child, two generation family. Patients with repeated hospitalization in the public system may also be extruded. The strength of the extrusion in the family seems to be related to the number of hospitalizations the patient has had and to the ability of the patient to maintain employment. At times, it seems that the patient is a residual of a system that has changed from one organized around the patient's symptoms in bygone times, to one which has reorganized differently and must now deal with the patient as an aftereffect.

In working with the extruding family, you can sometimes get improvement by shifting the goal from reorganizing the family to include the patient to the goal of building a linkage between the patient and one or two family members. In doing so, the task is to normalize the functioning of the patient as well as possible, and then work toward connecting the patient and family members in a noncaretaker away.

While family types may result in some of the problems you describe, a more critical factor may be the professional context of the inpatient unit itself. Inpatient units frequently fall into the same mold since they must meet standards for accreditation. These influence not only the physical facilities of the unit but also the number and kinds of staff that work there, and the procedures that must be followed for admission, medication, records, and the like.

Most often, the procedures and staff interact to produce a context that is likely to defeat family therapy. Admitting the patient to the unit validates the position of the patient as patient and creates an almost impossible problem for the therapist who tries to redefine the problem as a family one. Reality is on the side of the family. Compound this problem with medication and other unit procedures and treatment will encounter difficulty. In particular, attempts to define or redefine the problem will be counteracted by a continued or heightened focus on the patient. Some interventions into interactions between the patient and other family members require continuity if they are to be effective. The possibility for continuity is decreased when the family goes home after a session and the patient stays on the unit.

One of the greatest hindrances to treating the family is the massive overlap among all of the treatments the hospitalized patient experiences. These may include, for example, individual therapy, chemotherapy, group therapy, and so on. On top of these, you may add the overwhelming number of staff, all of whom interact with the patient around the way he or she "should" be. Treating the family frequently becomes simply "another" therapy that is likely to conflict with other therapies, since the unit of treatment is not the patient but the family.

Those doing family therapy ordinarily expect change to occur and recognize that such change will frequently be accompanied by increased disturbance in the patient. Inducing such disturbance, however, directly counteracts the covert format of the unit, that is, stabilizing the patient. The emphasis is more or less on returning the patient to a condition of stability which is assumed to have existed before hospitalization. The move is backwards and is based on the idea of removing or cancelling out the forces leading to hospitalization. In contrast, the better direction may be forward and through the problem, not backward and away from it. If you try the progression strategy, you will likely cause the patient to become disruptive in some way which, in turn, will disturb the staff. It is likely that they will see you as different and may exert pressure on you to stop "upsetting" patients. At worse, they will label you as harmful to patients and extrude *you*.

There is an alternative way of working which leads to less frustration and which may do the family more good. It is best applied to nonextruding families. Rather than use family sessions to attempt change, you use them to plan discharge. The thrust of these meetings is to organize the family around the task facing it when the patient leaves the hospital. The tendency of the family may be to draw you into a discussion of symptoms or history. Although you may spend time on these as a matter of courtesy, the continued focus should be on the issues of what will happen after discharge. The sessions may take on the format of contingency planning and appear at times to the outsider as rather dull and boring. What you hope to achieve, however, is the bonding of the patient to the family, and a counteracting of the process of marking the patient as patient. The latter becomes feasible, particularly if focus is given to the types of problems the family members expect to have with the patient at discharge. As these emerge, you get an accurate picture of the interpersonal processes within the family and the interplay of forces which are being balanced by the patient's symptomatology.

Focusing on the issues of the patient's reentry into the family counteracts the tendency to diffuse issues as well as the tendency to stabilize around the patient's symptomatology. In order to maximize these results, it is important to follow-up with outpatient treatment, which may be done by return visits to the unit after discharge, or through some other facility.

ROSS E. CARTER, Ph.D.
Director, Family Center
Columbia Hospital
Milwaukee, WI

47. Family Therapy After Psychiatric Hospitalization

Question:

A number of problems frequently surface when a hospitalized identified patient and family have been in family therapy and discharge is imminent. Questions arise: Who should conduct the family therapy, the person who began it in the hospital or another therapist in the community? If the identified patient will be in individual psychotherapy and/or pharmacotherapy, what should the relationship be between the individual therapist and the family therapist? Should it be the same person? What happens to the therapeutic arrangement in the community if the identified patient requires rehospitalization? Who is in charge? Are the goals of the inpatient family therapy different from that of the outpatient family therapy, and if so how can the transition best be handled? In what clinical situation is family therapy most useful? What clinical situations suggest a relative contraindication to family therapy?

Discussion:

I conceptualize work with families in connection with an identified patient's hospitalization in three categories: 1) diagnostic, 2) counseling, 3) therapy. Diagnostic inpatient family meetings with the patient present are much easier to arrange than outpatient family meetings, either because the family is genuinely concerned about their hospitalized relative's welfare, or has been frightened and intimidated by the patient's destructive behavior. The family is eager to cooperate in the hope that the patient will be discharged sooner, perhaps to satisfy the family's need to have the identified patient back in the family system to play the "sick role" and maintain a pathological homeostasis. Or, perhaps the family may be responding to the ever climbing costs of hospitalization. These factors give the hospital family therapy a unique leverage to aid in involving resistant families, at minimum for one to several sessions to "help in better understanding the patient."

Given the painful family crises that often precede hospitalization, and the obvious disturbance of the identified patient, the family may be open at this time to suggestions of family meetings of a counseling nature (i.e., no contract for reflection or marked change in behavior by family members). The model of these meetings can be similar to that of the neurologist counseling a family who has an epileptic member, or a child guidance format. This is not usually experienced as threatening or intrusive by the family members because they save face in the fact that the identified patient is indeed very troubled and the focus of the family counseling sessions remains on the identified patient.

If, in the course of the diagnostic and/or counseling sessions, the inpatient therapist notes family phenomena that reinforce the identified patient's problems and/or discourage the identified patient's growth and separation, the therapist can tactfully point this out to the family members and gradually suggest, over at least three or more meetings, a contract for family therapy.

With regard to the question of whether the family therapy should begin in the hospital or wait until the patient's discharge, I find the following guidelines to be useful. If it is likely that the identified patient will require repeated hospitalizations—e.g., 1) a patient with rapid cycling bipolar illness who refuses lithium or other pharmacotherapy; 2) an identified patient who makes frequent serious suicide attempts; 3) an adolescent with one or several addictions (alcohol, opiates, etc.) who frequently endangers his/her or others' lives while intoxicated—the inpatient family therapist should continue the outpatient family therapy.

The individual therapist might best be involved in the family therapy in the following clinical situations: 1) when confrontation and reality testing are an important part of the individual therapy, as in people who are sociopathic, addicted, impulsive or infantile personalities, and 2) certain paranoid patients. The family meetings give the individual therapist valuable observations to counter the manipulative and/or psychotic distortions of the identified patient.

If it is decided that an out-of-hospital family therapist will conduct the family therapy, it is very useful to have at least two or three sessions in his/her office before the patient is discharged. This soothes the often intense termination anxieties around discharge and gives both therapists an opportunity to share observations that each can use in responding to the family's attempt to do any of the following: 1) split the therapists (he/she is a better therapist than you); 2) distort the communication of each therapist; or 3) pretend that all the family's problems were solved by the hospitalization. In consultation with each other, the two therapists can help the family distinguish the short-term goals of the inpatient family meetings (e.g., defining transactional problems) from that of the long-term outpatient family work.

The therapist-to-therapist liaison involves a good deal of professional time, and even more so if one or two individual therapists are also involved. But this effort avoids the serious dangers of the family's blocking the transition from inpatient to outpatient work, splitting or denying the need for further family work.

Continued family work is strongly indicated when the identified patient is living at home, in frequent contact with the family, and/or is financially dependent on them. An adolescent who is in the process of separating from the family might best attend the family meetings only occasionally, while investing his/her major therapeutic energies in individual psychotherapy and peer group therapy. Other relative contraindications to inpatient family meetings are when the identified patient is manic-paranoid, paranoid-schizophrenic, or has active homicidal impulses toward family members.

On occasion, in spite of the inpatient family work, the family may close ranks while the patient is in the hospital and impede his/her return to the family home. This possibility can be clarified by having the patient visit home prior to discharge and bringing this issue for discussion to the family meetings in the hospital.

If the patient requires rehospitalization, it is helpful for continuity's sake, and again to avoid splitting, to have the outpatient family therapist continue to meet with the family along with the inpatient family therapist, the two serving as cotherapists.

NORMAN I. MOSS, M.D.
Department of Psychiatry
Beth Israel Hospital-
Harvard Medical School
Boston, MA

48. Resistance to Change in Families with a Schizophrenic Member

Question:

I have been working with schizophrenic patients for many years and have experienced difficulties engaging families in therapy. I have often had trouble avoiding entanglement with the family's paradoxical logic: While asking me to help, they prevent all my attempts to help them change. I have often wondered whether it might be "provocative" behavior directed to test my ability to get in touch with their pain without exposing them to another failure. How can the therapist break the family's defensive barrier and activate real change for the patient as well as for the other members of the family?

Discussion:

Requests for therapy by families with a schizophrenic member are usually made in moments of crisis, when the system perceives a threat to its equilibrium. The fear of uncontrollable variations in the status quo coexists with a long-standing desire for change. However, although real change is desired, it is opposed by all of the family members because it seems too dangerous.

The family therefore enters therapy with the expectation that the therapist will help them to reconsolidate the system's previous equilibrium. "Basically, the family wants the therapist to perform an impossible task: to help them *to change a situation while adhering to the same rules of interaction that previously served to maintain the existing situation*" (Andolfi et al., 1980). Clinical experience has shown that these contradictory expectations on the part of the family often create a situation in which the therapist attempts to cure a family group whose members unite to demonstrate the futility of these efforts. "As a result, a rigid therapeutic system is formed, and family-therapist interactions tend to crystalize in increasingly static and predictable roles and functions" (Andolfi, 1980).

All differences and conflicts among the members of these families are disguised by the one issue on which they unanimously agree: that the sick member, the only one who needs treatment, is the identified patient. Being considered crazy, the identified patient is not conceded the right to make decisions, nor does he/she claim this right. In the sessions the identified patient's behavior tends to reinforce three basic characteristics of all family transactions: 1) the patient's symptomatology is of central importance to the system, apparently filling the family's entire world; 2) all of the patient's communications (even those that are fully appropriate) are denied any validity; 3) consequently, all efforts made by the family or by outsiders to modify the patient's behavior are doomed to failure.

The family's request, which is based on these premises, can be formulated as: "Help us to cure him by telling us what to do to make him normal." If the therapist fails to see the incongruity between the request for treatment and the more or less explicit definition of the patient's disturbance as incurable, any moves tried will prove ineffectual. The therapist will inevitably become trapped in the homeostatic mechanisms that have so effectively maintained the identified patient in the passive yet central role as the crazy member of the family.

How can a person unanimously considered incurable possibly be cured? If the therapist ignores the paradoxical message transmitted by the family system and openly accepts a therapeutic role, the question of the patient's curability will eventually become a battleground between the family and the therapist. On the one hand, the therapist will try to force the system to effectuate real changes; on the other hand, the family members will engage in a collective campaign to demonstrate its own good intentions and the failure of the therapist. The identified patient will be completely excluded from the whole process, and his/her inadequacy will thus be reconfirmed once more.

The approach I developed in the last six years at the Family Therapy Institute in Rome consists in considering the message transmitted by the family as a *provocation* and trying to formulate a therapeutic strategy that constitutes a *response* to this message.

This strategy is based on "a model of *relative contrasts*, set in stages, which addresses the interplay between the two major components of a therapeutic system—on the one hand the family, and on the other hand the therapist. Within each component there is a balance between the tendency to espouse homeostasis ('remaining the same') and the ability or tendency to transform, i.e., to change. The therapist modulates the extent to which he/she advocates or pushes for homeostatic behavior by the family in accordance with a) the homeostatic leaning of the family at the moment, and b) the particular stage to which the therapy has progressed" (Stanton, 1981).

To the family message, "Help us, even if it is impossible," the therapist responds with a counter provocation, "Yes, I will help you by not helping you." In this first phase of therapy, the therapist attacks the system by depriving the identified patient of the power to control family relationship by behaving "crazily." By redefining this behavior as logical and voluntary, and by supporting the identified patient's function as the acknowledged, indispensable and irreplaceable leader of the family (no other member could perform this function as well), the therapist destroys the family's rationale for playing its usual transactional game of maintaining a scapegoat so that the members can avoid open conflict.

The therapist's *counterprovocation* serves a twofold purpose: It divests the identified patient of the power to control the family, and it reevaluates him/her as a person capable of autonomous behavior. In other words, the therapist simultaneously *attacks the patient at the level of function and supports him/her at the level of self*. The patient will be able to accept the provocation if encouraged and supported in the desire to present him- or herself to the family in a more authentic way.

By redefining the patient's "crazy" behavior, the therapist also warns the family that any modification of the present situation would jeopardize the family's hard-won equilibrium. The therapist, through such a position, denies the utility of therapy (implicitly denying also his/her own role as an agent of change), thereby challenging the system, since *the therapist's* investment in the homeostasis appears greater than *the family's*. The therapist becomes more rigid, allowing, by contrast, the family to become more flexible.

As the behavior of the identified patient improves in the sessions, therapy enters the "strategically unacknowledged improvement" stage. In our experience we have noticed that severely dysfunctional families cannot easily accept individuation on the part of the identified patient, so they deny this improvement. The task of the therapist is to deny the positive change before they do, in order to reinforce it. Accordingly, the therapist persists in the strategy of provocation by instructing the family to maintain the status quo—just at the time when changes are beginning to occur. The therapist justifies this position by pointing out the potential risks inherent in these changes. Once again, the therapist attacks the system through the identified patient, this time on the question of improvement.

The therapeutic strategy is actuated in three successive moves:

1) *refusal to recognize any improvement*—the therapist behaves as if totally unaware of the first signs of improvement;
2) *redefinition of improvement as dangerous*—the therapist warns the family of the risks involved in change, thereby activating the family's own worst fantasies and fears. When the members are helped to envisage possible modifications of the system, change begins to appear less menacing. This actually encourages the process of change that is already taking place;
3) *prescription to not change*—the therapist prescribes behaviors intended to accentuate the system's dysfunctional rules (Andolfi, 1979; Selvini-Palazzoli et al., 1978), presenting the prescription as a necessary precaution to avoid change. This paradoxically supports the improvement taking place and creates a new sense of cohesion among the family members. The family must now struggle to demonstrate that it *is* capable of changing.

In the "restructuring" stage, the family begins to disagree with the therapist, stating that in reality things are improving. The therapist again challenges them, building up stress by repeatedly emphasizing that the family has not changed or *should* not change. The therapist claims not to trust them, exhorting them to "show me," cautioning them to "be careful," or claiming they are "crazy." The family then can take delight in proving the therapist is wrong; they can become active in order to work against him/her.

In other words, the therapist pushes the family to demonstrate that the changes they claim have taken place actually lead to verifiable results. These changes are to be verified first in the sessions and then at home. In this way the movement toward change will be reinforced and the therapeutic process will be amplified beyond the sessions.

Once the family has become more flexible, we can apply a typically structural approach, promoting new interactions among and within the various subsystems. Toward the end of this stage, the IP will become less central. The family members will start to behave as a group of *people* rather than a massively reactive system.

The final stage is that of the "therapeutic system schism." Now there is a balance between homeostatic and transformational tendencies, both within the family and between the family and the therapist. The family notes that things have changed and that they are able to continue to progress. They assert that they can make it on their own; the therapist asks them to demonstrate how they will do this.

Pushing the family to separate, the therapist is able to disengage from the therapeutic system because he or she is not needed anymore.

References

Andolfi, M. *Family Therapy: An Interactional Approach*. New York: Plenum, 1979.

Andolfi, M. Prescribing the families' own dysfunctional rules as a therapeutic strategy. *Journal of Marriage and Family Therapy*, 1980, *6*, 29-36.

Andolfi, M., Menghi, P., Nicolo, A.M., and Saccu, C. Interaction in rigid systems: A model of intervention in families with a schizophrenic member. In M. Andolfi and I. Zwerling (Eds.), *Dimensions of Family Therapy*. New York: Guilford, 1980.

Selvini-Palazzoli, M., Boscolo, L., Cecchin, G. and Prata, G. *Paradox and Counterparadox*. New York: Aronson, 1978.

Stanton, D. Strategic Approaches to Family Therapy. In A. S. Gurman, and D. P. Kniskern (Eds.), *Handbook of Family Therapy*. New York: Brunner/Mazel, 1981.

MAURIZIO ANDOLFI, M.D.
Director
Family Therapy Institute
Rome, Italy

49. Breaking the Paranoid Closed System

Question:

At the clinic with which I am associated, there is a consensus as to the advantages of the therapeutic approach which enables treatment of the psychotic patient together with the family in the community, rather than in the hospital. To this purpose a comprehensive community-based treatment model has been designed which places primary emphasis on intervening in the family and social environment of the patient. Treatment objectives include work with the family to change or neutralize whatever pathological family relationship appears to contribute to and maintain the patient's problems. In a parallel way, a social support network is mobilized to help the patient remain involved in his or her natural living situation.

In applying this program we have encountered a concrete stumbling block with paranoid patients. It appears that, for a high rate of patients with paranoid delusions, both the family transactions and the relationships with the support system are centered to an exaggerated degree around repeated arguments over the question of the truth or falsehood of the patient's paranoid allegations. Indeed, very often I find myself also invited to participate in the argument and act as an arbitrator to determine the precise boundaries between reality and imagination. As a result of this situation, no small part of the therapy time is wasted on debates between the patient and between the family and the social support group about the paranoid theme.

Do you have a practical suggestion with respect to techniques of intervention which could turn aside this sort of debate and the impasse to the progress of therapy?

Discussion:

The problem which you describe is well-known and widespread. One of the reasons why paranoid patients are considered very defiant and resistant to treatment derives from their impelling need to demonstrate that their delusional beliefs are true. As a rule, paranoids do not benefit from the sincere efforts of relatives and friends to convince them of the absurdity of their allegations. On the contrary, the attempts to make them see a different reality may lead to an unfruitful pattern of repetitive allegations and counterallegations, as patients usually react with more obstinate and elaborate arguments to overcome their contenders. This closed reinforcement system is clearly observed in cases of persecutory delusions or paranoid jealousy, in which the superhuman attempts of the accused individuals to prove their innocence appear only to intensify the paranoid distrust and the search for confirmation of the paranoid claims.

Undoubtedly, the incessant preoccupation of the family members with the paranoid theme and the turning of the paranoid interlocking engagement into the dominant family content serve in actuality as a smoke screen meant to conceal other distressing problems within the family. In this sense, there is no real difference between the function filled by the delusional system and that of many other clinical symptoms in nonparanoid families. In general terms, one can say that for both paranoid and nonparanoid families the presenting symptom often serves as a defensive cover to prevent exposure of underlying family problems.

However, there is an essential pragmatic difference between families with a paranoid patient and other dysfunctional families, which is revealed in clinical practice by the great difficulty the family therapist encounters in loosening the paranoid entanglement and transferring the focus of treatment from the delusional arguments to the relevant problems within the family relationships. Paranoid patients apparently lack the skills and capacity to stop transmitting their fixed paranoid messages. Within the process of treatment the therapist is also drawn into participation in the closed system around the delusional arguments.

One of the main reasons for paranoid patients' compelling urge to prove the authenticity of their claims is that they are not only convinced of the veracity of their allegations but, in fact, *they are right* in that there is always some objective truth behind their paranoid thinking systems.

Recently, I examined my findings in a group of 34 paranoid patients who received family therapy at the Kibbutz Child and Family Clinic. It turned out that in all our cases the paranoid patient was essentially right; convincing evidence could be found to at least partially confirm the existence of clear connections between the paranoid premises and concrete facts and events in the patients' past and present objective experiences. The patients undoubtedly react to events relevant to their paranoid system with focused attention, distortion and misinterpretation, but by no means does this contradict the irrefutable fact of an objective basis to their claims. Therefore, a primary reason why most of these patients are openly resistant to stopping the controversy around the delusional issue is that they have good reasons to counterattack in response to any statement intended to prove that their delusional beliefs are imaginary and unrooted in reality.

As a characteristic and well-known example, it is worthwhile recalling the case of the German judge, Schreber, who spent many years of his life and exerted great efforts to prove in his autobiographical memoirs the truth of his paranoid ideas, which were analyzed by Freud. Not many years after Freud published his conclusions, numerous connections were found between the delusional persecutory threats perceived by Schreber and the sadistic techniques recommended by his father—a noted physician and an "expert in child-rearing methods," who was revealed in his writings as a paranoiac personality absorbed in designing punitive procedures and techniques to raise perfect children, who would be the foundation for a new race.

In Schreber's case, as in other cases of paranoid ideation, the delusions are obviously founded on real living experiences and become egosyntonic, undeniable truths, reinforced by repeated "logical" refutations of significant others. From this it follows that the method of frontal counterargumentation usually proves ineffective and may even increase the patient's mistrust and resistance.

Paradoxically, in not a few cases, I have managed to overcome the resistance to treatment when, instead of using counterarguments, I affirmed that there are indeed elements of justice and truth in the delusional beliefs and that they are not just a product of wild imagination. The next step is to agree on conditions of a therapeutic contract which includes, among other objectives, seeking an alternative way to influence the surroundings in order to achieve the basic goals the patient is striving for—acceptance, basic security and respect of significant others, instead of criticism, rejection and suspicion. I make it clear that, since the patient failed to achieve these positive goals by the means he or she had been using, a new plan of conduct, agreed upon by the family and the therapist, must be sought. A truce in the war of arguments and counterarguments concerning unanswerable paranoid claims and a joint effort to elaborate an alternative plan for the attainment of the agreed basic goals should be achieved in order to reduce the patient's resistance to cooperation in family therapy treatment.

For example, I avoid denying the credibility of the delusional system. I give full credence to patients' complaints that people have a negative opinion of them and assume that they might be right in their allegations. Actually, in a number of cases of this sort in the kibbutz setting, I tell patients in a sincere, friendly way that it is not surprising that in their present state—socially isolated, totally absorbed in the task of divulging their complaints, working at a low level of productivity—they have become eccentric and undesirable people in the kibbutz. I then propose to search together with the families for a different way to present their claims, to gain the respect of the people in their surroundings, and to change the current situation which causes them nothing but misery.

The therapist's skill is manifested in the capacity to stop the excessive attention and concentration of family members and significant others around the paranoid theme. The absorbing quality of the paranoid engagement can be mitigated by recognition of the patients' right to *think and feel* in complete freedom, without criticism and external limitations, while behaving in accordance with the rules of society and seeking a more acceptable and successful way of getting an "objective examination" of their claims. Thus, the patients raise their chances of both attaining their goals and utilizing their skills and capacities in a more satisfying way. Family members should be repeatedly prompted to accept this line of action and stop their unproductive arguments about the delusional theme.

Sometimes we suggest a compromise by passing the patient's charges for inquiry and clarification to an agreed upon objective person or to a professional who is expert in the area concerned and will consent to cooperate in such an "investigation." The patient is then requested to wait patiently until the authorized person finishes the job of systematically clarifying the matters.

In my experience, this simple arrangement can substantially lessen the strength of a patient's impulse to prove the truth of the paranoid thoughts at every possible opportunity. Thus, we may achieve the desired truce from the endless discussions and go on to treat other relevant problems in the course of family therapy. My impression is that the very fact that the patient meets for the first time a positive and sympathetic approach of readiness to help examine the veracity of his/her charges, becomes an important factor in soothing him/her and reducing resistance to treatment. Thus, what I try to do is to reach an acceptable contract in which it will be agreed that the paranoid arguments are certainly worthy of consideration and therefore given over for objective investigation to an authorized agent. In addition, all sides agree to seek and plan together other more enjoyable activities and occupations.

When necessary, I use other techniques to take the edge off the patient's impelling need to prove allegations. For example, I might suggest the family recognize the patient's right to raise the paranoid theme, but only on fixed and agreed upon occasions, and then within a time limit. During the time deliberately devoted to the paranoid subject, the family members are requested to listen patiently while expressing a positive relationship, e.g., by a handshake, a hug, a kiss, or an affectionate remark, yet with total avoidance of response to the specific subject. If the patient demands an answer or raises the subject at times which were not agreed upon, the members of the family should react in accordance with the terms of the contract by switching the conversation to some other subject, by attending to some other occupation, or even by leaving the room.

I see deemphasizing the centrality of the paranoid belief in the family as well as in the patient's daily life within the community as a primary task in the course of family therapy. Reducing the fuel the patient receives from the repetitive arguments around the single delusional theme usually leads to a parallel reduction of the impelling urge to deal with the delusional idea. It is in this manner that the way is paved for changing the paranoid subject to more constructive alternatives in the content of therapy as well as in the content of daily life.

MORDECAI KAFFMAN, M.D.
Medical Director
Kibbutz Child and Family Clinic
Tel Aviv, Israel

50. Treating Schizophrenic Families in a Community Mental Health Setting

Question:

How do you get around the roadblocks to change in schizophrenic families?

Discussion:

Family therapy evolved from observations about the interrelationship of the behavior of the schizophrenic family member and the "pathology" of the family group. The notion of an interlocking pathology stimulated new hope in the treatment of schizophrenia. Early family therapists imagined that by treating the family as a whole they could interrupt the collusive group process which enabled the overt pathology to be primarily manifested in one of its members.

However, family therapy for schizophrenic families, even in the hands of the most skilled, has not been particularly effective. In order to account for this frustrating situation, it was suggested that the therapist was simply being "out-maneuvered" by the family. A "war" metaphor emerged readily out of family systems theory. The Selvini-Palazzoli team in Italy designed a playful-combat treatment approach in order to fight back. With humor and paradox as their major artillery, and with troops of therapists flanked behind a one-way screen, they ingeniously maneuvered to outwit the family into getting better.

While these heroics illustrate refreshingly new therapeutic strategies and make good stories (see David and Goliath, James Bond movies, and Selvini-Palazzoli et al., 1978), they are neither practical nor widely applicable. The lot and challenge of the treatment of schizophrenia rests largely in the hands of community mental health centers. Alternative yet practical approaches need to be evolved. What follows is a description of how a multifamily group has been utilized with some success to overcome the roadblocks presented by one particular schizophrenic family. The advantages of this treatment format will be discussed.

Laura, a 41-year-old divorced mother of a 16-year-old daughter,

Karen, came to our clinic in June 1978 complaining of "headaches and hearing voices." She was accompanied by her mother, Mrs. M., age 76, with whom she lived. The notion of an "interlocking pathology" was suggested by the following history. Laura's daughter Karen suffered from obesity, defiance, marginal school performance and occasional physical abuse of her grandmother. When Karen was 14, Laura was hospitalized for a psychotic episode. Karen went to live with the family of her mother's brother, Don (Mrs. M.'s only other child). When Laura was discharged, her brother and sister-in-law refused to return Karen on the grounds that Laura was an incompetent mother. A court battle ensued. Karen ended up in a foster home for a year before returning to live with her mother and grandmother in 1976. Since that time, all communication between the two families had come to a bitter standstill. They had not as much as spoken a word to one another, despite the fact that they lived within several miles. The presenting problem, the other family problems, and the family's history appeared to be intricately interwoven. The family was stuck. They joined a multiple family group in hopes of getting unglued.

The family appeared to be precariously stabilized around Laura's dysfunction. She was started on antipsychotic medications. Her voices stopped. However, she continued to lead a marginal life doing little more than watching television. Mrs. M. functioned in both the roles of mother and grandmother. She cooked, cleaned, shopped and chauffered the family wherever was needed. Mrs. M. bitterly and continuously complained about this situation. Laura and Karen resented her complaining. Karen resented having two mothers. Laura resented Karen's defiance and was ashamed of her obesity and poor school performance.

Laura's capacity for regression was highlighted when she refused to drive her mother's new car because it was different from the old one. One evening the multiple family group became activated to cut through this behavior. The group joined arms in an all-out effort to get her to drive before the session ended. There were protests, but it was a surprise attack, and the family was caught off guard. Before the forces of resistance could be marshalled, Laura and I were heading for her mother's car in the parking lot, while excited faces peered through the window cheering us on. Laura, of course, drove the car with ease. As we walked back into the room, we were greeted with a standing ovation. Laura now does almost all the driving for the family.

A similar but even greater effort was needed to get Laura to apply for a sheltered workshop program. She repeatedly agreed to call the rehabilitation counselor, but did not follow through. Another group member was given the task to call Laura several times during the week to ensure that she would stop procrastinating. The group member called her. Laura called her counselor. The workshop was set up.

The greatest group effort was invested in getting Mrs. M. to make contact with her son. With the full support of the group and the family's minister, Mrs. M. sent her son a letter. The precise wording was carefully gone over in the group. Briefly she stated that she wanted to get beyond the bitterness of the past and to resume contact with him and her grandchildren. When he called her several days after receiving the letter, no one was more stunned than Mrs. M. It became clear that the resumption of contact would depend on the initiative of Mrs. M. The group provided a critical advocacy role in getting her to take and sustain this initiative. Calling Don on the phone to speak with him directly was her most difficult step. This was approached in the group like a job interview situation. The roleplay was rehearsed over and over again. She made the call. The contact resumed. Mrs. M. and her son now meet regularly for dinner. This breakthrough appeared to have a positive ripple effect on the family. The daughter, Karen, too, became less passive and withdrawn. She got a job and began a diet, which were very significant steps for her. Mrs. M. joined a Golden Agers Club which made regular trips into Boston. The family has participated in the multiple family group for the past one and a half years. Their progress, as in most therapies, has occurred in spurts, but it has occurred and it has been sustained.

In this approach, the multiple family group is given the collective responsibility and challenge to see that everyone in the group improves. If the family does not follow through on the therapist's directives, the other group members become involved to see that they are done. This variously allows group members to be in a care-giving and care-receiving role. The advantages of a self-help group and professional help are blended and synergized while the limitations of each approach are minimized. The group also provides an important socializing experience. This past holiday season was celebrated by the multiple family group with a party to which friends were invited and a Christmas "grab." Both these events were organized by Laura and Kelly, a 12-year old from another family. This interfamily interaction is central to the effectiveness of the group. The positive interaction between Laura and Kelly modeled through displacement the kind of mother-daughter relationship they longed for in their own family. As these families live in the same community, they frequently run into one another at school or shopping. These interactions outside of therapy help to translate the idea of community mental health into a concrete reality. What is more: these relationships will carry on long after the therapy is over.

Unlike the paradoxical approach of the Selvini-Palazzoli team, the communication mode in this setting is straightforward and sincere. Schizophrenic families appear to get stuck perhaps more frequently and more intensely than other families. The challenge to the therapist in this setting is to shape, channel and utilize the group members' longing for well-being and connectedness so that these roadblocks can be overcome. Rather than requiring a superhuman effort by the therapist, a multihuman effort is needed. A multiple family group provides such a setting.

Reference

Selvini-Palazzoli, M., Boscolo, L., Cecchin, G. F. and Prata, G. *Paradox and Counter-paradox.* New York: Aronson, 1978.

BRIAN L. ACKERMAN, M.D.
Fitchburg Clinic Director, North Central Mass. Mental Health Center; Associate in Psychiatry, University of Massachusetts Medical School Worcester, MA

51. Establishing a Multiple Family Group With Families of Schizophrenics

Question:

I work in a large Community Mental Health Clinic. A large proportion of our clients are young schizophrenics who are living with their parents. Recently we attempted to set up a program for these patients and their families. After considerable efforts to persuade them to attend, four families came to our first meeting. We intended to teach them some behavioral approaches such as contracting, goal-setting and reinforcement strategies. After two sessions, two of the families dropped out of the group and we decided to abandon the program. Although discouraged, we have not given up and would like to attempt a further behavioral educational multiple-family group. What can we do to engage the families more successfully? Is a multifamily group the best format for these families? How much structure should we impose on the group? What would be the ideal number of families to start with?

Discussion:

The problem of establishing a good therapeutic relationship with a young person suffering from schizophrenia, and his or her family members, is a difficult one that requires considerable planning as well as therapeutic skill, enthusiasm and, above all, persistence. You appear to have initially engaged families in the multiple family group but were unable to sustain the working alliance with some. This possibly reflects a lack of effective planning of the group. Several steps may be followed in the planning phase. They include: 1) assessment of the needs of the target population; 2) formulation of treatment objectives; 3) planning the structure of the group; and 4) planning the specific interventions.

Assessment of the needs of the target population. The first step in planning an effective therapeutic intervention is to carefully evaluate

238

the needs of the group you wish to treat. Without such information your treatment is clearly hit-or-miss. You have already identified that a large number of your clients are young, live with their families and suffer from schizophrenia. That is an excellent start. The next step might be to conduct interviews with the patients and their family members and explore their individual strengths and weaknesses as well as their reports of family transactions. This can be accomplished through a series of interviews with each household member. If the family is involved in the therapeutic process from the time of the patient's intake to the clinic, there will be less difficulty encouraging them to increase their level of participation at a later date. After the initial assessment of family behavior and attitudes, you may find it helpful to meet with the whole family to examine their interaction. A home visit is often very revealing and less threatening for the family.

While evaluating the needs of individual families is stressed, there is a substantial literature on the family factors associated with schizophrenia. There are several detailed reviews, but perhaps the most readable is by Lansky (1979). The experience of people who have developed treatment programs for schizophrenia, or who have studied the family problems of schizophrenia, may provide further information on the potential needs of this population. Several studies of family factors in schizophrenia have suggested that living with the family is detrimental to the young adult suffering from this illness. However, although these studies have suggested that negative family attitudes appear to have a dramatic effect on the course of the illness, the majority of families studied provided positive support which appears to enhance the prognosis (Vaughn and Leff, 1976). A substantial proportion report considerable difficulty coping with the behavior disturbance associated with florid schizophrenic symptoms. These families may be helped to learn more effective, less emotional responses to the patient's inappropriate behavior, or to any other family member's inappropriate behavior for that matter. Much has been made of the overprotective, symbiotic bonds between the parents and the child with a schizophrenic illness. There is less evidence that moderate dependency is detrimental, but in its more extreme forms there is a need to assist both parent and patient to achieve greater independence. This becomes a particular problem in adult persons suffering from chronic schizophrenia, who are living with aging parents.

A further area where the provision of services to patients and their families are reported deficient is in providing a clear understanding of the symptoms, causes, prognosis and treatment of schizophrenia. Hatfield (in press) surveyed a large group of families and found that their most frequently expressed need was to increase knowledge and understanding of the patient's symptoms of schizophrenia. Other types of help requested included talking to people who have been through the same experiences, the provision of alternative care to relieve the family from time to time, and having the patient change his or her place of living. Each sample of families may have different needs specific to the subculture which they inhabit.

Formulation of treatment objectives. A thorough assessment of the needs of the families and patients makes the task of formulating specific treatment objectives relatively easy. The main concern is to decide upon goals that can be readily attained through the multiple family group. Several community programs that involve family participation in the rehabilitation of schizophrenia have been reported. Some have a clear objective to separate the patients from their families (Dincin et al., 1978), while others aim to educate and support the families while they are caring for their disabled relatives (Lansky, 1979). In addition to considering the needs and goals of the families, it is essential to coordinate family programs with other existing services. For example, there is little value in aiming to reduce the need for drug therapy unless the psychiatric service providing the medication has similar objectives; or encouraging families to find alternative living arrangements for patients in an area where affordable alternatives are scarce. A systems approach is crucial to the success of any such community program.

There are several objectives that have been identified in most families with members suffering from schizophrenia. These include: educating the family and patient about the illness; maximizing interpersonal communication skills; improving coping behavior; obtaining support from the social network; and helping the adult patient gain independence. You may decide to focus on one or more of these objectives in the family group. Family therapy cannot provide all the interventions the patient and family may need to overcome the handicaps of chronic schizophrenia. In combination with other interventions such as drug therapy, vocational and leisure counseling, and social skills training, family therapy may make a major contribution to improving the long-term outcome of this disabling condition.

Planning the structure of the group. The choice of a multiple family format as the primary mode of therapy is of interest. Before definitely opting for this structure it may be important to check that it is conducive to therapy with the target population. Clearly, some of the needs of the families and patients may be well suited to the multiple family group, e.g., obtaining education about schizophrenia, sharing experiences and learning ways of coping with behavior difficulties. However, specific family communication and problem-solving tasks are more effectively dealt with in more intimate individual family sessions. Family therapy with both single and multiple families requires considerable therapeutic skill. Emotional intensity frequently runs high and becomes difficult to control. However, although the multifamily approach helps reduce emotional levels, when they do begin to rise, the therapist may have even less control over the situation. Regardless of the nature of the specific intervention strategies employed, skill in the nonspecific elements of family therapy may be crucial to establishing a sound treatment alliance.

Once the decision to develop a multiple family group has been made, the number of families to invite, the frequency of sessions, the time and place of the meetings, and any specific group rules can be considered. There is no empirical evidence to guide the therapist on these practical issues. Four or five families is probably a maximum. My preference is for three, where two parents and one or more adult children attend. If you plan considerable didactic presentation, a larger number could be accommodated. The frequency of sessions will again depend on the treatment objectives. A support group that aims to provide adjunct parental participation to a community rehabilitation program may meet once a month, while an intensive group that aims to change family interaction may meet twice weekly. For most families, the early evening or late afternoon are the most convenient times for meetings. Attendance may be poor if a mutually convenient time is not negotiated. Provision of light snacks and beverages creates a hospitable environment, particularly when the evening meal is delayed by the meeting. If the group is small, families may offer to host sessions in their own homes. In this setting therapists may be concerned that the sessions will become less structured and more social. However, if the aim is to enlarge the families' social network, such a move may be supported.

Several therapists who work with the families of adult schizophrenic patients have elected to work with the parents only. If the therapist is attempting to enhance family interaction and problem-solving on issues concerning the patient, the full participation of the patient is indicated. Behavior change will be most effective if it is mutually contracted between family members. But at times the parents may be seen alone to discuss issues such as their marital or sexual relationship. Although patients may distract group members, I prefer that they be invited to participate fully in a behavioral group. Aberrant behavior serves as a stimulus for teaching families the coping techniques that they may use at home. One technique that has proved extremely useful has been to teach patients and family members to use self-initiated "time out." Group members are instructed to politely excuse themselves when they feel excessive tension, telling the group when they intend to return, e.g., "I'd like to go out and take a walk for five minutes, O.K.?"

For many families the support they need may extend beyond the relatively brief duration of the group. Therapists may wish to structure their availability to provide around-the-clock consultation and to encourage families to call whenever they have serious crises which they have been unable to resolve. At these times the family may be prompted to employ behavioral strategies they have rehearsed in the group. This contact outside the session can thus enhance generalization of newly acquired skills.

- *Planning the specific interventions.* Several specific therapeutic interventions may enhance involvement. First, in the initial phase of the group, it is helpful to maximize the strengths and assets of the group members. Positive interaction and attempts at coping are reinforced with attention and praise. The behavioral approach assumes that an individual's response at any time represents the very best alternative he or she knows to cope with that specific situation, given the constraints operating at that point in time. Or, more simply, a person is always doing his or her best. The behavior that therapists describe as maladaptive or inappropriate may be a person's best or only choice from his or her point of view. Delusional beliefs and perceptual disturbance may severely limit a person's behavioral responses. Confronting the inappropriateness of these responses is usually counterproductive, and empathic understanding may prove more effective. Until family members feel supported and are capable of attempting alternative responses, it is wise to avoid confrontation of negative issues. Encouraging group members to work cooperatively, to provide praise and attention for appropriate behavior, hastens the development of the optimal environment for change.

A frequent theme of families with members suffering from schizophrenia is parental guilt. Frequently this results from a lack of clear understanding of the illness. The commonly asserted belief that a child's upbringing is at the root of *all* mental illness, along with overt or covert reinforcement by mental health professionals, results in parents believing that they have caused schizophrenia. Fear that the family group might lead to further accusations may result in avoidance of the experience. We have found that a few sessions devoted almost entirely to teaching the families about schizophrenia have greatly reduced parental guilt and improved their understanding of many of the patient's difficulties.

Effective behavioral interventions will depend on the varied assets and deficits of family members. Communication training with role rehearsal, modeling, feedback and social reinforcement may be taught. Reinforcement strategies to promote appropriate behavior and to reduce undesirable responses can be employed as indicated. Techniques of problem-solving and stress management may prove useful. In our program at the University of Southern California, a wide range of specific behavioral interventions are employed during two years of family treatment. Over this period families show considerable change. Dramatic improvement is infrequent and most gains derive from a persistent positive commitment to the patients and their families.

References

Dincin, J., Selleck, V., and Streicker, S. Restructuring parental attitudes-working with parents of the adult mentally ill. *Schizophrenia Bulletin*, 1978, *4*, 597-608.

Hatfield, A. Help-seeking behavior of family care givers of the mentally ill. *American Journal of Community Psychology*, in press.

Lansky, M. R. Research in family therapy. In E. A. Serafetinides (Ed.), *Methods of Biobehavioral Research*, New York: Grune and Stratton, 1979.

Vaughn, C. E., and Leff, J. P. The influence of family and social factors on the course of psychiatric illness: A comparison of schizophrenic and depressed neurotic patients. *British Journal of Psychiatry*, 1976, *129*, 125-137.

IAN R. H. FALLOON, M.D., M.R.C. Psych.
Assistant Professor
Department of Psychiatry
University of Southern California
School of Medicine
Los Angeles, CA

52. Evaluation and Treatment of Affect Disturbances Within a Family Context

Question:

When encountering depressive and/or manic behavior in members of a dysfunctional family, how does one distinguish cause and effect?

Discussion:

Whether such behavior causes family dysfunction or vice versa may be the wrong question. Posing it may indicate failure to assess such problems from a general systems orientation. Without such assessment, there is no intelligent treatment. For this discussion, let us define depression and hypomania as mood disturbances, whether or not of sufficient degree to be diagnosed a major unipolar or bipolar Affective Disorder (APA, 1979). (Capital letters will be used to refer to major disorders.) New knowledge of neuroendocrine regulation of mood in health and disease establishes Depression and Mania as preeminent psychosomatic illnesses. Nevertheless, clinicians of every discipline still become mired in dualism; they emphasize soma (psychophobic attitude) or psyche (biophobic) and neglect the patient's surround (sociophobic).

Engel's (1979) biopsychosocial model of disease is useful here. Dysfunction occurs on one or more hierarchical levels, from brain cell receptor site to community. If not contained on one level, dysfunction spreads intersystemically, up or down. For example, genetic predisposition to Affective Disorder directs a psychobiologic disruption of the person, with impact upon his/her interpersonal networks. A major corporation moves out of state, creating a ripple effect upon those in its employ. In either case, it is important to examine the function which altered mood of one member serves in the family emotional system.

Whatever the levels impinging upon it, the family emotional system is an important level at which affect disturbances may be reinforced or ameliorated, and thus a level at which to treat. But when a family therapist notes that one or another member of a family is always depressed, it is naive to assume that homeostatic family processes necessitate this, without *also* looking at the psychobiologic makeup of each member and at extrafamilial influences. Comprehensive diagnosis must be made at the outset and whenever developments in treatment suggest incomplete formulation. Diagnosis occurs at three major levels:

1) *Individual*—Includes biomedical variables, psychodynamics, and specific psychiatric syndromes.
2) *Family*—Observe the extent to which the dominant mood is depressive or a defense against depression. Look at current transactions, past generations, special legacies (e.g., inherited diseases, other dark secrets, holocaust).
3) *Larger Contexts*—How do they contribute to the losses and disruptions known to precipitate depression?

Let me discuss these levels further. The emotional lability of a member with a major Affective Disorder has a centralizing effect upon the family emotional system. When other members are also vulnerable, a contagion of depression and marital dissatisfaction may lead to divorce or recurrent crises and impaired family organization. Biochemical variables account in part for the increased incidence of depression in women: monoamine oxidase levels are higher than in males and increase with age. Losses in childhood predispose to depressive character structure. In the adult, self-esteem regulation is crucial to understanding depression in its intrapsychic and transactional manifestations. Feldman (1976) describes marriages wherein one spouse is self-depreciating and the other spouse maintains self-esteem by dealing with the first spouse's self-depreciation. This schema is useful for heuristic purposes and in treatment planning, but problems in practice are seldom so simple.

Let me illustrate. Alice, 45, presented with catastrophic dreams, tears and panic attacks, particularly when premenstrual. She was dreading her son's departure for college and her daughter's two years later. They were the only "dividends" from a destructive marriage. Past history was consistent with a diagnosis of agoraphobia with panic attacks (APA, 1979; Liebowitz & Klein, 1979). Psychotherapy had helped, but she remained susceptible to attacks when threatened with loss. Alan, her husband, knew how to trigger them. His sexual avoidance increased her dysphoria. Imipramine relieved her depression and prevented the desperate panics (which, at times, are symptomatic of depression). After their son departed, Alan drank more; at home, he either raged or withdrew. He had his own therapist, but a crisis made it possible to get him in with her. Alan's personality was cyclothymic; depression and suicide were prominent in his family history, as revealed by Alice. In the session, when not belligerent, he wallowed in shame and self-depreciation. Intoxicated, he bellowed and sobbed. Alan was clearly the identified patient, to his wife's satisfaction. Though she often countered his self-criticism, she also triggered it. Their interaction confirmed my impression of a highly sensitive self-esteem system, a seesaw with one up, the other down. Alan's reaction to their competition for my support was to stop drinking a quart of whiskey daily. By their third session, Alice was more depressed, while he reported soberly on her pathologic behavior. Alan refused conjoint treatment but remained in a productive, mildly Hypomanic state (not requiring lithium) until fall, while Alice continued in therapy to mourn the loss of their son (for both parents). When, in October, Alan returned to alcohol and depression, the change seemed biologic due to a history suggestive of seasonal cycles. But this isolated man was most dependent upon his work system for self-esteem, and sales had fallen off. To complete the picture, the day he began to drink was the very day Alice (active and off antidepressant medication) started a responsible, well-paying job. With Alan so regressed and dependent that he moved in with his widowed mother, I was able to engage him in family therapy. When sober again, his depression proved responsive to imipramine. These and later developments (and past and family history) established a diagnosis of mild, previously undetected Manic-Depressive illness.

So here was a couple, each with exquisite psychobiologic susceptibility to Affective Disorder, each able to relieve their own depression by triggering it in the other. Their support network consisted of aging parents, lovers and friends, therapists, and children. The son showed signs of adolescent depression; his talented sister vigilantly defended against it with adaptive activities and sarcastic wit. In college, the son tried to tune out with girl friends and pot, but made a suicide gesture and returned home. Intensive individual and family therapy emphasized self-awareness, the avoidance of destructive triggering, and differentiation from extended family. As mother and father took more responsibility for self, son and daughter were freed from pathologic triangulation.

A therapist helping families with such lability must track events throughout their network; otherwise, he/she may confuse reversals (first order change) for system (second order) change. The richer the therapist's repertoire in communicating with people in their emotional tongue (the words and the music), the better he or she can both join and restructure a variety of families. The therapist must sometimes *be with them* through their turbulence, and sometimes take charge and protect them from overwhelming affects and destructive behavior. A family therapist may need to bellow to be heard; other times he/she serves the family best by articulating their shared despair. To experience the blaming, pessimism and destructiveness in these families is heavy. Sufficient training and personal resources are needed to sustain a therapeutic role in the face of such powerful induction. Cotherapy is useful here, adding energy and a built-in therapist support system. Davenport et al. (1979) describe the value of cotherapy with a couples group where one spouse has Manic-Depressive illness.

For an integrated family therapy approach when one or more members require specific medication for an Affective Disorder, it is best that one of the regular therapists be a psychiatrist. My preferred option is family cotherapy, with one therapist being a psychiatrist experienced in *both* family therapy and the latest nuances of psychopharmacology. The next best option, if only one family therapist is available, is such a psychiatrist. The third best option is a nonpsychiatrist family therapist, plus a psychiatrist as consultant, *provided* this consultant is part of the formal or informal colleague network of the family therapist. It is important that the consultant be conceptually and personally compatible with the family therapist and readily available when the family therapist, mindful of complex issues regarding medication, might seek advice. This is more feasible when both work at the same setting. The least desirable option, in general, is a nonmedical family therapist and a nonpsychiatrist physician as consultant. Alan and Alice had been treated (without benefit) by an agency as character disorders with a "sadomasochistic marriage." In such cases, a biophobic or otherwise unaware family therapist might miss biologic factors, without whose diagnosis and treatment the good results of family therapy are unlikely.

The single parent with mood disturbance is most central to the family emotional system. One such mother with chronic Agoraphobia became more phobic, depressed and obese as her three children grew into adolescence. In more mature ego-states, she agreed to our contract to help them individuate. But when such changes increased her separation anxiety, she sometimes bound them closer as phobic companions. Thanks to improvement of her Depression and Agoraphobia with imipramine and desensitization, we could sustain our goal of differentiation for all members. The middle son, at first defiantly, led the way beyond their enmeshed, extended family. The eldest daughter, a somber girl who was both parental child and parentified by mother, felt encouraged to lead the life of a teenager. She broke a collusion with mother that both remain obese, losing 60 lbs. while mother gained. When I returned from vacation, the mother's anxiety had increased to panic; she clung to her youngest daughter. Though these events are most comprehensively understood on the level of family-therapist system, there were relevant pathophysiologic changes in the mother: In a pseudoindependent, angry move she had secretly discontinued imipramine during my vacation. Metabolic consequences of her recurring agitated Depression and of increased weight put her diabetes out of control, creating a vicious cycle of infection, somatic symptoms and dysphoria. This increased parentifying pressures on the children to worry about and look after mother. After restarting imipramine and beginning insulin, mother's health improved. Only then could family therapy with this single parent family make progress.

Let us survey a case in which the IP was in the generation most prone to depression. A grandmother of 70 presented with insomnia, weight loss, irrational pessimism about her cardiovascular problems and a wish to die. For years, she and her husband had been high achievers despite his ulcer and her heart disease. But as her stoic husband continued his prominent career into his seventies and in other ways overfunctioned as patriarch over three generations, she became more depressed. As the couple's surviving siblings and friends retired and moved away, she became more isolated. When he was home from work her symptoms abated. Grandmother's suicidal wishes, spoken to husband and relayed to her daughters, mobilized a support system within this family, to her benefit. As family therapist, I amplified this message. However, denial in the larger family was great; they needed grandmother's depression as conduit for their psychological problems and were not available for system change.

In the above family, grandmother's depression served a function (albeit conflictual) for both husband and daughters. By tracking events in three or more generations, one notes the skip-generation phenomenon: A child and/or grandparent manifests the symptoms of a disturbance resonating through the generations. A patriarch dies, his grandson develops school phobia and sulks at home. Once father gets his son back to school, he has anxiety spells, becomes morose, stays home from the family business he now heads, and drinks. Caught in a squeeze play between their adolescent offspring and aging parents, middle-aged parents are at risk nowadays. From a systems perspective, their treatment benefits each generation.

References

American Psychiatric Association. *Diganostic and Statistical Manual of Mental Disorders, Third Edition* (DSM-111). Washington, D.C.: American Psychiatric Association, 1979.

Davenport, Y. et al., Manic-depressive illness: Psychodynamic features of multigenerational families. *American Journal of Orthopsychiatry*, 1979, *49*, 24-35.

Engel, G. The biopsychosocial model. *General Hospital Psychiatry*, 1979, *1*, 156-165.

Feldman, L. Depression and marital interaction. *Family Process*, 1976, *15*, 389-395.

Liebowitz, M. and Klein, D. Assessment and treatment of phobic anxiety, *Journal of Clinical Psychiatry*, 1979, *40*, 486-491.

LAWRENCE GROLNICK, M.D.
Assistant Professor, Family Studies Section
Department of Psychiatry
Albert Einstein College of Medicine
Bronx, NY

53. Family Therapy When
an Affective Disorder Is Diagnosed

Question:

What is an appropriate family treatment strategy when the marital or family problem is complicated by the presence of an acute affective disorder in one or more members?

Discussion:

Diagnose and treat the affective disorder, usually depression, concurrent with or before instituting marital or family treatment. The rationale underlying this strategy is that the symptoms of depression can prevent interpersonal change. The disordered mood can be a debilitating irritant and, as such, interfere with inclination, motivation and/or well-intentioned plan for interpersonal behavioral change. The dysphoric mood or loss of interest or pleasure in almost all activities can, at the very least, take the zest out of interchanges with family members. The cognitive set of depression, so well described by Beck (1976), including an unrealistic view of one's self as inadequate and unworthy, misinterpreting current situations in a negative way, and anticipating future failure, defeat and deprivation, clearly interferes with interpersonal enjoyment and growth.

Case Illustration

One of the authors (IDG) recently treated a couple, both of whom suffered from recurrent depressive disorder. Mr. A was a 46-year-old lawyer and his wife, Dr. A, was a 45-year-old physician. They had three children, ages 12, 9 and 6. The couple was referred for marital treatment (as a last resort) because of dissatisfaction with the marriage, so that divorce was seen as the only solution. Over the last year there had been an intensification of fighting (and mutual blaming) between the couple that had dated back to the beginning of the marriage some 20 years earlier. The areas of conflict focused on money and childrearing. Dr. A's need for control of the relationship was evident in financial and parenting issues, while Mr. A was attempting unsuccessfully to combat her domination. To accomplish this, he would criticize his wife's attempts in both areas. For example, she would discipline the children; he would say she should not have been so tough on them. When she did not discipline them, he would proclaim that she was negligent.

Their past history revealed that both had been brought up in Europe in what they described as chaotic households, with parents who were also fighting more than their peers' parents. Each of them had a parent who had experienced depressive episodes. The history of past treatment attempts revealed that both husband and wife had had separate, classical psychoanalyses which they described as "helpful but not sufficient to end the marital fighting." Diagnosis for both was Major Depressive Disorder, Recurrent Type.

When family treatment started both were so depressed—manifesting symptoms of loss of interest and pleasure, low self-esteem, and lack of energy—that treatment sessions were centered around mutual blaming. Three sessions led to no improvement. At that point, antidepressant medication was instituted. After six weeks, they both experienced considerable improvement in mood and activity level.

This change afforded the therapist with two tactical advantages. Most obvious was the fact that with the mood improvement in cognitive set, the couple could now conceivably begin to deal with behavioral interactions that might build a viable relationship. Secondly, the therapist was now viewed as an expert who could prescribe tasks (e.g., taking the right medication) that were effective, and thus was in a position to prescribe interpersonal tasks to change the previously described negative feedback systems—such as Dr. A's control, Mr. A's criticism, their resulting morass of further depression and lowered self-esteem. At this point, the therapist took advantage of this position by guiding the couple to interpersonal changes that led to further marital improvement.

This case is an illustration of our experience that whenever possible, when treating an initial or recurrent, acute depressive disorder in one or several members of a family unit, a combination of chemotherapy and family therapy was the most efficacious treatment strategy.

Further Comments

The affective disorders appear to be a heterogeneous group of disorders with diverse etiologies related to biochemical, intrapsychic and interpersonal factors. There is a growing literature dealing with interpersonal factors in depressions, and more specifically with marital discord and the depressions. This literature is especially intriguing and relevant to the marital and family therapist. Primary affective illness occurs more frequently in divorced samples than in controls (Briscoe and Smith, 1973). Depressed women are more likely than normals to have marital relations characterized by friction and hostility (Weissman and Paykel, 1974), and marital difficulties are the events more likely to be reported by depressed women prior to the onset of depression (Paykel et al., 1969). Therefore, we are arguing here for a type of marital intervention that is flexible in its conception of the heterogeneity of causes of depression and in its strategies of marital therapy.

Some clinicians would argue against early treatment of the symptoms of depression since the discomfort of the symptoms can motivate an individual or family to seek or remain in treatment. If the symptoms are removed right away, they argue, it takes away the patient's motivation for working in therapy and getting at the intrapsychic or interpersonal causes of the depression. We believe that ameliorating *some* of the acute symptoms still leaves plenty of symptoms and marital and family dysfunction to change.

The strategy in the case presented was based on the assumption that marital therapy would not be effective on the interpersonal plane while both partners had the affective disorder which prevented them from making the necessary changes in their marital interaction.

In summary, then:

1) Depression is probably a heterogeneous group of disorders with different combinations of causative agents. Those depressions that are more endogenomorphic are most likely to respond to antidepressant medication, and this treatment modality should not be ignored even though interpersonal causes or effects resulting from depression are most obvious when doing marital or family therapy.

2) Treatment of the symptoms of depression is not synonymous with treatment of the interpersonal difficulties, even though the two may have an intimate connection, even a causative one. Klerman and his colleagues (1974) have demonstrated, for example, that the effects of chemotherapy—reduction of depressive mood, etc.—are different than the results of individual psychotherapy. As soon as the therapist makes this distinction, he or she is faced with the strategic choice of the timing of these interventions.

3) If antidepressant medication has some likelihood of success, it should be utilized early in the treatment for the appropriate indi-

vidual or individuals in the family system. The early use of such medication provides the therapist with an initial positive change in mood that lays the foundation for further interpersonal changes.

4) Some neophyte family therapists worry that chemotherapy of one person in a family system puts the therapist's seal of approval on the family's projective mechanisms and reinforces the patient role for one member. The present writers believe this risk must be taken and, if it occurs, handled with the appropriate therapeutic strategies. If the therapist understands clearly the biological, intrapsychic and interpersonal aspects of depression, strategies to frustrate such scapegoating will be readily apparent. Once the somatic treatment is instituted, the therapist can focus the intervention on the interpersonal plane and make clear to all involved the repetitive familial interaction (Feldman, 1976) that perpetuates the depressive symptoms.

References

Beck, A. T. *Cognitive Therapy and the Emotional Disorders*. New York: International Universities Press, 1976.

Briscoe, C. W. and Smith, J. B. Depression and marital turmoil. *Archives of General Psychiatry*, 1973, *29*, 811-817.

Feldman, L. B. Depression and marital interaction. *Family Process*, 1976, *15*, 389-395.

Klerman, G. L., Dimascio, A., Weissman, M. et al. Treatment of depression by drugs and psychotherapy. *American Journal of Psychiatry*, 1974, *131*, 186-191.

Paykel, E. S., Myers, J. K., Dienelt, M. N. et al. Life events and depression: A controlled study. *Archives of General Psychiatry*, 1969, *21*, 753-760.

Weissman, M. and Paykel, E.S. *The Depressed Woman*. Chicago: University of Chicago Press, 1974.

IRA D. GLICK, M.D.
Professor of Psychiatry
Cornell University Medical College;
Associate Medical Director for Inpatient Services and
Director, Family Therapy Program
Payne Whitney Psychiatric Clinic
The New York Hospital-Cornell Medical Center

and

JOHN F. CLARKIN, Ph.D.
Associate Professor of Clinical Psychology
Cornell University Medical College;
Associate Director, Family Therapy Program
Payne Whitney Psychiatric Clinic
The New York Hospital-Cornell Medical Center
New York, NY

54. Marital Therapy for
Borderline Personality Disorders

Question:

Patients with borderline personality disorders usually have such difficulty forming a working alliance even in individual treatment that I have trouble imagining how they could withstand couples therapy, where they would get only "half" of the therapist. Can someone suggest some basic guidelines for doing couples therapy with one borderline partner, especially in terms of how to give the patient enough, yet not end up treating only the identified patient?

Discussion:

One of the most basic problems in doing any form of psychoanalytically oriented therapy, whether it be individual, group or family, with borderline patients is the theoretical underpinnings which determine the goals for treatment. "Giving the patient enough" seems to be based on the older theoretical model concerned with deprivation of oral supplies, with the implicit need to make up for past deprivations in the patient's childhood. In recent years, object relations theory, which is based more on a developmental-relational model, seems to offer greater promise and fewer pitfalls than the libidinal model for working with borderline patients.

Winnicott was perhaps the first to note that, due to the lack of responsiveness in the mother, the child's omnipotent fantasies of fusion with and control over the mother in terms of the child's needs, are not formed. The child does not experience what Winnicott terms "good enough mothering," and the mother does not serve as a "transitional object" to provide this symbiotic state that is the foundation for basic security and trust. Internalization of the good mother function does not occur, thus disrupting the individuation and separation process. Thus, borderline patients persistently feel distrustful that their needs will be met; this results in excessive demands and the need to control the nurturant others such as the therapist or spouse. Others are not seen as separate individuals with separate motivations, but are viewed as all good or all bad in egocentric terms of whether or not they meet the patients' needs. This lack of trust, the need to establish a symbiotic relationship, and the type of primitive defensive mechanisms employed become the areas to be worked with in treatment and not simply the deprivation itself.

Kernberg has enumerated these primitive defenses as splitting (seeing objects as all good or all bad), primitive idealization, and the use of projective identification. Unlike the neurotic patient who uses projection onto the therapist, which determines simply how the other is perceived, these more disturbed patients use projective identification onto the therapist, which attempts to actually induce the other to respond behaviorally. There is an attempt to provoke or shape the other's responses to fit the internalized mental object in the patient. This attempt by borderline patients to induce responses in the therapist has resulted in greater interest in countertransference reactions. Many current psychoanalytic clinicians working with borderline patients have broadened the classical definition of countertransference to include these reactions in the therapist that come from the patient and not simply from the therapist's own unresolved conflicts (i.e. transference).

My own work has stressed that more disturbed, nonneurotic patients themselves have been induced in the family, via projective identification, into certain behavioral, cognitive and emotional patterns. These include borderlines (Slipp, 1977), schizophrenics (Slipp, 1973), and depressives (Slipp, 1976). The patient's use of projective identification comes from identification with the types of defenses employed in the family and is not solely from an intrapsychic origin. The family's defensive style reinforces these primitive defenses. In essence, the borderline attempts to induce behavior in others just as was done to the patient in the family. I have termed this particular type of countertransference "dissociative" (Slipp, 1976).

In working with couples and families, there is a greater possibility of being sucked into a countertransference reaction than in individual therapy; the complexity of the field and presence of a triad tend to foster splitting. The therapist may feel empathic toward one spouse and judgmental of the other, which interferes with the role of objective observer and interpreter of interactional patterns and behaviors. On the other hand, by seeing the couple together, the intensity of the borderline's transference in treatment is diluted. In addition, a good deal of the intense transference is already being acted out with the spouse. The tendency of the therapist in marital and family therapy to be more active than in individual therapy also tends to diminish the transference.

One of the most difficult problems with borderline patients in treatment is the intensity and fragility of the transference, which creates problems in developing a working therapeutic alliance. The observing ego of the patient is deficient, causing difficulty in joining the therapist in looking at his or her own motivations and behavior. Borderline patients have a lack of impulse control (poor tolerance for anxiety and hostility), a tendency to act out, and poor self-esteem which causes them to view interpretations as devastating criticism. By diluting the transference and focusing on the interaction, rather than the borderline patient's individual pathology, hopefully some degree of a trusting working alliance can develop.

Since the borderline patient tends to act out intrapsychic pathology in the interpersonal sphere, it is especially helpful to include the spouse in joint treatment. Either by selection of the mate to fit internalized objects or through shaping of behavior via projective identification, the patient's old conflicts from the family of origin become reenacted in the marriage. The therapist can join in an alliance with the couple to look at their interactions in a parallel fashion. Because there is less transferential distortion of the therapist, this approach may at times be even more successful than in working with the borderline patient individually. It may be that the original work in conjoint family therapy started with more disturbed, nonneurotic patients, since a therapeutic alliance may be more possible to attain.

Before proceeding further, it is important to discuss the goals of teatment of the borderline patient and the spouse. These will often depend on the needs of the patients, their motivation, the flexibility of their defensive structure, as well as the ability to develop a therapeutic alliance. The skills, training and theoretical foundation of the therapist also play a crucial role. As was shown in our study of outcomes of family therapy (Slipp, 1978a; 1978b), the less-skilled therapist may be just as effective as the trained therapist in short-term problem-solving approaches. In the problem-solving approach genetic factors and deeper unconscious motives are not touched, but the couple is helped directly to resolve conflict. Suggestions, advice giving, direction and emotional support come into play to produce change. However, in insight forms of family therapy the skill and training of the therapist are crucial.

Other approaches that do not attempt to produce structural change within the patient, but that produce changes in the couple's interaction, are restructuring the family system or paradoxical instructions.

In both these approaches, the therapist uses his/her dominant role to change family interaction. In structural family therapy, the power structure is more equalized, allowing for greater communication and hopefully freer ego functioning. In paradoxical or strategic family therapy, the family's resistance to change (to preserve the homeostasis) and their opposition are harnessed in the service of change. In the paradoxical instruction given the family, a reverse double-bind is prescribed, with the family explicitly told not to change but with the implicit message being to change. Change becomes necessary since the motives or secondary gain from the symptom or behavior are revealed.

If the therapist wishes to work within a psychoanalytic framework with couples, greater self-awareness by the therapist is mandatory because of the problems of countertransference. The therapist must develop an observing ego concerning his or her own reactions to the patient, since acting out the countertransference only reinforces the patient's pathology. This greater self-awareness and the therapeutic use of one's own reactions require that therapists undergo psychoanalytic psychotherapy or analysis to be in touch with their own feelings, fantasies, and conflicts. These have become integrated within the ego and can be observed and dealt with in a controlled fashion. The therapist is then better able to differentiate his/her own neurotic conflict from that projected by the patient. In addition, the therapist who wishes to work in depth with the borderline and the spouse needs to be acquainted with object relations theory, with the work of Bowen, Lidz, Wynne and myself, as well as the literature on countertransference such as that of Racker, Kernberg and Langs.

One of the most important issues that needs to be worked with is the patient's lack of differentiation, the fluidity of ego boundaries, and the need to establish a symbiotic relationship with others and the therapist. Lidz feels the establishment and resolution of this symbiosis may be one of the essential elements producing curing in the schizophrenic. Borderline patients also attempt to establish a symbiotic relationship (Slipp, 1973; 1977). As Wynne has pointed out, the patient gives up autonomy to sustain a relationship. However, as I have previously noted, the borderline expects others to do likewise. The patient tries to behave, think and feel as the other wishes in order to sustain and control the relationship, but also demands the same in return. I termed this the "symbiotic survival pattern," wherein fusion serves to sustain dependency, to control the other's responses and to serve as an interpersonal defense against one's own insecurity and rage.

Autonomy is equated with abandonment and lack of survival, since the fixation in development occurs during the symbiotic phase (as described by Mahler and elaborated by Jacobson and Winnicott). Borderline patients do not trust the responsiveness of others, and hence, to survive attempt to control others by giving up autonomy and functions according to what they perceive as the others' demands. This creates considerable rage, as well as fear and jealousy, that others will be disloyal and betray them.

This need for excessive control and distrust coupled with a great deal of rage and jealousy often brings couples, where one or both are borderline, into treatment. These dynamics need to be brought into conscious awareness and traced back to their genetic origins; how they find expression in the couples' current interpersonal relations needs to be explored. As pointed out by Kohut, the therapist needs to be active, warm, empathic and supportive just as in individual therapy. However, if the therapist gives into the patients' demands, the demands may intensify to the point where the therapist will be trapped into only giving support and thus be unable to form a therapeutic alliance to explore the reasons for behavior. In addition, the primitive defenses have to be worked with and the patients helped to become more aware of their rage and jealousy and its origins, as discussed by Kernberg.

Some of the guidelines in working psychoanalytically with couples where one or both are borderlines are as follows:

1) Focus more on interpersonal relations than on intrapsychic pathology, especially in the beginning phases, to develop a trusting therapeutic relationship.
2) Take an active, empathic and unbiased position.
3) Be keenly aware of your own countertransference reactions so as not to be sucked into acting them out, thereby reinforcing pathology.
4) Do not simply gratify the patient's demands to make up for past deprivations, but foster a therapeutic alliance so that the couple can join in exploring and becoming aware of their insecurity, distrust and needs to control and their historic origins.
5) Help the couple not to perceive the other including the therapist simply from the egocentric position of whether or not the other gratifies one's needs or demands. Help them each become aware of the other's independent motivations and needs. Help them accept an interpretation without taking it personally as a devastating criticism.
6) Help them give up the defense of splitting, of seeing others and self as all good or all bad.

7) Help them get in touch with their rage and jealousy, how it is manifested and where it originates. Help them integrate their ambivalence and anxiety about binding.

8) Encourage their autonomy and work through their fears of destruction or lack of survival if they function separately.

9) Help them work through denial of conflict with their parents, so that it need not be projected transferentially into current interpersonal relations and acted out.

10) Help them see how their individual psychopathology has meshed in the past, and help them work out a new and healthier relationship for the future.

11) Recognize resistance and fears of change, be supportive of efforts to risk new behavior.

12) Provide emotional understanding that permits catharsis and working through.

Finally, once the interpersonal acting out of conflict has subsided, and the borderline patient has a working relationship with the therapist, transition to individual psychoanalytic psychotherapy might be considered.

References

Slipp, S. The symbiotic survival pattern: A relational theory of schizophrenia. *Family Process*, 1973, 12, 377-398.

Slipp, S. An intrapsychic-interpersonal theory of depression. *J. Am. Acad. Psychoanal*, 1976, 4, 389-409.

Slipp, S. Interpersonal factors in hysteria: Freud's seduction theory and the case of Dora. *J. Am. Acad. Psychoanal*, 1977, 5, 359-376.

Slipp, S. Difficulties in family therapy evaluation: I. A comparison of insight vs problem solving approaches; II. Design critique and recommendations. *Family Process*, 1978, 17, 409-422. (a)

Slipp, S. Does family therapy produce change? An overview of outcome studies. *Group*, 1978, 3, 23-34. (b)

SAMUEL SLIPP, M.D.
Clinical Professor
Department of Psychiatry
New York University
Medical Center
New York, NY

55. Combined Couples and Individual Treatment of Borderline Lesbians

Question:

I am a family therapist whose private practice includes quite a number of borderline patients. Because I am a woman, I am often sought out by lesbian patients who are seeking help with their primary relationships. A complex problem arises when both partners are borderline lesbians and require couples as well as individual therapy. My question has to do specifically with the issue of how to decide whether to see the couple along with my original individual patient and refer her lover elsewhere, or to see both members individually as well as in couples therapy. I realize the issue is complicated because of the particular intrapsychic problems of these women and may be additionally complicated by my being a woman therapist. My intention in posing this problem is to communicate with other practitioners with similarly difficult cases, with the hope of establishing criteria for deciding interventions best suited to the interpersonal as well as intrapsychic needs of this rather special group.

Discussion:

The problem you present certainly addresses an increasingly identified issue for family therapists, that is, the relationship between the intrapsychic and interpersonal approaches. It has been my experience that this interface is particularly problematic when treating borderline couples, and unique and subtle issues arise if all three members of the triangle are women. I have worked with a number of such couples in my practice and have repeatedly faced the problem you describe. Perhaps a brief description of "Sara and Ann" and a discussion of my evolving treatment ideas will be helpful.

Sara, age 30, was my original patient. I initially met her while she was hospitalized in a psychiatric ward of a general hospital for acute anxiety attacks, drug abuse and alcoholism. After discharge, she requested referral to me for individual therapy. At that time, she was married, with a baby boy; but due to severe marital and sexual problems, she again resumed drug and alcohol use, began making suicidal threats, and her whole adjustment deteriorated. I referred her first to an alcoholism treatment program, then to a long-term hospital. During this period, she became divorced, acknowledged her lesbianism and met her present lover, Ann. Subsequent to these developments, she again requested therapy with me and has continued in outpatient treatment for more than three years. Despite these difficulties, she has been drug- and alcohol-free except for one brief period and has been admitted to a drug and alcohol counselor training program. She has also managed to handle her visits with her son with marginal competence.

Sara is a bright, talented, sensitive woman who has never been able to differentiate from her family of origin. Her father is a successful but passive, alcoholic man whose life has been lived in the shadow of his dominant, artistically successful wife. Sara's connection with her mother is ambivalent and highly sexualized, no doubt due to the mother's blatant, high-pressure attempts to keep the patient emotionally shackled to her.

Ann is a severely depressed, angry, suicidal 28-year-old woman. She also has a long history of hospitalizations and has been committed for violent acting out. Although she has not been hospitalized in the past three years that she and Sara have been in therapy, her functioning has been only marginal. She is also an intelligent, talented and sensitive young woman who has never differentiated from a sadistic and rejecting father or from her mother, the "good" parent, but one who appeared totally oblivious to her simplest feelings. For example, when she was 10, her father had three of her animals in succession put to sleep for illness, but her mother appeared not to notice the effect of this loss on Ann. She also seemed unaware of the fact that Ann did not speak to her father for four years after this event. The underresponsiveness of the system as a whole has been important in determining Ann's suicidal stance as "a way of getting a response."

These young women have come from complex family systems which have given rise to confused intrapsychic structures, which, in turn, have created another interlocking system which constitutes their relationship. Consequently, the following situation developed in their therapy with me. Sara had requested couples therapy with Ann after their mutual discharge from the hospital, in addition to her individual therapy with me. (By the way, I have found that institutions which regularly offer family therapy to other couples are often reluctant to do so with lesbians.) I began couples therapy and referred Ann to another therapist for individual treatment. The couples treatment seemed to go well and offered both some much needed help in sorting out their projections, encouraging limited separation, and allowing them some intellectualization of their overwhelming feelings.

Individual therapy with Ann had always been a failure, although she had seen three highly skilled therapists. Both patients gradually developed a powerful fantasy that I was the best therapist and the only person who could help Ann out of her plight of years of hopeless depression. Although there was a certain appeal to my grandiosity in this request, I resisted an urge to gratify this and refused to see her. There is a good deal of theoretical backing for this position and at first I felt quite comfortable in maintaining this stance.

I will attempt to outline the treatment complications that arose because of my rigid position. When I continued to resist Ann's wish for individual treatment with me, she became enraged, spiteful, jealous and quite intent on destroying Sara's relationship with me by trying to depict me as the bad mother with the same sadistic intent to destroy that Sara had perceived her own mother to have. The situation also played into Ann's tendency to project her sadistic father and unresponsive mother onto me. As a result, therefore, she was not able in her own psychotherapy to get behind her anger to the necessary mourning phase.

Sara, on the other hand, was caught between her need on the one hand to perceive me as the good mother with the phallic power of her own mother, and on the other hand by the perceived wish to destroy her bad mother. This conflict, of course, clashed with her need for Ann as a real object and as a source of intimacy. This split mirrored her own developmental failure to integrate and successfully reconcile the good and bad mothers and left her in the intolerable position of all borderlines. If I, as a therapist and the good mother, turned bad, she would lose the only object on which she could project all the good split-off parts of herself and thereby identify with these split-off parts. Because of Sara's lack of sufficient separation developmentally and her lack of ability to maintain internal as well as external object constancy, this woman was devastated by the possibility of my being "bad," thereby leaving her nothing useful with which to identify and use as a base from which to go forward. The crisis in Sara's therapy caused by Ann's jealousy happened just at the point when Sara was beginning the process of forming a whole and seeing herself and her mother as both good and bad. This delicate work of resolving the contradictions of "good" and "bad" objects could not proceed in the face of Ann's jealousy and sibling rivalry.

This destructive but dynamically understandable interaction functioned on two levels. It put an intolerable strain on the couple's relationship and on their therapies, no longer allowing them the emotional freedom to project onto the therapist all the withholding, unloving, punitive, rageful characteristics they perceived in each other, hence preserving their relationship, or providing them the chance to use me as a neutral, but good mother. The explicitness of the gender identity of the three participants creates a more primitive situation than with a heterosexual mix. With heterosexual couples, the rivalry over the yearned-for good mother is likely to become somewhat overwhelming, but does allow that need to be externalized instead of contained within the triadic relationship.

If the couple's therapy deteriorates because of a three-systems breakdown, the pressure on the couple or the individuals to remain functional may be too much. I, therefore, reversed my position and agreed to see Ann individually. This reversal was based on the premise that to continue to separate the interpersonal from the intrapsychic was artificial and in fact hurtful in this particular case. People with such severe family and ego deficits do not need, nor can they tolerate, further externally-imposed frustration that repeats the rigid triangles of their families of origin. The flexibility of the therapist to join one, then the other, then both patients, was essential and has allowed them greater freedom to experience other than angry feelings.

Both Ann and Sara were delighted at my decision and approached the situation with new hope. At last the magical mother had been seduced and one could again hope for a perfect union with her. The gradual abandoning of that hope has allowed the therapeutic work to continue. Ann has been able to face the loss of a yearned-for good mother and go beyond anger and suicidal fantasy to a real state of mourning over her many losses. Her need to destroy Sara's relationship with me has subsided and, in fact, appears to be of little interest to her. The stage has been set for both to acknowledge and respect the intrapsychic problems of the other, while seeing how they themselves influenced the system. More importantly, they have been able to creatively investigate their family systems, generational transmissions and the present expressions of this historical material. Both have been able to use me as a consultant and guide rather than as an object to be possessed.

As I became flexible, this flexibility was expressed in the systems interactions of the couples. My rigidity, supported by theoretical notions of individual and systems thinkers, threatened the destruction of the system as well as the component parts. It is clear to me at this point that working with a severely dysfunctional system necessitates reevaluation of treatment principles that work so well with healthier people. I have found this model most useful in my work with borderline lesbian couples and would be delighted to discuss it further.

BLAND D. MALONEY, A.C.S.W.
Faculty, Family Study Center of Connecticut
Faculty, Department of Psychiatry
University of Connecticut Medical School
Faculty, University of Connecticut
School of Social Work
Hartford, CT

56. Responding to Presenting Complaints in an Alcoholic Family

Question:

A family presents itself for therapy with a child-focused problem as its chief complaint. As the assessment proceeds, it becomes clear to the therapist that a second problem also exists: one of the parents has a serious alcohol problem. The therapist now faces a difficult choice, whether to recommend that the alcohol problem be addressed first, or that the focus remain on the family's presenting complaint.

Discussion:

It would be our position that unless the family's presenting complaint indicates the family is facing a "red-hot" crisis, if a serious alcohol problem exists in a family, it is this issue that *must* be addressed immediately in order for successful family therapy to take place.

Although alcoholism in families is often assumed to lead to disruptive, chaotic behavior, the more typical situation is one in which alcoholism is associated with relatively stable, albeit rigid, patterns of interaction. For this reason, alcoholism frequently goes unrecognized by the family clinician. Even when recognized, its impact on family life is systematically *unestimated*.

Because alcohol use and intoxicated behavior are often incorporated as part of a family's coping strategies and significantly color the family's daily routines of living, we contend that the alcohol issue must be understood and tackled *before* the therapist can fully appreciate the dynamics of the family's presenting complaint.

Consider the following case:

A couple was referred for treatment because of severe marital difficulties. An initial interview revealed an anxious wife with serious intentions of leaving the marriage and a depressed husband who wanted the marriage to stay intact. Their 17-year relationship had been riddled with stresses, including financial overextension, multiple moves (including international assignments), domestic violence, lack of fulfillment in their sexual life and extra-marital relationships.

The alcohol history was as follows: The wife drank only on social occasions; the husband, however, drank daily, starting at dinner, would consume amounts up to five highballs or five glasses of wine followed by two or three beers, and would then fall asleep in the early evenings. The therapist identified alcoholism as a problem based both on the quantity/frequency index of alcohol consumption *and* on the behavioral-social effects of drinking reported by the husband (which included marked reduction of energy interspersed with periodic aggressive outbursts). Keep in mind that the couple did not list alcoholism as a problem nor had it been addressed during the husband's previous individual therapy. It was the family therapist's review of the intrusion of alcohol into the couple's daily life, the husband's work and its contribution to husband's violent outbursts that alerted him and the couple simultaneously to the critical nature of alcohol for this family. Alcoholism was therefore labeled by the therapist, accepted by the couple, and given first priority for treatment.

This clinical stance, and the treatment approach to be outlined below, are based on a clinical model applying family systems concepts to the problem of alcoholism. The core concept is the notion of the "alcoholic system" (Steinglass, 1976). It is proposed that alcohol, by dint of its profound behavioral, cultural, societal and physical consequences, might assume such a central position in the life of some families as to become an organizing principle for interactional behavior. Behavior during intoxication may be particularly important in maintaining homeostasis (Jackson, 1957). In this sense, alcoholism contributes to stability in such families, but at a very high price.

How does this theoretical formulation translate into therapeutic strategies and what are the implications for clinical practice? What function does alcohol perform for the family, and how does it work to organize the family?

The initial treatment effort with the family has to be the labeling (diagnosing) of alcoholism by the therapist and the acceptance by the *family* of this diagnosis. It is obviously critical that the therapist couch this diagnosis in systems terms, e.g., "Alcohol is clearly a problem for your family." With the transformation of alcoholism into a family-level problem, additional resources become available and can be capitalized on in order to eradicate the alcohol. For example, a mother states she will stop drinking. This is something she is giving up for herself and the family. What can the family do to help her through this stressful period? In a typical case, the children might offer to assist with domestic chores, while the husband would take responsibility for seeing to it that all alcohol was removed from the house. In other words, the family would be actively involved in a set of tasks designed to maximize coping strategies. This is particularly critical during the first phase of treatment, the removal of alcohol from the family system. Alanon and Alateen, in addition to AA, can be important resources for the family during this time.

Failure of family members to follow through with assigned tasks can be anticipated by the therapist and becomes valuable clinical material. Suppose, for example, husband does *not* remove alcohol from the house as promised, but instead offers a host of excuses for his behavior. The therapist can use this data to make clear to the family how invested it is in maintaining the alcoholic homeostasis and how difficult it is to give up old, well-used patterns. In revealing to the family the overwhelming pull towards reestablishing their former state, the therapist is able to predict possible "slips" in the future and to identify the struggle the family is experiencing.

Once alcohol has been removed from the family system, treatment enters a second phase. The period following sobriety often unveils a family with poor interpersonal relationships and few resources for nurturance. Feelings of emptiness, loneliness and alienation, previously masked by the family's use of alcohol as an organizing principle for behavior, now gush to the surface (Usher et al., 1979). In the past, alcohol use and its consequences had served to mask this emotional impoverishment. Alcohol had been the solution to explain away the family's isolation from each other.

The task for the family now becomes facing the emotional distance that exists between members and beginning to deal with overwhelming feelings of emptiness. This is usually the final phase of treatment.

What has happened to the original presenting complaint in this process? In all likelihood, the presenting complaint can be understood as a signal of stress within the family, created by the rigidity of behavioral patterns adopted by the family in conjunction with the management of chronic alcoholism. This rigidity, a sort of sacrificing of long-term growth for short-term stability, has left the family vulnerable to the stresses created by normal developmental issues, such as the typical child-focused complaint in our original question. In such instances, changes in family functioning following recovery from alcoholism will allow the family to deal with this other problem with minimal assistance from the therapist.

References

Jackson, D. D. The question of family homeostasis. *Psychiatric Quarterly Supplement*, 1957, 31, 79-90.

Steinglass, P. J. Experimenting with family treatment approaches to alcoholism, 1950-1975: A review. *Family Process*, 1976, 16, 97-123.

Usher, M. L., Jay, J. and Glass, D. *A Family Therapy Approach to Restricted Emotional Interaction Following Initial Sobriety*. National Council on Alcoholism. Washington, D.C., May 1979.

MARION LAZAR USHER, M.S.S.W.

Assistant Clinical Professor
Department of Psychiatry and
Behavioral Sciences
George Washington University
Medical Center

and

PETER J. STEINGLASS, M.D.

Associate Professor
Department of Psychiatry and
Behavioral Sciences
George Washington University
Medical Center
Washington, DC

57. Managing the Violent Family

Question:

At a recent meeting of professionals from several community mental health centers, a psychologist from one center began to talk about one of his most difficult current cases involving a violent family. The relationship between the husband and wife was characterized by threats, several incidents of injury, and the presence of guns in the house. In the last session, the husband became quite angry, stated that he had a gun in his car and was going to shoot his wife. I suddenly realized that my graduate school had not provided any practical training in how to handle such situations. I certainly don't want to specialize in this area, but I know my work in a community health center may involve me in one. Help!

Discussion:

Graduate training programs in psychotherapy do not give much attention to family violence, despite the extensiveness of the problem. Our most substantial knowledge comes from research on the most violent act, murder. For the past 10 years, approximately 70% of all murders have been family dispute-related (FBI, 1970-79). Studies of assaultive violence have found physical aggression to be a problem in one out of every four or five families (Gelles, 1972). Traditionally, most family violence has been dealt with by the police, where the situation has proved risky and requiring repetitive interventions. The majority of police time and on-duty injuries result from family dispute calls, not from apprehending criminals. Increasingly, however, such cases are being sent, after the initial intervention, to the community health system. The psychotherapist and family therapist are now involved, whether or not they have been trained or are prepared to deal with the problem.

With what experience base does the therapist approach such cases? Most trained therapists have had an inpatient and emergency clinic rotation where assaults and threats have been a part of the clinical picture. This beginning is excellent, but the population can be very skewed. A rotation in a jail or large hospital emergency room will quickly demonstrate the number and severity of cases that never make it to the mental health center. Further, the therapist, in working with severely disturbed inpatients, does not see many of their threats materialized. In a unique study, MacDonald (1968) set up an experimental inpatient ward for "threat to kill" patients. In his follow-up of the 100 admissions, only 5% committed a homicide after discharge. If the percentage is that low in such a highly specialized ward, the average general inpatient ward percentage would be extremely small. Thus, the therapist would have a strong tendency to discount the possibility of assault threats becoming reality. This tendency is reinforced by the therapist's need to believe that such destructive behavior is not possible with his or her patients. Citing the above experience base, however, is of little consolation to the friends and relatives of the victims murdered by the 5%.

Therapists respond far more effectively to another destructive behavior, suicide. Therapists hear many threats of suicide, but completed acts are relatively few. Yet, such thoughts, gestures and attempts are handled carefully and with a great deal of planning. The clinical experience process is similar in both suicide and assaultive behavior, but the treatment attitudes remain different.

In dealing with the suicidal threat, therapists use the factors of impulse delay and increasing alternatives. In dealing with the assaultive or homicidal threat, these factors will also be prominent, but complicated by the interaction of multiple individuals with different motives and actions. To examine the practical issues in therapeutic strategy, let's divide the problem into two broad areas: managing an event outside the therapy session and managing an event inside the therapy session.

The case usually comes to the therapist after a threat or event has occurred outside therapy. If one member of the family is visibly angry or upset at the start of the first session, it is important to acknowledge these feelings, but also to reinforce positive aspects of control—"It must be difficult to control such feelings." This sets the stage for gradually learning to verbalize anger within limits, rather than acting out the anger. Explanation of the circumstances that brought the family in should come after the above step has been taken. As this explanation is taking place, the therapist should be mindful of the well-documented three stage cycle of family violence: 1) tension building, 2) acute assaultive incident, and 3) remorseful/consoling behavior by the violent member of the victim (Davidson, 1978; Walker, 1979).

The family will answer direct questions about this repetitive cycle, but will usually not volunteer complete information. The victim is very much involved in this cycle, sometimes precipitating the acute incident to control the timing, get it over with, and move to the remorseful/consoling stage. The family therapist's awareness of such dynamics, however, can be viewed by the victim and by victim shelter agencies in the community as excusing the violent act. Care should be taken to explicitly state that this behavior is not acceptable, and that if the family cannot manage the problem, the police or courts will. Therapy cannot proceed effectively without consensus on this by both the therapist and the family.

The next step is to take an aggression and impulsivity history of each family member. What are the personal, cultural and family supports for expressing anger through action? When has violence worked for you? When has it not? What impulse delay is shown in the events described? What would cause the member to break a promise about violent expression? The family knows this material is important, and will feel supported by the therapist's direct and straightforward inquiry. This inquiry continues to reinforce the overall therapeutic goal of verbalizing anger within limits, instead of acting it out. The therapist will not complete this aggression and impulsivity history in the first session, for at least half the session must be reserved for arranging a contract to prevent future violence.

For example, no matter how clear the clues of building tension or how severe the anticipated violence, most families will not attempt to leave the house until the very last minute. The combination of ego and magical thinking will overcome rationality almost every time. So the therapist must sanction that it is both OK and necessary to leave the house when the first clues to violence appear. Sensitizing the family member to both physical symptoms of tension as well as behavioral clues is one of the longer term directions in therapy, but this, unfortunately, is not enough. If, for example, the wife is going to leave by car, but has to find the keys, go through three house doors, open the garage door and back the car out, she will not be able to leave the house successfully. Exiting the house must be a simple, highly sanctioned and attractive alternative if it is to challenge the established pattern of not leaving.

To complete this contract, the family members must determine where they will go after leaving the house. Frequently, the initial response is to go to a best friend's or relative's house, the first place the assaultive member is likely to look. The best friend or relative may now be placed literally in the middle of a risky situation. A location unknown to the assaultive member is preferable, but if this is not possible, the best friend or relative must be knowledgeable of the risk and willing to promptly call the police to handle any confrontation. A cooling off period of six to 24 hours is desirable, with a telephone call to check out the situation before returning home.

Finally, after the exit from the house, family members involved must separately notify the therapist. Thus, the therapist has 1) helped the family to recognize the problem, 2) established a practical plan for impulse delay, 3) defused retaliatory anger for exiting the house, and 4) increased alternatives for problem management. If this cannot be agreed upon and the anger remains very high, temporary separation of family members may be necessary until the next session.

The presence of weapons in the home creates a serious additional issue. Most people have approach/avoidance attitudes towards guns and other potential weapons. The therapist must support the avoidance component and the individual's positive efforts to control the anger. A way has to be found to get the weapons out of the home, without threatening the individual's ownership of the weapons and without the therapist or institution being the depository. One procedure is to have the individual store them with a friend. The friend should be told, "We're having some family problems and we're seeing a doctor named Johnson at the community hospital." An alternative procedure is to put the weapons in a pawnshop and have the friend hold the pawn ticket. Although I recommend against it, exceptional situations have been noted where the pawn ticket was held for a very short time by a cotherapist or other professional at a hospital. Properly approached, creating such an impulse delay by managing for weapons removal is far less difficult than the inexperienced therapist might guess.

Sometimes a family member may threaten to harm another individual not present or involved in the therapy. Until recently, the emphasis in such situations was upon the maintenance of the confidential relationship between therapist and patient. This emphasis was based upon a combination of legal protection against intrusion in the relationship and ethical standards about the therapist initiating release of any information. This combination of law and ethics is rapidly being modified by the courts. In California, Tarasoff vs. The Regents of the University of California now requires the therapist to notify anyone who is at risk. Cases in New Jersey and other states have produced similar changes in the law. The definition of "at risk" will soon be made by succeeding court cases. Because there are major differences in the law from state to state, therapists must investigate the law in their state. The greatest difficulty comes when therapists confuse a legal requirement to notify with an ethical objection to breaking confidentiality. The courts are increasingly clear about the primacy of the notification rulings. Therapists should carefully consult several colleagues on the record if they choose to proceed on other grounds.

The second major problem area is managing an event inside the therapy session. A number of weapons, primarily guns and knives, are brought into health care settings. They are present as a means of defense for a frightened, confused individual as a part of a subcultural norm, or as a potential means of aggression against being "mistreated." Annually, the emergency rooms of large urban hospitals collect substantial numbers of such weapons. For mental health crisis teams working with emergency rooms or crisis clinics in high crime areas, this is an occasional problem for which they have a procedure. For most other therapists, this problem has not yet occurred and no planning has taken place.

When the referral information contains evidence of violence or weapons, preplanning can be done. The best procedure varies due to differences in office design and availability of police support. A common procedure is to employ a space larger than the usual interview room, having more than one exit, often with one door open, with a desk button to summon assistance, and a security or police arrangement for assistance. Having security assistance sit in during the initial evaluation session is an option, but will not work in a therapy course. Additional separate space should be designated and available if separation of family members becomes necessary. Always let family members know that it is OK to leave the room if they feel they cannot control their anger. Most families simply do not know that this is OK.

Occasionally, the possible presence of a weapon may become apparent only after the therapy session has started. Usually this will begin with a family member's rising agitation or increasingly labored attempt to control such agitation, followed by a hint or threat of what might happen if this continues. At this point, the therapist needs to ask what is meant, and what could be changed right now that would make things more manageable. If this does not work and the threats continue, the therapist needs to ask if the member ever carries a weapon around, and, if the answer is yes, if he or she is carrying one today. If the answer is yes to the second question, the family member is usually both relieved that this fact is out and that the therapist is able to face it, but frightened of losing face and unsure of what is going to happen next.

The therapist is extremely uncomfortable, too, and should not attempt to conceal it. It is important to acknowledge this shared concern, but add structure by not being immobilized by it. The therapist is concerned, even scared, but knows what to do about it. The therapist must honestly state that he or she cannot work under these conditions. However, the therapist must not be involved in a direct exchange of any weapon, must not be in the middle of such a direct challenge. A common procedure, telegraphing each move carefully, is to exit the family to another room, exit yourself, and then exit the remaining individual, having him/her leave the weapon on the table. Security or police support should take possession of the weapon.

Reading the above is enough to raise anyone's anxiety. However, the translating of these or another set of procedures into reality requires consensus by therapists in the clinic, and roleplay rehearsals. Intellectual knowledge is not sufficient. While problems with such violent families should continue to be a very rare event in the therapist's practice, they do exist and warrant careful thought and training.

References

Davidson, T. *Conjugal Crime*. New York: Hawthorn, 1978.
FBI Uniform Crime Reports. U.S. Government Printing Office: Washington, D.C. 1970-79.
Gelles, R. J. *The Violent Home*. Beverly Hills, CA: Sage, 1972.
MacDonald, J. *Homicidal Threats*. Springfield, IL: Charles C. Thomas, 1968.
Walker, L. E. *The Battered Woman*. New York: Harper & Row, 1979.

CHRIS HATCHER, Ph.D.
Assistant Clinical Professor and
Director, Family Therapy Program
Langley Porter Institute
University of California
San Francisco, CA

SECTION V

Separation, Divorce and Remarriage

58. Transition from Marital/Family Therapy to Individual Therapy Following Separation or Divorce

Question:

What happens to marital or family therapy when a couple decides to separate and/or divorce? Should the therapist ever see one of the spouses in individual treatment after the separation/divorce?

Discussion:

The decision to divorce and/or separate is typically painful and problematic for a couple. Even when, perhaps through therapy, both individuals agree that it's the right thing, a legacy of ambivalent feelings usually follows. It is rare for the "work" of marital therapy to be concluded at this point. However, the question of continued therapy and the format of such treatment raise problems and issues for both the therapist and the client: Does one continue to treat the family as a unit? Does the family therapist see one or more of the family members in individual therapy? Should some or all of the family members seek out a new therapist? Do the family therapist's own feelings cause problems in helping with such decisions? These and other questions are explored below in an attempt to guide the decision making of the therapist and the family in such a situation.

Toomim (1972) has elaborated the differential emotional response patterns that usually follow a separation/divorce decision. Often, there is the "leaver," who makes the active, spoken decision to leave the marriage and the "leavee," the person who perceives him/herself as being left. The leaver often initially experiences a sense of mild well-being and/or relief at having come to a decision about the marriage; the leavee often initially experiences anxiety, depression and/or rage. Over time, these feeling states typically reverse; the leaver may begin to feel guilt or increased ambivalence over his/her decision and the leavee may feel some relief and a heightened sense of mastery over having survived a psychologically painful experience.

The differential *initial* affective response to the fact of separation/divorce, however, strongly affects decision making by the couple. It is more likely that the leavee will want to continue therapy, partly as a result of his/her greater psychological pain. The most common issue regarding treatment following a separation/divorce decision is whether the one spouse will continue in therapy with the original family therapist or seek a new, different therapist with whom to begin individual therapy. There are good arguments both for staying and for switching. The present author believes the critical factor to be that of the original therapist's feelings toward the outcome of family therapy, namely the decision to dissolve the marriage.

If the therapist's treatment goal was helping the couple to stay together, and he/she feels a sense of failure in this regard, it is likely such countertransferential feelings will carry over in continued contacts with one or both spouses. The therapist's feelings of failure can easily compound the spouses' perception of having failed in the marriage. A negative synergy can then result between therapist and clients. This compounding can happen at the very time when therapy might be most useful in helping one or both clients to work through their feelings of failure and its common accompanist, guilt.

The sense of failure is often a subtle one for the therapist. Anyone who works therapeutically with couples realizes that many will or have already decided (perhaps covertly) to get a divorce. For a couple that comes to the therapist with the expressed purpose of help with the divorcing process, the potential for the therapist to a sense of failure is diminished. This is also generally the case when the decision is made early in the course of marital or family therapy. However, when (a) the couple comes to therapy with the desire to enhance their relationship and (b) therapy proceeds along these lines for more than a few sessions, the potential is increased for the therapist to have a sense of failure when a subsequent decision to separate and/or divorce is made.

In such instances, the therapist needs to examine carefully and work through his/her own feelings of failure before proceeding to treat one or both individuals in continued therapy.

Another risk of post-family therapy individual treatment of one spouse with the same therapist occurs because the therapist may come to be perceived as the ally of that spouse. This can cause problems if the couple express a wish to renew conjoint sessions, either to work through issues in the divorce process (e.g., custody or financial arrangements) or to explore a reconciliation. It is important to explore carefully any feelings on the part of the spouse who has not been in individual treatment toward the other spouse's individual therapy experience. If there are ambivalent or negative feelings, two modes of remedy are possible. The therapist may wish to meet with the (second) spouse for one or more individual sessions to help provide a more equitable situation vis-à-vis the individual treatment experience with the therapist, or a cotherapy format may be suggested, with the cotherapist available to be perceived (at least potentially) as an ally of the second spouse. The latter solution is a more natural one if the family was in cotherapy originally, in which case the original cotherapist would then rejoin treatment. However, an "agreeable" cotherapist may not be available or the financial consideration of paying for two therapists may work against the feasibility of cotherapy as a solution.

Despite the risks and problems elaborated above, the present author generally favors offering an opportunity for continued individual treatment for one or both spouses with the same family therapist. (It is a more difficult task therapeutically if both individuals want continued individual therapy but, as noted above, usually only one spouse is desirous of this option.) If one or both spouses are desirous of continuing, the main rationale in support of this option with the same therapist is "don't switch horses in midstream." The family therapist is familiar with the spouse and his/her experience and, hopefully, a therapeutic alliance (Smith and Grunebaum, 1976) has been established that will lead to a more efficient continuing of individual therapeutic work. The offering of this continuing treatment option implies, of course, that the therapist sees him/herself as comfortable working in both the family and individual therapy modes, with their somewhat different goals and areas of emphasis (Rice, 1977).

References

Rice, D. G. Psychotherapeutic treatment of narcissistic injury in marital separation and divorce. *Journal of Divorce*, 1977, *1*, 119-128.

Smith, J. W. & Grunebaum, H. The therapeutic alliance in marital therapy. In H. Grunebaum and J. Christ (Eds.), *Contemporary Marriage: Structure, Dynamics, and Therapy*. Boston: Little, Brown, 1976.

Toomim, M. Structured separation with counseling: A therapeutic approach for couples in conflict. *Family Process*, 1972, *11*, 299-310.

DAVID G. RICE, Ph.D.
Professor
Department of Psychiatry
University of Wisconsin
Medical School
Madison, WI

59. Transition From Marital Therapy to Divorce Adjustment Therapy

Question:

I am concerned about marital therapy in which divorce looms as the probable outcome for a couple. Many couples come into therapy as a "last-ditch" effort to save the marriage. As a therapist, I try to help them see and evaluate all their options and deal with their feelings about these so that they can make choices they understand. A couple will often choose initially to work on the marriage and invest a certain amount of energy in this choice. If, however, they subsequently decide on divorce, they often terminate therapy, perhaps feeling that they can negotiate this option alone or that they cannot afford further therapy. I have concerns about how such couples approach divorce, especially when children are involved or when it seems one or both of the clients need continued therapy. Do you have any suggestions about the therapist's role and responsibility in this kind of situation, or techniques for motivating clients to focus on the divorce adjustment process that they will soon be in?

Discussion:

The problem you raise is confronted by many family therapists. Dealing with it is complicated by several factors: the therapist's own values regarding divorce, the therapist's feelings about the couple and their efforts in marital therapy, and, most importantly, the therapist's degree of clarity regarding the professional's helping function when divorce becomes the choice.

The question of personal and professional values around divorce is one that the therapist must constantly scrutinize. Is there a tendency to see divorce as a sign of personal failure or as the failure of the therapist to help enough? Does the therapist hold a balanced view of the divorce process, seeing it as no panacea, but as the difficult, painful, yet potentially growth-producing process that may be the healthy choice for some persons? In addition to these issues, the therapist's own personal experience with divorce (or lack thereof) can be a factor in how s/he defines the helping function with couples deciding to divorce. These are some of the factors that a therapist must be constantly aware of and evaluate in regard to personal and professional values.

The remainder of this discussion will focus on the role and function of the therapist as the couple moves from working on the marriage to the option of divorce.

The primary task for the therapist is to carry out an immediate assessment of the couple's (and each individual's) ability to acknowledge the divorce decision, to act upon it, and to deal with its aftermath—all this is an adaptive manner. Although the therapist may believe that most clients will need further therapy for the divorce process, a general suggestion to continue in therapy may not be convincing.

When one or both partners indicate their decision to divorce, the therapist should consciously shift focus to start a new assessment of the situation. One should communicate openly and directly about the need to delve further into the decision and its meaning for the couple. The therapist who knows about the divorce process and its impact on people can use this knowledge to explore how clients are likely to meet the crisis and future challenges brought on by the divorce. Although the couple may wish to terminate therapy immediately, the therapist should insist on at least one session after their decision to divorce so that a new assessment and recommendations can be given.

Various techniques are effective in getting the assessment and divorce adjustment therapy underway. The therapist can adapt them to his/her own unique approach to conducting therapy. The following are specific activities that I have found useful:

1) Explore with the couple the reasons for the decision and how they arrived at it. It is critical to determine the extent to which it is a conscious or rationally derived decision as opposed to a gesture or decision by default of one or both partners. In other words, to what extent are they assuming responsibility for the decision?

2) Explore the extent to which both partners want the divorce. They should be helped to verbalize their deepest feelings in all their complexity. This is critical to accepting the divorce decision and being able eventually to move ahead to new goals and purposes. If one partner feels betrayed, coerced or convinced that it is the wrong decision, these feelings need to be dealt with, or they are likely to control that person's future relationship with the ex-spouse, children and even others.

3) Review the actions taken thus far by the couple or individual partners in terms of acting upon the divorce decision. Have they con-

sulted attorneys, has one partner moved out, who has been told what about the decision, e.g., children, relatives, friends, etc.? Exploring these facts is necessary for the therapist to decide how to proceed; the degree of rationality versus emotionality in the couple's actions are critical indicators of their prognosis for adjustment to the divorce.

4) Explore both persons' hopes, fantasies and fears about what divorce means for them as individuals. A technique to get at these is to ask the person to close his/her eyes and imagine what life as a divorced person will be like. This should be presented in an open-ended manner at first, but the client may need encouragement to consider both positive, neutral and negative aspects of this projected image. What the client produces, in conjunction with what the partner produces, will also be important data for assessing the person's abilities to cope with the divorce process. Obviously, as these kinds of data begin to emerge, not only is assessment underway, but also the divorce adjustment process has begun.

5) Focus on the impact of the divorce on the couple's children. They should be asked to explore their feelings about this and then to discuss specifically how they expect to and would like to explain the divorce to their children. Again, initially the therapist should approach this topic with an open-ended question, but should probe for details—who is going to tell whom what, when, where, under what circumstances. As clients confront the reality of these details in therapy, they will have to come to terms with some of the most painful aspects of divorce. Through this confrontation, they will express their feelings and degree of understanding of the tasks that lie ahead of them; in so doing, they will reveal to themselves and the therapist their abilities to cope with the problems in an adaptive manner.

6) Share knowledge, as needed and appropriate, with clients about typical reactions people experience in the divorce process as well as guidelines for dealing with the crisis. When children are involved, the therapist should also use this opportunity to assume a proactive stance relative to their welfare and healthy adaptation to the divorce process (Woody, 1978). The couple's interactions during the divorce process and afterwards and the quality of their continuing relationship with their children will probably be the most important variable in the adjustment of the children to the divorce. Concern about the welfare of the children is likely to be a pressing issue for couples with children. The therapist has the responsibility to assess the partners' abilities to face the issue in all its complexity and to begin to help them find ways of dealing with it in a healthy manner.

7) Bring up other realities of the divorce process that couples often

avoid in the early stages or approach in an irrational manner. For example, some partners do not want to deal with the reality of the economic issue, saying instead: "I don't care how the money or property is divided. I just want out!" The facts are, however, that these issues become important during the divorce process and are often a source of continuing hostilities among postdivorce families. Partners need to verbalize and explore their feelings about money, property, personal possessions, and how much agreement they can reach together and how much will be negotiated by their respective attorneys. It is irrational and maladaptive for a person not to care about his/her future welfare and economic security or to approach these issues in a haphazard manner. Although feelings of helplessness or not caring may be common during the early stages of arriving at the divorce decision, the therapist should help clients assess their ability to act on the decision in a rational manner.

8) Share the assessment regarding each partner's abilities to cope with and adjust to the expected divorce process. Since the therapist has helped the clients deal with specific divorce issues, the conclusions and recommendations will be meaningful and convincing. Although it is acknowledged that powerful feelings of loss, sadness, hopelessness and a certain degree of irrationality are to be expected, the therapist should continue to emphasize that healthy adaptation and future growth for both adults and children will hinge on working through these feelings and moving into acceptance and rational planning for future goals. Continued therapy is often indicated to help clients reach this stage.

Reference

Woody, J. D. Preventive intervention for children of divorce. *Social Casework*, 1978, *59*, 537-544.

JANE D. WOODY, Ph.D., M.S.W.
Associate Professor
School of Social Work
University of Nebraska
Omaha, NB

60. The Unit of Treatment in Divorce Therapy

Question:

Although I understand there is impressive evidence that conjoint marital therapy is more effective than individual marital therapy, I've heard it said that individual treatment is best for divorce therapy. What is the best unit of treatment for persons who have decided to end their marriages vs. those wanting to improve them?

Discussion:

Since divorce therapy is a relatively new subspeciality, we hope you won't be too disappointed to hear that there is no definitive answer to your question. We have found no published research which specifically compares individual and conjoint forms of *divorce* therapy.

From a theoretical and practical standpoint, we think there is certainly something to be said for individual treatment, particularly after a definitive decision to divorce has been made. Since some of the most important goals for divorcing persons are the development of a separate identity, self-esteem, and an autonomous life style, individual sessions may be most facilitative. Conjoint sessions have the potential of allowing couples to remain inappropriately attached and nurturing reconciliation fantasies in the persons who oppose the divorce. These persons, many therapists argue, need individual attention to help them cope with rejection and give up their "investment" in a relationship from which there is no "return." Likewise, the "leaver" needs personal attention to work through guilt and overresponsibility for the other party.

Two studies are most frequently cited to support these popular notions. Cookerly (1973) investigated the records of 773 former marriage counseling clients who had been seen for at least three sessions by one of 21 therapists. Cases were coded as divorced with "poor," "moderate," or "good" outcomes; or married with "poor," "moderate" or "good" outcomes. Individual and conjoint counseling were compared along with concurrent and group approaches. Cookerly's most striking finding was that conjoint (couple) interviews achieved the best outcome for those remaining married but had the *worst* record for those obtaining divorces. Individual therapy was ranked second only to conjoint (couples) group therapy as leading to best outcomes for the divorced clients.

The massive Family Service Association (Beck and Jones, 1973) follow-up of cases seen at member agencies demonstrated once again the superiority of conjoint over individual therapy for marriage counseling. However, Beck (1976) went on to point out that these findings applied only to intact families. Among a subsample of separated couples, change scores were strikingly higher for individual than conjoint interviews. Beck interpreted these results to mean that ". . . once separation has occurred, the partners need the one-to-one-relationship with the counselor to sort out, cope with, and integrate the traumas and anxieties stemming from the separation experience" (p. 440).

We personally believe, however, these studies have had more influence than they merit on the question of the unit of treatment in divorce therapy. In the first place, they have some serious methodological limitations. Cookerly's investigation was a retrospective analysis of client records at one private practice agency. There were no controls for such important factors as age of client or therapist, type or severity of problem, level of therapist experience or theoretical orientation of therapist. By Cookerly's (1976) own admission, the study is best thought of as only a pilot study. The Beck study was also retrospective and there was no random assignment to treatments or control for therapist variables. Although the overall sample was quite large, the specific comparison of separated couples receiving individual versus conjoint treatment was based on a very small sample. In fact, only six separated couples were in the group receiving conjoint treatment.

But perhaps more significant for this question is the fact that there is no evidence that either study investigated couples who were participating in divorce therapy *per se*. The available methodological details suggest that the clients were individuals and couples receiving marriage counseling who were separated and/or went on to divorce. Hence, it is not implausible that factors like frustration and disappointment contaminated the results. If, for example, a person wants to save his/her marriage and his/her partner wants out, conjoint therapy (for reasons I already mentioned) may be frustrating for both. In addition, self-selection may have been involved. Persons trying to hold on to their partners may have pushed hard for conjoint sessions thereby making the method appear to be the source of the unsatisfying results rather than the persons who chose it. Remember, there was no random assignment in these studies and therefore alternative explanations abound.

Interestingly, Cookerly (1976) did another study at the same agency which gives a different slant to his original finding. A mail questionnaire was responded to by 117 former clients, who had not received subsequent counseling for one to three years. On the criterion of remaining married, the most successful form of therapy was the conjoint interview (63%) and the second to least successful (of six forms of therapy) was the individual interview (45%). An earlier study by Graham (1968) in a conciliation court setting also found conjoint counseling superior on the reconciliation criterion—in this case to a combination of individual and conjoint sessions as well as to a randomly assigned control group. We are left with the odd situation, then, where a form of therapy deemed questionable for people who go on to divorce appears to be the best divorce preventative. These results are not necessarily contradictory, but they do point out the need for a careful weighing of just what is being measured in these studies.

Previous research is of limited value, then, not only because of its methodological weakness but also because it does not test divorce therapy. As Brown (1976) reminds us, it ". . . differs from marriage counseling in that it does not focus on improving the husband-wife relationship; but on decreasing the functions of that relationship with the goal of eventual dissolution of that relationship" (p. 410). And, as Gurman and Kniskern rightly point out, "Conciliation is not equivalent to reconciliation nor does divorce necessarily constitute evidence of ineffective therapy" (1978, p. 881). Studies of marriage counseling or of divorce *prevention* offer at best, indirect, and at worst, misleading evidence.

What, then, would we suggest in the absence of definitive research?

1) First, recognize that divorce is a process that proceeds in stages and that different units of treatment may be more appropriate at certain times. We demarcate three stages and use *primarily* conjoint sessions in the first, individual sessions in the third, and a balance of the two in the second stage if the parties are willing.

There seems to be the least debate in the literature about the value of conjoint sessions during the time prior to at least one partner making a firm resolve to divorce. It seems reasonable to label therapy before this point as "marital evaluation" and conjoint sessions will be enormously valuable for some of the same reasons they are the treatment of choice for marriage counseling. The therapist can assess interactional patterns and their responsiveness to change as well as the partner's level of caring and commitment to the relationship. If it becomes apparent that one person wants a divorce, it may be necessary for the therapist to "orchestrate" (Kressel & Deutsch, 1977) the other's motive to divorce. This may be done through an honest (yet hopefully caring) confrontation between the partners. The emphasis on conjoint sessions here, of course, doesn't preclude individual sessions (for example, to help the partner who is "left" avoid "pursuit" or "doormat" behavior).

The second stage (and the stages may overlap) centers on the tasks of working out separate living, financial, child management and social arrangements, as well as the legal aspect of divorce. Here, the use of conjoint sessions is more controversial. Some therapists believe it works against the goal of autonomy, and others think it entails something for which they feel unqualified or do not like—the mediation of divorce settlements (Kressel & Deutsch, 1977).

If both clients are willing to stay in therapy (persons primarily hoping the therapist will save their marriage often drop out when this hope vanishes), we think sensitive conjoint work can have significant benefits. It can facilitate the timing and arrangements for separation, blunt the impact of the adversary process through helping the couple negotiate as much of their own settlement as possible and hence have a sense of "ownership" of it; provide an opportunity to gain an understanding of what was not working in the relationship; and perhaps most importantly, offer a setting where the couple can deal with unresolved feelings. These will include not only anger, disappointment and grief, but also appreciation for what was good in the relationship. Ongoing disputes over such issues as finances, custody and visitation are often convenient disguises for the couple's failure to say good-by.

The final stage of the divorce process, the long term growth and recovery phase that follows separation and/or litigation, most often centers on issues like coping with loneliness, regaining self-confidence, and rebuilding social relationships that are dealt with individually. Of course, ongoing issues regarding children may suggest couple or family sessions. In a controlled study, Margolin (1973), for example, showed rather dramatically the value of conjoint sessions when problems of visitation arise.

2) Recognize that divorces, like marriages, vary enormously. If a couple have no children, a good understanding of the dynamics of their relationship, and share equally in the desire to terminate it, the value of conjoint sessions is minimized considerably—especially if the marriage was brief and of the parallel rather than the passionate variety.

Where there are children involved, an expanded treatment unit is most essential. Divorce does not end families but only changes their form. The only real choice ex-spouses (as parents) have concerns the quality (not the existence) of their relationship. The significance of this relationship will only be magnified as joint custody arrangements become more popular and encouraged by law (as was recently done in California). We always include the children in some sessions to minimize their fears, assure them of their parents' ongoing love, and facilitate the transition to new living arrangements. We work hard to get the kids' trust and maintain an "open phone" as well as "open door" policy for future contact. Usually the time following their parents' disclosure of separation is most crucial, but family sessions even well after the divorce are useful if their adjustment is not good or problems, such as visitation, arise.

Before winding up we might mention that what little evidence we have suggests that most of the good things we've said about conjoint (couple) divorce therapy may also apply to couples group divorce therapy. Intergenerational and social network approaches also make theoretical sense but there is no formal evidence.

We'll close by modifying Paul's (1967) famous dictum. We hope we will one day have better evidence to say what treatment unit is best for which divorcing couples under these particular sets of circumstances.

References

Beck, D. F. Research findings on the outcome of marital counseling. In D. H. Olson (Ed.), *Treating Relationships*. Lake Mills, Iowa: Graphic Publishing, 1976.

Beck, D. F. and Jones, M. A. *Progress on Family Problems: A Nationwide Study of Clients' and Counselors' Views on Family Agency Services*. New York: Family Service Association of America, 1973.

Brown, E. M. Divorce counseling. In D. H. Olson (Ed.) *Treating Relationships*. Lake Mills, Iowa: Graphic Publishing, 1976.

Cookerly, J. R. The outcome of the six major forms of marriage counseling compared: A pilot study. *Journal of Marriage and the Family*, 1973, *35*, 608-612.

Cookerly, J. R. Evaluating different approaches to marriage counseling. In D. H. Olson (Ed.) *Treating Relationships*. Lake Mills, Iowa: Graphic Publishing, 1976.

Graham, J. A. The effect of the use of counselor positive responses to positive perceptions of mate in marriage counseling. *Dissertation Abstracts International*, 1968, 28, 3504A.

Gurman, A. S. and Kniskern, D. P. Research on marital and family therapy: Progress, perspective, and prospect. In S. L. Garfield and A. E. Bergin (Eds.), *Handbook of Psychotherapy and Behavior Change: An Empirical Analysis* (Second Edition). New York: Wiley, 1978.

Kressel, K. and Deutsch, M. Divorce therapy: An in-depth survey of therapists' views. *Family Process*, 1977, *16*, 413-443.

Margolin, F. M. *An approach to resolution of visitation disputes post-divorce: Short term counseling*. Unpublished doctoral dissertation, United States International University, 1973.

Paul, G. Strategy of outcome research in psychotherapy. *Journal of Consulting and Clinical Psychology,* 1967, *31,* 109-118.

DOUGLAS H. SPRENKLE, Ph.D.
*Associate Professor of Marriage
and Family Counseling
Department of Child Development
and Family Studies
Purdue University*

and

CHERYL STORM, M.A.
*Ph.D. Candidate
Department of Child Development
and Family Studies
Purdue University
West Lafayette, IN*

61. Guidelines for Separation Counseling

Question:

As a marital therapist, one of the most difficult types of couples for me are those who are angry with each other and who separate two or three times, or more, during the course of counseling. Often therapy is disrupted during this splitting up process and all gains seem to be lost. I want to treat these couples with respect, high regard for their intellect and trust in their ability to grow in therapy, but they don't seem to respond. Although intelligent people, they don't seem to use their heads. Unconditional regard seems to go right by them and is lost somewhere in their emotional needs, apparently to be in conflict with spouse. They run out and have affairs during the separation, they go home to parents, or they retreat into depression of some sort. Can you suggest some guidelines to help me be more successful with these couples?

Discussion:

I spent nearly 20 years struggling with this problem before discovering a method that couples could profit from rather immensely. This method also freed me from the emotional binds I found myself in when trying to help these people "the old way."

First, I realized that in the last 50 years our society had developed in much of its married population what I call the *Ladies Home Journal* mentality, namely that togetherness of couples is the preferred ideal and that separateness is a "no-no." The rest of the world recognizes that marriage is only one part of life, a rather realistic part of it at that. To be apart during stretches in the marriage does not mean that romance is gone; in fact, separateness can enhance romance, while too much togetherness can kill romance. Separating couples, then, need to be reminded that spending time apart for a while could be the best thing that they could do for their marriage.

Second, I realized that these couples were separating repeatedly but were not getting the good out of it, because they were separating out of rage, anger, disappointment and other primitive emotional reactions. They were both feeling guilty about it and so was everybody else—all the laws, in-laws, and outlaws—so all the irrational emotional processes in the system were pushing them back together again. Emotions ruled, reason had no chance to operate, and personal, family and social guilt forced them back together again—too soon.

Third, nobody was paying attention to individual differences, to the fact that people vary in the amount of time they want or need to be alone and in the amount of time each person could spend in the presence of another without feeling a need for distance.

Fourth, I realized that couples who characteristically used separating as a means of managing marriage problems were:

(a) usually immature personalities—what Bowen refers to as lower level of differentiated self;
(b) using emotional reactions as a way of life rather than using their heads to solve any marital issues;
(c) using separation as a means of either getting their way in the marriage or of proving the partner wrong;
(d) using going home as a means of obtaining temporary relief from the rational demands of living with a spouse and/or children under adult/demand conditions (when they were too immature to take it);
(e) repeatedly separating (and feeling guilty about it) for years; and
(f) finally, they wound up divorcing only when one or both got tired of the separating process *and* when they found someone they thought they would just never separate from—they were so in love!

Fifth, over the years it appeared to me that couples were going through separations in much the same ways. It was as if they had talked with each other and were following the same rules. They were making the same mistakes:

(a) They separated in anger and they stayed mad at each other, as if this were the only way to separate. This is fusion, in Bowen's terms, and represents a low level of differentiation of self.
(b) They often "went home to mother" who welcomed the opportunity to shield them from a cruel spouse (fusion), or they avoided any contact with the family of origin for a variety of reasons (emotional cut off).
(c) The separation was usually only partial, in that they were in contact all the time through phone calls, letters, notes, messages sent through the children, family, friends, attorneys, counselors or whoever would cooperate with the triangling process.

(d) They often took the opportunity to develop or to exploit an affair of the heart or go full bore into a sexual affair, thus avoiding differentiation of a self.
(e) They stayed busy, running from one thing to another, getting no satisfaction from the new activities, or they stayed home and moped, blaming the spouse.
(f) They either talked to everyone or no one about what was happening, resolving nothing because, for one thing, everyone's advice was different. Nothing worked.
(g) They spent most of their time in counseling talking about the separation and the marriage, but spent little time dealing with themselves and their contribution to the failures in the relationship.
(h) And always, they went back together too soon—before problems were resolved.

In time, it became apparent, due to partial successes (and sometimes complete successes) in some of my clients who would listen to my sense of direction in some of these matters, that as a marriage counselor I needed a plan, a full-scale plan. I needed to become a separation counselor, if you will. I had to believe that separation for some couples is a necessity and a good thing—an opportunity for personal and marital growth. Some couples had simply had too much of each other; some people need a good deal of distance between self and spouse.

These separating couples had a great deal of unfinished business with their families of origin and each spouse could benefit from some kind of "going home." They had brought too much of the emotional "junk" from their own families and expected their spouses to accept it lock, stock and barrel.

The Plan

The separating couples should be separated completely. That means they should not be in contact during the separation. To be in contact in *any* way is to vitiate the reasons for separation and the psychological work that needs to be done during that time.

They need to spend time alone, (a) thinking about themselves and how they contributed to their problems, and (b) learning how to change themselves and their own goals in line with what is important in life: What do I really want and what price do I wish to pay for it? Do I really wish to be married to this person and he/she to me?

Armed with experience and with these concepts, I developed a plan for separation counseling. There are several steps, each of them probably equally important theoretically and not to be skipped over by the counselor or client without running the risk of failure.

1) This is an educational plan, so the entire plan is explained to the clients. What the counselor knows, clients can learn. They are given this *Discussion* to read.
2) Only one spouse need agree to the plan for it to work, but it is obviously best to have the full cooperation of both spouses.
3) As a rule and ideally, couples need about three months of complete separation for the plan to work well. Any less time is a compromise to emotion and tends to defeat the purposes of working through some of the vital issues of leaving home and assuming the roles of adult/reasoning person/spouse/parent, etc. The absolute minimum amount of time for young married couples is six weeks, but it crowds everything they are doing too much. Some people can stand on their heads for six weeks and not change at all! One spouse in most couples will object to three months, while the other spouse is more eager for it and can see the reasons for it. The spouse who wants that time has to have it and, one way or another, will get it. I explain the reasons for time and space between them.
4) During this time apart there is absolutely no reason to see each other, visit, make telephone contact, write notes or exchange messages in any way. Only death, fire or flood might bring them together. Otherwise, they are not taking the matter seriously—their emotions are in charge when they violate the command to separate completely. Children, dogs, rent money, etc., can be arranged for without seeing each other. If nothing else works, get an attorney to handle these matters—in which case, predict failure.
5) Have the couple read Bowen's *Family Therapy in Clinical Practice* (1978). This is very important. I like to have them read Chapter 21 first and then Chapter 16. Of course, some people can't or won't read; in those instances I teach Bowen's theory to them, one or two concepts at a time. They are also to use this time apart to learn how to get in touch with their family (of origin) systems and learn how to begin to collect factual information about mother, father, grandparents, other relatives and generations past. Differentiation of self work is begun and it is explained that this is a life-long endeavor. The only rush is to get started.
6) During the separation, they are to spend some time every day alone, preferably over half an hour. An hour or more is better. Ideally, they should lie on the floor on their backs with doors closed, no

noises, no radio, no T.V., no company, no one; only their own thoughts, thinking about how to make life (including marriage) better. Most of these people have spent very little, if any, time alone with time to think. They have lived off their emotional reactions to others all their lives.

7) They are to cease and desist all "outside" relationships during this time. The same binding rules under 3) and 4) above must apply to any and all other sex interests. No dating, no lunches, no dinners, no sex, no affairs *during this time.* These detract from the task at hand. When a spouse will not do this for six weeks to three months, there isn't much of a personal reason to continue the marriage. Toomim (1975) disagrees and recommends dating others during separation, but that is like trying to get a person to learn to eat straw while feeding him/her champagne and caviar. Many clients like that kind of advice, but it can only emotionally complicate an otherwise emotionally complicated relationship. Couples who have followed my direction in this invariably tell me that they learned as much about themselves from giving up the "other" as from following the rest of the plan. Some of them, on the other hand, have made the decision to divorce and marry the "other." This was done with decisiveness and in a more rational and straightforward way than they had thought possible, once they followed the plan of total separation.

In system terms, separation demands mean that a new balance is being signaled—positive feedback. One partner usually "loves" more than the other and holds on with some desperation. Both can often tolerate a time-limited separation with some counseling, even perhaps a great deal of counseling. Like divorce counseling, separation counseling is a form of crisis counseling, in which case the counselor assumes more authority and a greater leadership role in structuring the separation.

Total Separation

The philosophy of Total Separation is based on the beliefs that a) couples who separate almost always go back together too soon; b) the lack of understanding of the causes of the separation must be faced by the one who doesn't want the separation if the marriage is to work; and c) some individuation in the pair leads to a stronger relationship.

The partners are asked to participate in a series of mini-contracts which spell out the terms of the Total Separation. They are asked to:

1) agree to counseling regardless of how the relationship goes;
2) agree not to see each other for at least six weeks or longer;
3) agree not to communicate with each other in any form for the duration of the Total Separation;
4) develop separate relationships with the children;
5) agree to tell their children separately about the Total Separation (frankness is the best policy);
6) disrupt the children's lives as little as possible;
7) agree to write (journal style) daily about their relationship and how the writer contributes to its failure;
8) agree to take responsibility for how the relationship developed from the beginning;
9) agree to see the counselor about once a week during the Total Separation in order to evaluate and estimate how best to make the marriage work. During sessions the counselor focuses on: (a) personal growth needs (differentiation of a self) vs. (b) relationship adjustment needs, and, (c) minimally, the couple's reactions to the separation.
10) agree not to form, or attempt to form, outside affectional or sexual relationships. These can only confuse and confound what is going on in the primary relationship. Before the Total Separation they are encouraged to express and to explore fears of affairs and other relationships. They agree to learn to stand on their own feet and to become more responsible for themselves as individuals.

Partial Separation

When the Total Separation is over and both agree, then they can go to a Partial Separation as follows:

1) They agree to date each other, i.e., meet on neutral ground, such as a restaurant or park, for a talk and just for fun.
2) When anxiety (tension) runs high, either can leave (distance) any time without fault or feelings of guilt.
3) They can get together with the children every week or so for a few hours.
4) They continue the "no sex" rule during at least the first week of Partial Separation.
5) Sex by mutual agreement after first week—but not required. Sex adjustment counseling may be indicated at this time, but probably not before.
6) Normally the Partial Separation should be about six weeks.

7) The second week of Partial Separation and weekly thereafter, a problem-solving date is advisable to discuss matters such as finances or children's needs. "Talk it over rationally" is learned.

8) The second to fourth week can include a fun date. Of course, it can also be awkward, unless one or both partners deliberately takes the lead and/or the responsibility for its success.

9) Remember, most couples go back to living together too soon! The reluctant spouse must be the guide as to how long the separation will be.

10) Separation can cause shock reactions for weeks, even months. There are various emotional and physical reaction symptoms as in any loss. Emotional reactions are likely to occur in cycles.

11) They should make good use of nutrition, sleep, exercise and fantasy along with the daily journal writing.

12) It is a good idea to write all kinds of poetry.

13) They must avoid drinking, pills or other excesses which only delay focusing on the problems inherent in the separation and in the relationship.

In separation counseling, the counselor must have a sound rationale and a definite plan for action; otherwise, the counseling is likely to drift, wander and deteriorate into failure. When the counselor is confident of his/her approach, clients tend to respond very well.

References

Bowen, M. *Family Therapy in Clinical Practice*. New York: Jason Aronson, 1978.
Toomim, M. Structured separation for couples in conflict. In A. Gurman and D. Rice (Eds.), *Couples in Conflict*. New York: Aronson, 1975.

CLINTON E. PHILLIPS, Ph.D.
Director
California Family Study Center
Burbank, CA

62. Dissolution of Homosexual Relationships

Question:

In the past few years many homosexuals have come out of the closet, to such an extent that they have become an identifiable group of society and are beginning to be visible in all the aspects of society which are familiar to heterosexuals. The services of marriage and family therapists are in great demand among heterosexuals, therefore, it is expected that homosexuals will begin seeking the services of marriage therapists when discord develops in their relationships. I am a marriage, family, child counselor who has been in practice five years. I have attended several workshops and seminars on human sexuality. The subject of homosexuality has been introduced in the educational settings; however, no attention has been paid to counseling homosexuals for "marital discord." My question is whether there is a difference between counseling homosexuals and heterosexuals for marital discord and, if there is a difference, what are the best available approaches to counseling homosexuals whose relationships are dissolving?

Discussion:

Whether homosexual or heterosexual, the cause for the breakup of couples can usually be traced to several general reasons. The manifest problems which breaking up couples cite merely describe their particular circumstances and would not be significant in the absence of fundamental deficiencies in the relationship. The most common of these deficiencies is the lack of effective communication, which includes no, or a limited amount of, dialogue or a generous amount of dialogue without frank or genuine expression of feeling.

Lack of communication permits the second general cause for the breakup of unities and marriages, which is manifest when the action of one mate or spouse causes important principles of the other to be violated. The principle is important when the violation causes visceral change. For example, when being on time is an important value to one mate to such an extent that being late causes internal physical discomfort, the other mate's continual lack of promptness will cause marital discord. Moreover, if the first spouse has failed to communicate the degree of his or her feeling about punctuality, the other is likely to be late and thus bring about the circumstances of marital or unital unhappiness.

When a unity or marriage is built upon transient factors, the third most common cause for discord and breakup is inherent. Such factors include qualities which are of themselves temporary in nature, such as occupational position, as well as qualities which are held in temporary esteem by the individual. Lasting relationships are those built on viable qualities such as mutual appreciation of values, self-respect, friendship and individual autonomy in the pursuit of mutual goals and interests.

The parasitical nature of many close interpersonal relationships helps explain a problem commonly encountered in therapy, which is the client's inconsistency in describing the mate in vicious terms on the one hand and affirming his or her desire for the mate on the other hand. In a parasitical relationship, at least one of the participants feels incomplete without the other. The dependent individual has a poor self-concept, is unaware of his or her own stimulus value, and is overly concerned about the mate's opinion and feelings about her or him. When a breakup occurs, whether between homosexuals or heterosexuals, the individual who feels abused defends his or her ego by derogating the mate. The victimized heterosexual describes the mate as the perpetrator of all the negative attributes of the opposite sex; whereas, the victimized homosexual describes the mate according to the negative stereotypes of homosexuals, i.e., he or she is abnormal and cannot be trusted. In this manner, the client justifies on a conscious level why he or she is fortunate to be rid of the mate. Like scratching an itch, however, this maneuver is comforting at first, but soon begins to hurt. As the parasitical individual consciously continues to villainize the mate, he or she subconsciously feeds the importance which the mate occupies in his or her thoughts and thereby reinforces the parasitical need for the mate. The main difference between homosexuals and heterosexuals in this regard is the greater intensity of manifestation among homosexuals and the projection of negative attitudes about homosexuality onto the mate.

An important distinction pertaining to homosexual and heterosexual breakups is that the homosexual has an ambiguous attitude toward homosexuality. There is usually an emotional acceptance of the negative stereotypes about homosexuality and an academic acceptance of the right to sexual preference. When a breakup occurs, the balance of these feelings is upset and the victimized mate views him- or herself from the academic point of view while the mate is viewed from the emotional point of view. Consequently, the homosexual has a complexity of weapons to use against the mate. He or she has all the arguments which heterosexuals usually apply to the opposite sex as well as the prejudices which heterosexuals have about homosexuality. The crisis of the breakup will invariably involve a crisis of sexual identity and the therapist must deal with conflicting attitudes toward homosexuality as well as inappropriate attitudes toward the mate.

Before venturing to approach therapy, there are several preliminary do's and don't's. The first word of caution is to the therapist who does not feel comfortable with homosexuality. He or she is advised to refer a homosexual client to another therapist, for polite toleration is easily unmasked. At the time of a breakup, the homosexual is more acutely aware of the negative connotations of homosexuality than at any other time. If the client detects insincerity on the part of the therapist, his or her ability to seek help from a qualified therapist is adversely affected and guilt feelings about homosexuality are reinforced. Part and parcel of the first precaution is the second, that the therapist should not use the therapy session as a forum for research or for gaining personal enlightenment about homosexuality, so that the client does not feel like an abnormality to be studied and cured. Third, in talking with homosexual clients, the therapist is advised to try to understand the client's feeling about terminology such as "marriage" and "mate." Attitudes among homosexuals about the use of heterosexual nomenclature vary but are usually intense, and the therapist must learn to think in the language of homosexuality. Fourth, the therapist is cautioned against rationalizing the homosexual breakup by the absence of those elements which are supposed to support long-lasting heterosexual marriages, such as children, mutual property ownership and legal sanctions. This is not a useful approach to therapy for the homosexual in addition to being invalid as a basis for maintaining heterosexual marriages. Finally, the therapist should keep in mind that the client is not seeking reversal of his or her sexual orientation; therefore, therapy should be focused upon the problem for which the client is seeking counseling.

Therapy is directed toward helping the individual examine his or her feelings about self, with the ultimate objective of helping the client become an independent free agent. Once the therapist has determined whether a parasitical relationship exists and, if so, the role of the client in the parasite-host dynamic, he or she should then ascertain the client's perception of the problem and help the client examine the validity of that perception. The next step is helping the client to develop alternative solutions to the problem and to choose the alternative appropriate for his or her current circumstances. The latter phase is not as simple as it might appear because the homosexual will frequently articulate what is academically appropriate, including those conditions which heterosexuals claim strengthen family ties. In other words, if the homosexual poses impossible solutions, such as, "if we had children," the therapist must lead the client away from these obstacles toward functioning within the reality of homosexuality.

In those cases where the client and the mate wish to work out their differences, the mate should be interviewed to ascertain his or her perceptions and attitudes toward the client and the relationship. This is effectively done using the Taylor-Johnson Temperament Analysis, the criss-cross evaluation in particular. Although not a diagnostic tool for marital discord, the Taylor-Johnson profile is a useful inventory for comparing and contrasting the individuals' perceptions of themselves and of each other. It is also useful as a catalyst for opening dialogue between mates in a relatively threat-free situation similar to that of a table game. The results of the interview and Taylor-Johnson analysis will help the therapist determine if in-depth evaluation is needed, using an instrument such as the MMPI. The therapist should be cautious, however, in interpreting the MMPI results since homosexuals tend to score higher on the schizophrenic scale than the general population.

When breakup is inevitable, three problems which require therapeutic intervention usually ensue. First is the client's concern with what other people will think. A frequent complaint is, "People will think there's something wrong with me that I can't keep my mate." There is also the client's wish to "show up" the mate as verbalized in, "I'd like to see his face next year after he's fallen flat on his face and I'm living in clover with a new mate." The therapist's task is to help the client incorporate as a part of his or her personality an attitude of, "so what and who cares" in response to these kinds of concerns about what people might think.

The second problem associated with breakup is the tendency of clients to retell their dilemma over and over again to both friends and enemies. Friends who are sympathetic at the first telling are eventually alienated by the unvarying sad theme. The client should be advised to take his or her troubles to the therapist rather than to friends and, if there is something he or she cannot wait to say, write it down in a note to the therapist which may be mailed or held until the next session. Third, therapy must deal with the hate syndrome, which the client uses to relieve the pain of depressive neurotic feeling. The analgesic effect lasts only as long as the hate can be maintained, which is not as long as a lifetime. Helping the client learn to live with the pain of the loss of a loved one fortifies him or her for similar situations which might occur in the future and removes the need for the client to consult a therapist each time there is a disappointment in his or her life. To combat the hate syndrome, the therapist should help the client accept that the mate was inappropriate for him or her but may be ideal for another person, in a positive sense.

References

Baisden, M. J. *The World of Rosaphrenia: The Sexual Psychology of the Female.* Sacramento: Allied Research Society, Inc., 1971.

Baisden, M. J. *The Dynamics of Homosexuality.* Sacramento: Allied Research Society, Inc., 1975.

Baisden, M. and Baisden, J. A profile of women who seek counseling for sexual dysfunction, *The American Journal of Family Therapy*, Spring, 1979, vol. 7, pp. 68-76.

MAJOR J. BAISDEN, JR., Ph.D.
Co-Director, Allied Counseling Center
M. Div. Program, SFTS
San Anselmo, CA

63. Family Systems Theory and Child Custody Determinations

Question:

What contribution can family systems theory and therapy make to child custody determinations?

Discussion:

Child custody determinations can be among the most highly emotional events in family life. Although many such determinations are arrived at amicably with or without legal and mental health professional intervention, many do become bitter disputes. In the bitter disputes, the unresolved emotional attachment in the marital dyad becomes focused on the custody of the child. This struggle for continued attachment to a child can absorb unresolved feelings of anger, guilt, resentment and depression regarding the dissolution of the marriage. The intrafamilial, adversarial process can extend beyond family boundaries to include social friends as well as the legal and mental health professions.

Partially because of the lack of family law theory and the constraints of the legal canon of ethics to represent only one client in the proceedings, the legal profession traditionally deals with these custody disputes and questions in an adversarial manner. A mental health professional who offers an opinion regarding one side or the other in these disputes does little to reduce the adversarial nature of the proceedings and possibly fosters the lack of resolution of the attachment in the marriage. A theoretical approach which focuses only on individual psychological functioning will likely foster one side to the exclusion of another. A family systems approach which emphasizes balanced mutuality in family relationships is most likely to promote intergenerational continuity and resolution in relationships.

A family systems approach to child custody disputes acknowledges that children are part of an emotional universe that comprises not only parents and children but also grandparents, aunts and uncles. Divorce and custody disputes are considered part of a developmental change in the family in which the marital relationship recedes but the parental relationship continues. Although these marital dissolutions can be highly conflictual, experience shows that the more the spouses, rather than the lawyers, do their own negotiations, the more likely a spouse is to adhere to the agreement.

The family systems approach asserts that a child should be placed with that parent who is more likely to grant access of the child to the other parent and to both extended families. This principle is based on the idea that family emotional ties persist beyond divorce and that, specifically for children, emotional ties are retained in fantasy if not reality. Continued contact can help deal with the emotional pain of separation from a parent and can give a child ongoing knowledge about his/her place in the family's history. Additionally, continued contact provides opportunities for balanced reciprocity in a caring parent-child relationship and tends to avoid situations where the child is simply the recipient of parental attention with no opportunity to reciprocate. Therefore, visits should be designed in a manner that allows the child to see the noncustodial parent in the actual role of parent. While it is true that this arrangement has the potential of accentuating divided loyalties in the child, the alternative of little or no contact tends to foster the child's fantasies and encourages the child to adopt the custodial parent's view of the noncustodial parent. In general, the more realistically the child can be helped to appraise his/her situation, the better the child will function.

Good parenting is not defined by a single quality but by a range of capabilities. Moreover, there is no single quality that would exclude a parent as custodian except the case where a parent systematically and in an ongoing way is involved in abuse or neglect of the child. A history of mental illness in a parent does not by itself exclude an individual from being a custodial parent. The view of one parent as unfit must be examined in the context of the entire family relationship system. The critical issue is to what extent an individual's dysfunction influences his/her interaction with the child.

A child's preference, especially an adolescent's, is relevant insofar as each individual within the family is a participant in the decision making process. However, child custody determination is a parental function and should not be abdicated to the point that a child's preference alone determines custody. Leaving such decisions only to children maximizes their loyalty conflicts.

There are a number of service delivery systems that come in contact with divorce and custody related problems. These systems of evaluation and treatment range from public and private clinics to private practitioners to court-connected services to special demonstration projects funded by grants. The majority of these services are oriented to evaluating individuals or the individual within a family context. Few of these services evaluate divorce and custody problems as a family systems phenomenon.

An appropriate intervention model exists in some court-related programs that provide pre-, post- and divorce-related counseling. Custody determinations can then be made as part of the ongoing mental health and legal investigatory process. However, the far more common experience is when a private practitioner or clinic receives a call from a lawyer or perspective patient and is interviewed regarding his/her views on divorce and child custody determination. The essence of this inquiry is for the lawyer or client to determine if the mental health professional will evaluate his/her situation and make a recommendation regarding custody. If the evaluation is favorable regarding custody, the lawyer will use this information to support his/her side of the adversarial proceeding. If the evaluation is unfavorable, he/she is bound by the canon of ethics not to use it, since it would be detrimental to his/her client's chances of winning in the adversarial process. A mental health professional who accepts a referral on this basis may knowingly or unknowingly become a participant in the adversarial process. Declaring an individual to be a fit parent in isolation from the other parent does little more than increase the likelihood that the other parent will obtain a mental health professional to do likewise.

A more appropriate and potentially more objective method of evaluation involves interviewing both spouses and other members of the family as indicated. Efforts at mediation are initially appropriate. While evaluating the family decision making processes, the mental health professional can provide feedback regarding this process or facts regarding custody arrangements which may allow the spouses to make their own decision. Efforts should be made to strongly encourage divorcing spouses to arrive at their own decision regarding custody. In general, a court imposed decision functions no better than one negotiated by the divorcing couple. If mediation and negotiation fail, the family therapist can provide an opinion directly to the court regarding the best interest of the family as a whole. This opinion will be one among many that the judge will have available with which to make his/her decision.

The emotional attachment is a concept describing the process of emotional influence between any two people, and family relationships reflect how emotional attachment among all members are managed. In providing an opinion for the court, the family therapist should describe the patterns of management of relationships within the family and make predictions, if possible, about how the divorce will or has modified these patterns. Previous patterns of management plus the degree of acute and chronic stress experienced by any of the individuals can be an index of the manner in which custody decisions will be made. A thorough examination of the decision making processes within the marital dyad and between each parent and his/her family of origin gives clues as to how families will make and cooperate on child custody decisions.

Factors to be considered in the decision making process include dating and courtship behavior, length of courtship, length of time between marriage and birth of first child, degree of emotional involvement with the child, decisions regarding discipline, degree to which the child occupies the emotional focus of marital disagreements and the intensity and chronicity of marital conflict. Identification of these processes allows a tentative formulation about the decision making patterns in the marital dyad, the events that activate the patterns and the factors that influence the patterns. Clinical investigation in child custody determinations should focus more on what people in fact have done in the past, rather than on what they say they will do in the future. Although custody evaluations and decisions are among the most difficult ones in forensic psychiatry, information derived regarding the above-mentioned family processes will be useful in providing a family focused approach both for the family and the court to the child custody decision making process.

EDWARD W. BEAL, M.D.
Clinical Assistant Professor
Georgetown University Medical School
Washington, DC

64. The Family Therapist
   in Child Custody Cases

Question:

From time to time I am asked to offer testimony about custody
and/or visitation arrangements. Frankly, I'm a bit ill at ease with
the idea of leaving my role as a family therapist and becoming
a decision maker—at least I sense I would have to say that one
parent is more suited than another to have custody. I would welcome ideas about how to enter into or stay out of these custody
and visitation matters.

Discussion:

You have put your finger on a critical question: How can one be a
therapist and a legal advocate at the same time? There is no easy
answer, but I believe that professionals have a social obligation to offer
expertise in any manner that will be beneficial to people. We cannot,
therefore, limit ourselves to activities that are always comfortable. Let
me offer you some ways to maintain your identity as a therapist, yet
enter into custody proceedings.

Most basically, it is important to let the parents (and children) know
that you are speaking on behalf of what is in the best interest of the
family. Most states have adopted the Uniform Child Custody Act as
statutory law, which holds that the best interests of the child be the
criterion in custody determination. This has led some professionals,
such as Goldstein, Freud and Solnit (1973), to assert that the child's
interests are beyond any rights of the biological parent (as opposed to
a psychological parent who could better aid the child). From a legal
point of view, this is now true (such was not the case in the past, when
children were seen as chattel of the father and later as automatically
belonging to the natural mother, regardless of what the natural parents could or could not offer them). My approach is to urge that a child
and family advocacy stance should be maintained (Woody, 1978a).
After all, the family is responsible for fulfilling all sorts of societal
functions that the individual—child or adult—cannot, and the child

must exist at least to adulthood in some sort of family framework, even if it is a single-parent family.

The traditional therapist role is not incompatible with advocacy. Indeed, I have participated in a number of child custody cases where both parents, even the one that I was "opposing" (more will be said about this in a minute), achieved psychological growth through the courtroom confrontation with their commitment to and abilities for effective parenting. There are also legal precedents supporting that, in certain situations, social welfare must come before personal welfare, e.g., the *Tarasoff* (1974) case held that confidentiality and privileged communication had to be subjugated to protecting others. This social responsibility should, of course, be communicated in a therapeutic manner to members of the family prior to and throughout custody legal proceedings.

The legal arena is far different from the therapy room. While the most desirable approach would be for both parents to recruit your participation in the custody and visitation decision making, it is most likely that there will be a decision to separate and divorce and that you will then be requested by the attorney for one of the parents to speak on his/her behalf. The parent and attorney who approach you want to win a decision from the court. They will be paying your fee. But you, of course, are faced with maintaining privileged and confidential communication (although if both parents were present in the same sessions, the information will not be proscribed) and hoping (at least in some cases) that you will not destroy your therapeutic potential for future contacts with the family. There is no easy solution to this dilemma. The best you can do is try to be totally honest and consistent in adhering to the concept of the "best interests of the child and family." Your professional responsibility to society and to each member of the family requires your participation—ethically, you should not try to avoid it.

Research I have conducted reveals that professionals are not always reliable and valid in the professional information that they offer to child custody legal proceedings (Woody, 1977a). Sexism can certainly creep in (Woody, 1977c; 1978b). Factors such as professional discipline, gender, age and personal marital/parental background hold the potential to influence expert opinions (Woody, 1977a). My position is:

> Every professional involved in child custody determinations should be able to specify the criteria used, the definitions thereof, the academic rationale for selecting them, the reliability and validity of the evaluations, the safeguards against bias and unjustified subjectivity, and the best methods for interpreting and communicating the data. (Woody, 1977b, p. 264).

Stated differently this will mean that the professional has:

1) developed a professional stature that will allow involvement without personal ego needs dictating actions: 2) worked through any personal experience (such as possibly a divorce and custody dispute within his/her personal life) that could potentially shape opinions; 3) established an academic rationale for criteria deemed to be important; and 4) the capability of utilizing evaluation methods that are reasonably objective (Woody, 1977a, p. 17).

In addition to your own awareness of the criteria for decision making in child custody proceedings, you should orient the attorneys and the parents (and the children whenever it is reasonable to do so) to what factors are important, how they can contribute to garnering data on these factors, and who they can bring into their legal strategies (such as other experts). I have summarized research on these matters and offered guidelines for the layperson elsewhere (Woody, 1978c).

Finally, it is important that you prepare yourself professionally for involvement in child custody and visitation matters. Too often family therapists lack familiarity with the law to the degree that would complement their efforts. There is no shortcut. It would be preferable if all professionals had an academic exposure to the relevance of law to their discipline throughout their formal preparation. Every professional training program should structure the curriculum to encompass the psychological and social factors in child and family theories that would find application in child custody proceedings, the sociopolitical and organizational aspects of the American legal system, and the methodologies required for effective participation as an expert witness. Regrettably, to date few programs are offering courses on the forensic aspects of the discipline. Workshops and self-directed reading may pave the way to on-the-case learning.

Although perhaps surprising, I have found that extending my role as a family therapist into the courtroom can yield many of the same benefits my clients and I gain in the treatment room. Like it or not, divorce and custody proceedings are a reality that many families must deal with. It can be helpful for all concerned to have the family therapist as an active participant in the child custody and visitation legal proceedings.

References

Goldstein, J., Freud, A., and Solnit, A. J. *Beyond the Best Interests of the Child.* New York: Free Press, 1973.

Tarasoff v. Regents of the University of California. 13 Cal. 3d 177, 118 Cal. Rptr. 129, 529 P.2d 553 (1974).

Woody, R. H. Behavioral sciences criteria in child custody determinations. *Journal of Marriage and Family Counseling,* 1977, *3,* 11-18. (a)

Woody, R. H. Psychologists in child custody. In B. D. Scales (Ed.), *Psychology in the Legal Process.* New York: Spectrum, 1977, 249-267. (b)

Woody, R. H. Sexism in child custody decisions. *Personnel and Guidance Journal,* 1977, *56,* 168-170. (c)

Woody, R. H. Family counselors and child custody. *International Journal of Family Counseling,* 1978, *6*(2), 81-88. (a)

Woody, R. H. Fathers with child custody. *Counseling Psychologist,* 1978, *7*(4), 60-63. (b)

Woody, R. H. *Getting Custody: Winning the Last Battle of the Marital War.* New York: Macmillan, 1978. (c)

ROBERT HENLEY WOODY, Ph.D., Sc.D.
Professor
Department of Psychology
University of Nebraska
Omaha, NB

65. Joint Custody Conflicts

Question:

I have been seeing an increasing number of couples whose marriages have broken down and who are at the point of separation or have already separated. The concern in helping them work out plans for reorganizing their family life is usually focused on what is best for the children. There are conflicting views expressed by authorities about custodial plans, that leave me uncertain whether it is helpful to present optional plans to my clients for custodial care for the children. The typical recommendation prompted by legislation is that mother is awarded sole custody. The traditional view that mothers are the nurturing parents appears to be supported by divorce lawyers, judges and, I believe, many therapists. However, I work with many couples where both mother and father have participated in parenting the children. Some people (e.g., Goldstein et al., 1973) support the "sole custody" tradition based on the premise that the child should be in the custody of a single "psychological parent" who has the legal authority to remove the other parent from contact with the child. Others (e.g., Roman and Haddad, 1978) point out that the latter arrangement effectively disposes of the noncustodial parent as parent, denying the right of both parent and child to continue their relationship. I am very uncertain whether joint custody can work or whether the thesis that sole parenting, preferably by mother, is the safest plan for children.

Discussion:

One of the major issues in a separation/divorce process is how to continue the functions of parenting with as little lapse as possible. Ideally, continuity of parenting should involve both parents. Coparenting provides not only for the needs of children, but also preserves the social and emotional satisfaction for each parent of his/her relationship to the children. Both parents, whether in the intact family or the separated/divorced family situation, have vital tasks in the growth, development and sense of well-being of the child. For families who experience separation/divorce to be deprived of parent-child relationship adds to the trauma. The father's role-loss is frequently overlooked.

Fathers who leave the marriage have to adapt to a whole new lifestyle. They lose marriage, family life and daily parenting. There is no assigned role for the noncustodial parent with visitation rights. Fathers have reported that they need help in learning how to retain a significant parent role with their children when they see them for only brief periods. The tendency is to try to fit a tight activity schedule into the infrequent visits. Fathers report that, in their desire to make the visits pleasant, they tend to treat the children as guests, to entertain them; there is little intimacy when they are visiting together rather than living together. The more the visitation rights are fixed by appointment the less intimate the involvement between parent and child. The visits begin to feel contrived and burdensome to all concerned.

Certainly our prevailing social assumptions as well as common legal arrangements declare the mother to be the preferred parent. These assumptions are inconsistent and outdated for those fathers who have been actively involved in their children's development and growth and in many instances share the primary care of their children. This is being reflected by the increase of fathers who are contesting custody as well as many fathers who report that they were not aware that there were alternative plans to sole custody. Therapists have a useful role in helping couples weigh the advantages to all concerned of alternative approaches to child care. When couples can be helped to separate their marital conflicts from the rights of each parent to continue to parent the children, the threat will be reduced for children that parental separation will mean the loss of a parent.

I believe this reassurance for children must be offered them at the time that they receive information that the parents are going to separate. Ideally, plans for continued parenting and living arrangements should begin prior to parental separation and before the legalities of financial settlement begin. Too frequently hassles around finances become emotional issues, hostilities escalate and children can be used as tools for parents to punish each other by depriving them of rights to the children. Studies of children of divorce strongly indicate that children need continuing contact with both parents in the interests of their own psychosocial development and emotional stability. The parent leaving the household also needs this continuing contact to insure his/her own emotional stability and parental role. A role for therapists can be to help both parents restructure their family life with each parent assuming joint custodial rights and responsibilities.

An additional comment on joint custody is that the large majority of divorced persons remarry. In the interest of a second marriage, when children are able to resolve successfully their continued relationship with both parents, they will more easily be able to make room for another adult in authority in their lives, who will not be displacing their biological parent. This makes the entry easier for the new partner in the marriage. For the noncustodial fathers who remarry, frequently they do poorly in setting up relationships with their new partner's children due to their sense of depriving their own children of significant parenting.

Another benefit for each parent who remarries is that it leaves more time for the couple relationship when children are able to move comfortably from one parental home to the other.

The concept of joint custody is too new to predict its popularity. However, to date the complexities have been highlighted more than the benefits assessed. As therapists, we would do well to help each separating couple assess whether they can agree that continued sharing in the parenting of their children is in the best interest of all members of the family.

References

Goldstein, J., Freud, A. and Solnit, A. *Beyond the Best Interests of the Child.* New York: Free Press, 1973.

Roman, M. and Haddad, W. *The Disposable Parent: The Case for Joint Custody.* New York: Holt, Rinehart & Winston, 1978.

LILLIAN MESSINGER, M.S.W.
*Chief Social Worker, Community and
Social Psychiatry, and
Principal Investigator, Remarriage Project
Clarke Institute of Psychiatry
Toronto, Ontario, Canada*

66. The Divorced Family:
Whom to Include in Therapy?

Question:

As a family therapist in an outpatient mental health center, I deal primarily with symptomatic children. For several years, I have been working with an increasing number of families in which the parents have divorced. This circumstance presents me with a problem in determining which family members should be involved in treatment. In the past, I would have seen the custodial parent only. It often turned out, however, that in the course of therapy, I discovered the noncustodial parent was a crucial missing piece in my understanding and treatment of the problem. Under what circumstances, therefore, is it appropriate to include both divorced spouses in treatment when the presenting problem involves a child they have in common? How is this accomplished?

Discussion:

This issue is directly relevant to an increasing number of family-oriented clinicians. As the frequency of divorce has increased, there has been a corresponding increase in the number of people living in family situations who do not fit the traditional structure of mother and father with children born of their marriage. When a child of divorced parents develops symptoms that lead the family to seek help, the question is raised, Which members should be involved in treatment? Shall the therapist see the custodial parent and child, or all persons living in the same household, or all original, predivorce family members? This decision will be explicitly or implicitly determined by how the divorced family is defined by the therapist. It is a critical decision, for it will shape the ensuing therapeutic process.

I take the position that in the cases of adults who divorce but continue to share parenting responsibilities, it is critical to include both former spouses as part of a treatment plan. This stance is based on a conceptualization of divorced families as systems within the formal paradigm of general systems theory (Rubin and Kim, 1978) and is

313

consistent with recent research and clinical data (e.g., Hetherington et al., 1976; Suarez et al., 1978). Within this paradigm, divorce does not automatically mean family dissolution; rather, divorce entails an initial family disequilibrium which, over time, resolves itself into an altered family system. All of the original family members may (and often do) continue to play significant roles in the new family system. Particularly when both parents continue to participate in child rearing, mother, father and children continue their predivorce interdependence, with change in one family member affecting all the others. Thus, exclusion of either divorced parent from your treatment plan severely limits the extent to which you can understand and treat a divorced family system with a symptomatic child.

The following exemplifies what can happen if you do not include both parents in your treatment plan. Let us say the presenting problem is acting out behavior in a ten-year-old male child as reported by the school. Mother calls you on the school's recommendation. Because the mother and father are divorced (and mother has custody), you decide to see only the mother and the children. If you exclude the father from your sessions, what you do not know is that he never wanted the divorce and, in fact, is still very attached to his former wife. What emerges in therapy is that mother sets limits on the child but backs down because she is insecure about her ability to rear her children alone. In such instances, when the mother sets limits on the child, he often runs off to father's house. Father uses this opportunity to make contact with his former wife and "rescues" her by giving her advice on how to take care of their child. This, in turn, supports her idea that she can't cope on her own and still needs him. Thus, by acting out the child functions as a homeostat in the system. He keeps his parents tied to one another. If therapeutic efforts are exclusively directed toward getting the mother to control the child and indeed the child's acting out is reduced, significant stress may be placed on the father and on the relationship between the former spouses. Without a full understanding of this situation, the likelihood exists that the father (and possibly the other family members) would sabotage the gains made in therapy.

Sometimes, the divorce crisis does, in fact, result in a single-parent family. This occurs where one parent has given up child rearing responsibilities and the children have only a single parent. Here, therapy should focus on the single parent and child. Even in these instances, however, it is important to find out about the role of the former spouse. I have found sometimes that the single parent will first say that their former spouse is not at all involved with the children, but as therapy progresses, it turns out that the other parent is much more involved than was first described. It is useful to ask directly about the other parent's involvement in early contacts with the family. Here, the children are a good source of information. Be prepared to alter your assessment of the parenting situation as well as your decision about which family members to include in treatment, as therapy progresses and new information emerges.

In addition to the single-parent postdivorce family, there are also remarried family situations in which new family members (e.g., new spouse/stepparent) must be considered part of the postdivorce family system. While a full discussion of the remarried family system is beyond the limits of this discussion, it is important to recognize that the remarried family situation does not negate the importance and the feasibility of including former spouses who participate in parenting, in addition to the new family members, in a treatment plan (Suarez et al., 1978).

When the divorced family system includes both parents and you do involve them in your treatment plan, you are opening the possibility of working on their relationship as a critical area for therapeutic change. There may be times when it is possible to free the child from the conflict between the parents and reduce symptomatology without actually working out the conflict between the parents. Just as in non-divorced families where the marital relationship can be important in working out the child's presenting problem, so too in the divorced family, the relationship between the divorced parents may be the key to effective intervention. Therefore, to be successful, treatment may often focus directly on the relationship (e.g., continued hostility and/or emotional entanglement) between the divorced parents. This is best accomplished in a therapeutic structure in which both divorced parents are seen. Family therapists have learned in many other situations that even though it may be possible to obtain information about an absent family member from one who is present in the therapy, it is far better to have the person involved in the therapy than to learn about them through another.

Once you have decided to include both divorced parents in your treatment plan, the question becomes how to do it. I will describe some general strategies that have worked for me with these families. Any strategy that you have found effective in bringing in resistant family members in other family situations may be applied to the divorced family situation as well.

Just as I would explain to family members where divorce has not occurred that I need to work with all family members, so, in this situation I explain to the divorced parents that because they are both involved with their children, I need their help to understand and treat the problem. This treatment strategy often requires extensive telephone conversations with each parent before the first session. These discussions largely focus on the parents' anxieties and resistance to becoming jointly involved. I find it is important to emphasize that it is their relationship as coparents which is critical, that the sessions will be problem focused and that the joint therapy will be time limited rather than open ended. Above all, I try to make clear that the purpose of the therapy is not to reunite them.

If the parent who called me is open to my plan, I have that parent contact the former spouse. If the former spouse is resistant, I suggest s/he call me to talk before the first session. If there is resistance to calling me as well, I will make the call. In other cases, the resistance of the parent initially calling me is so high that it is necessary to meet for several sessions without including the other parent to develop trust and diminish anxieties about including the other. Often, after several sessions, the other parent may be contacted.

When either parent refuses to be seen with the other or when there is a great deal of hostility between the former spouses, it makes sense to meet with each of them separately. Only when the resistance and/or hostility has diminished over the course of therapy will it be constructive to see them together to work on coparenting issues relevant to the presenting problem. In fact, even when resistance is not an issue in working with divorced families, it makes sense to develop a structure for each session which reflects the problem you are working on but supports the clear boundaries necessary in a divorced family system. For example, when working on behavior control with an acting-out child, it is best for both parents to be involved with the children. When, however, the therapeutic issue involves the mother developing new dating relationships (so as to free her son from a "spousal" role), it is clearly inappropriate to include the former spouse in the same session. A flexible structure in which different combinations of family members can be seen in different sessions is most appropriate for dealing with resistance and working on problems in the divorced family situation.

My experience is that, in addition to the resistance of family members, resistance on the part of the therapist often inhibits success at including both former spouses in treatment. Therapists sometimes feel that it is inappropriate to meet together with two people who have divorced. In actuality, recent data show that the vast majority of former spouses who both participate in child rearing continue to have direct, although episodic, contact with one another postdivorce (Goldsmith,

1979). This contact is often not limited to child rearing matters, but may involve friendly relating (e.g., talking about old friends in common). Therefore, chances are that getting the divorced parents together in your office will rarely be the first time these people have been together since their divorce and will not be an unusual situation for them.

In summary, involving both divorced parents in therapy requires ingenuity, flexibility and perseverance. However, by providing the most complete picture of the family system and by offering greater opportunities to directly change it, this approach maximizes the likelihood of therapeutic success with divorced families.

References

Goldsmith, J. *Relationships between former spouses: descriptive findings.* Paper presented at the National Council on Family Relations Annual Meeting, Boston, 1979.
Hetherington, E. M., Cox, M. and Cox, R. Divorced fathers. *The Family Coordinator*, 1976, *25*, 417-428.
Rubin, B. D. and Kim, J. Y. (Eds.) *General Systems Theory and Human Communication.* Rochelle Park, N.J.: Hayden, 1978.
Suarez, J., Weston, N., and Hartstein, N. Mental health interventions in divorce proceedings. *American Journal of Orthopsychiatry*, 1978, *48*, 273-283.

JEAN BARNETT GOLDSMITH, Ph.D.
Staff, Center for Family Studies/
The Family Institute of Chicago
Northwestern Memorial Hospital;
Associate, Department of Psychiatry
and Behavioral Sciences
Northwestern University Medical School
Chicago, IL

67. Single Parenthood and Child Management Problems

Question:

Frequently we encounter in our child psychiatry outpatient clinic separated or divorced mothers who are feeling overwhelmed by the responsibilities of single parenthood and have great difficulty managing their children's oppositional behavior. The problem appears particularly acute when the departure of the father figure is recent and when the child or children involved are male. These mothers are often unable to enlist their former spouse's aid in child care, or are afraid to allow the spouse to become involved because he is seen to be antagonistic, abusive or unreliable. The relationship between the mother and son is often highly charged and volatile, especially if the son is in the Oedipal stage of his development or is a pre-adolescent. By the time these families come to our clinic, the mothers are frequently at the point of requesting out-of-home placement for the child. Are there specific ideas or techniques that are useful in working with these families?

Discussion:

These are extremely difficult families to treat, especially if the child involved is an only child and the mother has a limited or no support system. Three issues appear critical for the therapist to consider in working with these families: 1) the recent loss of a significant other; 2) the process of identification of the son with his father figure; and 3) the mother's own "emancipation" issues.

Although both mother and son must encounter these issues, what is often lost sight of is that they do so in quite different ways, based upon the different meaning these issues have for each of them. For the mother, the "loss" is often experienced as relief from a painful relationship and an impetus to greater autonomy and responsibility; while for the son it is the loss of a real, potential or fantasy caregiver, and an impetus to increased dependent, nurturance-seeking behavior.

318

For the son, identification with his father is a normal part of growing up but if the relationship with the father has been negative, or is described as such by the mother, confusion around this identification as a male results for the boy. This confusion may be increased by the mother's tendency to see her son as "just like his father," or by her continued and oft-spoken determination to keep him from this fate.

Finally, there is the issue of the mother's emancipation. Many of the single mothers we see in our clinic are women who have had little experience with being on their own. They moved impulsively into early marriages as a way to escape parental authority, only to find similar struggles arising in their relationships with their spouses. With the breakup of their marriages, these women again experience major concerns about their self-esteem and individual potential. Both out of economic necessity and the desire to "be one's own person," they may be seeking personal advancement through employment or education. Similarly, they may wish to go out with a variety of men as an opportunity for experiences previously not available to them. The children, however, may view any involvement of their mothers outside the home as a loss of the only caretaking adult they have left, and they may oppose such involvements through their negativistic and oppositional behaviors. Their mothers, in turn, may experience these oppositional behaviors as the same kind of attempts to control them that they have been trying to escape from with their parents and former spouses. The role reversal becomes complete when the child insists that the parent be home by a certain time and the mother "acts out" by refusing to do so.

In treating these families, we have encountered significant difficulty with the individual therapy approach. If the mother is seen individually, the therapy tends to focus on her personal gowth, and reinforces the view of her child as interfering with this growth. If the child is seen individually, his behavior may improve initially in response to the dependency gratification of the therapy relationship, but with this behavioral improvement the mother's involvement with her son may decrease further. This, in turn, often leads to a recurrence of symptoms and prolonged course of treatment, or to the parent's withdrawing the child abruptly from treatment because it is "making him worse."

The approach we have found most useful in working with these families is to see the mother and son together, taking as our primary focus the clarification of the *parenting role*. This is done particularly in the early sessions by discussing issues around parenting to the exclusion of other topics of concern to the mother, such as her schooling, career issues, dating, etc. This is done to promote the mother's efforts to achieve a sense of competence and self-worth *through* her role as a parent rather than in spite of it. The therapist explores in specific detail the ways in which the child's needs for caretaking are attended to throughout his day. Those times during the day that are known to heighten separation and nurturance concerns for the child (i.e., bedtime, meals, leaving for and returning from school, etc.) are carefully reviewed with the child and mother together. This is often done by asking the child questions such as, "Who takes care of you after school?" When there is a lack of clarity on the child's part, he is instructed to ask his mother to explain the arrangements to him. This approach both clarifies the nonreciprocal nature of the mother/child relationship (i.e., he does not have responsibility for taking care of her, nor can he set the rules) but also helps the child to learn to communicate to his mother his concerns about who will be taking care of him.

As this discussion occurs between mother and son, if either the mother or son begins to slip into the role reversal situation, in which the son sets expectations which the mother reacts against, the therapist can then intervene to block this shift in roles from occurring. Within this context, it is often useful for the therapist to point out to both the mother and son that although, as his parent, she is always responsible for his being cared for, this does not mean that she is always the one who will provide that care. The therapist thus promotes the child and mother seeing the other caretakers (babysitters, day care workers, designated neighbors, etc.) as direct extensions of the mother's caretaking role. These mothers are often reluctant to use other caretakers because they feel obligated to "make up for" the absent father by their own increased involvement. However, they then quickly find themselves resenting this increased involvement.

An example from our clinic illustrates this process. A mother, with some difficulty, arranged her work hours so she could be home when her six-year-old son returned from school. She did this so he would not have to go to a sitter's after school. However, two or three times each week she would stop on her way home to do some "brief" errand, and as a result, would not arrive home until an hour or more after her son returned from school. When she did get home, she would find him in the midst of a temper tantrum which would "spoil the evening" for both of them. With the therapist's support, she was able to "give herself permission" to delegate some of her son's afterschool caretaking to a neighbor and her resentment and his tantrums quickly decreased.

The second area regarding the parenting role which the therapist explores with the mother and son is the way in which the mother is taken care of. Often the child will attempt to "make up for" the absent father by adopting a protective, solicitous stance toward his mother, offering himself as a "shoulder to cry on" or someone to hug. His mother may promote this stance by referring to him as "her little man" or "her best helper," only to discover that her son takes this role increasingly seriously and sees himself as being responsible for her well-being. With the power implicit in this role, the child may become demanding and tyrannical around his mother, insisting that she confide in him all her plans and decisions. The mother, who understandably comes to resent this behavior from her child, may not be able to appreciate the way in which ventilating her feelings and worries to him when he is "warm and loving" promotes this sense of his being responsible for her.

Again, the therapist may get at these issues by asking the youngster, "Who do you think takes care of your mother?" When the role reversal becomes apparent in the boy's response, the therapist may direct him to talk with his mother about the topic. The mother may then, in this context, be encouraged to assert to her son her ability and wish to take care of herself and to see that her own needs are met. This is often a useful context within which to have her explain to him her intention to date and spend time by herself away from her son. Having the mother explicitly tell her son that she does not expect him to take care of her often serves as a useful impetus for the mother to more actively pursue the development of an adult support system for herself as a way of behaviorally demonstrating to her son her intent to care for herself.

In summary, the approach we have found most useful in working with single-parent mothers and their sons is one which focuses upon the interaction between the mother and son in such a way as to promote for both mother and son the clarification of her parental role.

RICHARD A. MINER, M.D.
Assistant Professor
Division of Child and Adolescent Psychiatry
University of Minnesota Medical School
Minneapolis, MN

68. How Therapists Can Help with Stepfamily Integration

Question:

More and more I find myself working with rather newly formed stepfamilies in our family service agency. Can you offer some guidelines about the most important things a marriage counselor or family therapist should know about stepfamilies, and identify the most common issues in their treatment?

Discussion:

The Need to "Know the Territory"

"The Music Man" opens with a song by a group of traveling salesmen testifying that the key to success is—"know the territory!" In therapy with stepfamilies you have to know what they are all about, what it feels like to be a stepparent, and what the stresses are for stepchildren attempting to deal with drastic changes in their lives.

A new kind of family has emerged which is demanding recognition and acceptance. Although precise demographic data are lacking, it is estimated that there are over 35 million stepparents in the United States today, and that one child in six under the age of 18 is a stepchild. There are half a million new stepfamilies being formed each year.

The members of the stepfamily exist in a cultural climate in which there are three myths which create difficulty for them:

1) Stepmothers are wicked. Even preschool children are influenced by the Cinderella fairy tale, and the new stepmother, try as she may, cannot avoid the label. In fact, the harder she tries, the greater the family pressure, and the more likely she is to fail.
2) Instant love occurs between stepparents and stepchildren because the adults love each other. . . . presto, you will love the child of your beloved! The fact is that love doesn't occur instantly, and can only grow and develop as a result of time and experience which overcome

fears and mistrust. In addition, for all members, getting along together takes work and negotiation.

3) Stepfamilies are just like nuclear families, and the "ideal" family is close-knit, without strong outside influences, and with intense interpersonal relationships among the members. In a stepfamily, there are structural differences which make this type of family impossible; stepfamilies usually are not as cohesive and harmonious as nuclear families. It is important to recognize that equally satisfying family life can result from looser ties and more casual and friendly relations.

Perhaps the most important message is that a stepfamily is not a "first family" or nuclear family. The most common mistake made by members of stepfamilies is an attempt to re-create their original family, hoping to "do it right" this time, and to prove through the success of the new family that the failure of the first marriage was not their fault.

There are six important structural differences which distinguish stepfamilies from nuclear families, and each of these differences may be accompanied by specific stresses and tasks.

1) A stepfamily is a family born of loss. Even when there has not been a death, after a divorce, love relationships have been lost, parents and children separated, and hopes and dreams have had to be relinquished. Mourning of these losses is necessary before new adjustments can be made.

2) All family members, adults and children alike, have their own family histories. Previous experiences and values gained in different settings result in expectations which may be at variance with one another. How to cook the spaghetti sauce, and how much T.V. is "good" must be negotiated if the family is to live together amicably.

3) Parent-child relationships precede the new couple bond. At times of family tension and crisis, there are pulls and loyalties which may destroy the fragile new couple bond unless special attention is given to preserving it. Forty percent of remarriages do not survive after four years, and the rate of dissolution is higher when children from previous marriages are involved. Remarried parents often feel that it is a betrayal of the earlier parent-child bond to form a new primary bond with the new partner; on the contrary, the survival of the remarried family usually depends on the establishment of a strong bond between the new couple.

4) There is a biological parent somewhere else. Even when the previous spouse has died, the influence of the ex-spouse on a new relationship continues. When there has been a divorce, children are often torn by loyalty conflicts, and they may become pawns in an unresolved struggle between the biological parents. If an amicable relationship can be established, at least insofar as the children are concerned, the children will be free to relate to both biological parents with positive psychological and emotional growth as a result.

5) The children are often members of two households. It is difficult for children to move back and forth between these two different worlds, and the transition periods are often times of stress. Each living place has different rules and expectations, and there may be different styles of parenting. These are different rather than "right or wrong" ways of living, and adults and children may learn how to adapt successfully if they can receive and accept this message.

6) There is no legal relationship between stepparents and stepchildren. Because there is no legal or societal support structure for the stepparent, this adult may have reservations about getting involved emotionally with a child who is not legally related, and therefore subject to future "disappearance." Society needs to understand and make legal provision for "stepparent rights" in order to have beneficial and stable environments for the growth and development of children.

Helping with the Stages of Stepfamily Development

Once they "know the territory," therapists and counselors can be of immense help to the stepfamilies that consult them. Often it is enough to provide them with information about the complexity and uniqueness of their situation, or to refer them to books on the subject. They need to know that they are facing a difficult adjustment which almost all remarried families find stressful and emotionally draining. They need to know that they aren't crazy, or bad parents and stepparents because they find the integration process so painful and consuming at times. Often, there are stepfamily organizations and groups which can provide the support through sharing and listening to the experiences of others. One such group is the Stepfamily Association of America, Inc., which has state divisions and chapters that provide a network of mutual help services, and educational programs.

Using conventional individual, couple or family therapy techniques, therapists can often assist in more complicated situations through help in the following areas:

1) Members of the family need help with their mourning of lost relationships and dreams.

2) Remarried couples need help to "get some glue" in their relationship, since a strong couple relationship is a key to the survival of the stepfamily. It is important to see the couple without the children until partners have been able to form a more cohesive and loving relationship, an opportunity they have often not had because of the presence of "instant children." Including children at too early a stage may have divisive and polarizing effects.

3) Because there are many differences in values and experiences, stepfamily members often need assistance in negotiationg and renegotiating what are to be the rules and traditions in this new family unit. Family "meetings," once they have had some guidance in the technique, may be continued without the therapists, but it is usually helpful for a few sessions to make the point that there are no "right or wrong ways," that everyone needs to be heard and respected, and what people agree upon can be discussed and changed again if needed. "Turf" and "chore responsibilities" are examples of issues which can often be discussed profitably by the family.

4) Because of the existence of a biological parent elsewhere, stepfamily members often experience a profound sense of helplessness. In this helplessness the individuals often beat their heads against the wall of "no control" rather than look for the areas of control they do have. For example, with help, many families have worked out successful ways of coping themselves with the times "the children are never brought back when promised," rather than spending hours of anguish trying to force the other parent to return the children exactly as had been agreed.

5) If the adults accept the deep need of the child to have access to both biological parents, they can escape the need to play a blame game. Then the children are more able to move back and forth comfortably, without the burden of being caught in the middle or feeling like a pawn in adult struggles. This reduces the guilt and the loyalty conflicts of the children, and as a result, the children often are able to relate more closely to their stepparents as well as to their biological parents.

6) Therapists may be able to help families to understand the importance of helping parents who feel like outsiders to become insiders. A parent who feels excluded, helpless, powerless and frustrated by the difficulty of trying to play a significant role in the child's development may sometimes remove him- or herself from the pain by becoming more distant and less involved. This is often very harmful

to children. New forms of sharing children legally have been developed. One of these is joint custody, which permits both parents to continue to have significant roles in the decisions concerning the child, and encourages both parents to remain involved.

Stepparents may be the outsiders trying to join an ongoing group, or the grandparents may feel cut off and excluded, or a child coming into a new home as the result of a change in custody may be the new person in the group. Making space so there is a comfortable spot for everyone within the new family constellation often requires the skill of an outside counselor.

Whom to Include

In therapeutic work, the complexity of stepfamily structure makes many subgroupings possible:

1) Stepparent couple. As previously mentioned, the bond between the couple in a stepfamily is usually crucial, and the therapist needs to be sure that the couple perceives this need for unity before other family members are brought in. This new alliance needs some trust and caring before individuals with longer relationship histories join the stepfamily group.

2) All adults involved with particular children. At the discretion of the therapist, and after consulting with the stepparent couple, it may be helpful to include an ex-spouse, with the focus being strictly on the needs of the shared child. It is usually not possible or wise to attempt to resolve difficulties between the adults. Since grandparents can "build bridges or build walls" it may be most helpful for them to be included if their understanding and cooperation can remove important roadblocks to better stepfamily functioning.

3) Ex-spouses. The therapist may elect to see an ex-spouse in order to improve communication for the benefit of the child. Major areas of discussion would be visitation and custody issues. If the two ex-spouses are to be seen together, the number of sessions is usually very limited and care needs to be taken to avoid excluding a concerned and involved stepparent. The more all the parental adults can work together, the better the growth climate for the children.

4) The whole family. If the therapist is skilled in family therapy, involving all the adults and children can be an enlightening experience. Children are often impressed to see that both of their biological parents are able to talk to one another without anyone getting killed! Children learn that they do not have to feel respon-

sible for protecting their parent, and that they do not have to feel "caught in the middle." Also, children have the opportunity to relate directly to each adult in the presence of others, to be listened to, and without being able to play one adult off against the other. Family therapists often remark how helpful it is to see a family together, where the dynamics are exposed and acted upon, rather than merely discussed. Sometimes stepfamily interaction is so complicated, however, that a cotherapist is needed to protect the sanity of the therapist as well as provide a sense of security for the family. Many times the cotherapists may each have met separately with certain subsets of the family groups. In such cases, when the full group meets together, stepfamily members may be more relaxed because "their" therapist is present. Such groupings are particularly feasible in clinic settings.

Guarding against Countertransference

As with any family, therapists need to be alert to the possibility of countertransference feelings which may impede the therapy. Distortions in the way the therapist perceives or "judges" the problem being presented will depend on the therapist's own experience and knowledge of stepfamilies. Deep feelings may be stirred by hearing a stepmother describe her jealousies towards her husband and his children, for example, and her reaction may be judged pathological unless the therapist understands that she is dealing in reality with a difficult situation with many experiential and structural roots. A therapist who has never had any contact with stepfamilies might not be sensitive to the insecurity of being an outsider attempting to wriggle into an ongoing system.

On the other hand, when the therapist is a stepparent, for example, there may be a tendency to overidentify with the stepparent in the family. As a result, the stepfamily may find the therapist pushing in directions that are not helpful for their particular family.

In summary, a stepfamily is a different type of family with its own unique challenges and rewards, and attempts to squeeze it into a nuclear family mold can produce heartache and dysfunction rather than its cure. Society still regards a mother, father, two children and a dog as the "normal" or "ideal" family, and it takes eternal vigilance on the part of therapists and counselors to remain sensitive to the fact that there is no longer a single pattern of family normalcy. Often it also requires much therapeutic skill to help stepfamilies view themselves as families in which there are predictable situational stresses, and emotional richness and diversity, all of which can lead to positive and satisfying personal growth for both the children and the adults.

JOHN S. VISHER, M.D.
Secretary-Treasurer
Stepfamily Association of America

and

EMILY B. VISHER, Ph.D.
President
Stepfamily Association of America
Palo Alto, CA

69. Common Problems in Stepfamilies

Question:

What problems can be expected when people with children remarry? Please discuss this from the point of view of the spouses as well as the children.

Discussion:

Stepfamilies are more complex than nuclear families, with many more possibilities for loyalty conflicts, jealousies and triangulation. The previously married partner has a continuing relationship with his/her former spouse, as does each child of that pair, and this affects the new marital partner. When both have been previously married and both have children from previous marriages, the complexity increases; it is maximal when both sets of children are living in the new household.

Couples enter a subsequent marriage with strong motivation for it to succeed; often they are more aware of the work required to maintain the desirable qualities in a relationship. They must confront a number of issues:

1) Issues arising from the neurotic and character problems of the partners: the leftover transferences and projections based on unresolved childhood attachments, expectations, disappointments and grievances, as in any marriage.
2) Specific issues related to life stage in personal development as that affects expectations of the new marriage and family life.
3) Conflicting images of marriage and of parenting arising from the experience with the previous spouse and differences in the families of origin, including ethnic value assumptions.
4) Coping with many more triangular relationships than exist in the nuclear family: the new couple and the former spouse(s); the child, the father and the stepfather; the child, the mother and the stepmother; parent, child and stepchild; and so on, all with their potentials for rivalry, competition, splitting of ambivalence and conflicting loyalties and role expectations.

5) Problems with the stepparent role: especially the idealized expectations of the stepparent (by the stepparent, the child, the spouse) and the negative parental image (the wicked stepmother, the cruel stepfather). Stepparents don't start off loving their stepchildren; love may or may not develop with time. They may find themselves very angry at the stepchild and feel guiltier about it than a biological parent would, since the anger may not be accompanied by love. In an attempt to ward off the negative image, stepparents may profess love for the child when they don't feel it or deny and guiltily suppress anger at the child, which then can be displaced onto the spouse. When a stepparent enters the situation expecting to "make up" to the child for his/her parent's presumed or real faults, unrealistic expectations lead to tension and disappointment.

Here is a case illustrating these problems. It is a composite construct, based on actual cases, but fictitious to protect privacy.

The Kaufmans were deeply in love with each other and were shocked and pained at the increasing level of verbal violence in their quarrels during the first year of a second marriage for both. Ethyl was from a highly Americanized, originally German Jewish family who had been settled in New England for many generations, for whom gentility, civility, rationality, emotional restraint and high achievement were cardinal values. Her father was a successful college professor, her mother (in Ethyl's eyes) an unliberated, overly submissive, undeveloped person who put her energy into childrearing and her social life. Ethyl's first husband was a disappointment to her; he was preoccupied with business schemes which generally failed, and ignored her. She put her energy into raising her three daughters and fell out of love with her husband. Affiliation with the women's movement affirmed her guilty resolution to end the marriage, and she did so. Before it was final she met Sam.

Sam Kaufman's parents were Russian and Polish Jewish immigrants who grew up in New York and gradually prospered through hard struggle in business. Sam was his mother's favorite, an eldest son and the delegate of his mother's ambition; he was a successful lawyer. His mother was the stormy emotional center of the family; he was enmeshed with her and cut off from his father. His first marriage had been to a fellow law student; they had one son together. His first wife resented the intrusion on her career which childrearing represented, and after several years of marriage began an affair. When Sam discovered it, he felt humiliated and betrayed and divorced her. After a series of brief affairs, he met Ethyl and they soon fell in love.

Therapy involved working with his mistrust of women and his defensive need to control and dominate his wife. These issues were related to his experience with his mother and first wife, his identification with his mother's style, and his rejection of his father. His defensive need to be the Ideal Father had been attractive to Ethyl at first; she had been Daddy's little girl in her family, and had been disappointed in her weak first husband. When Sam began responding to her daughters in a way that was a confusing mixture of nurturance, authoritarianism and flirtatiousness, this upset them and angered her. He was still enmeshed in the battle with his former wife, and his animosity toward her was beginning to carry over to his son Bob. Increasingly, he saw her traits in him; when Bob visited, he tended to command him or ignore him. In addition to the couples work, we had two sessions including Bob. In one, the boy's roleplaying of his father's style of greeting him when he came home from work really helped Sam see what he had been conveying to his son. We also had one session with Sam and his father, in which I encouraged his father to reminisce about his own childhood, which increased Sam's empathy with his father. There was a reduction in the tension and isolation in both relationships.

Ethyl had to overcome her fear of Sam's anger, which was intense, hot, dramatic and verbally unrestrained, unlike her family's style of cold, logical, submerged but relentless anger. I encouraged her to discuss separately with each of her parents their experience of their relationship starting with their courtship and the early phase of their marriage including what their hopes and disappointments had been. Her idealized image of her father and denigrated image of her mother gradually became more realistic. Sam and Ethyl explicitly discussed their differences of parenting style, and an agreement was reached that established clear boundaries between her daughters and Sam. He could begin to work out more genuinely friendly relationships with them after he stopped trying to be the kind of father he had thought he wanted as a boy. His relationship with his son became warmer. With these issues sorted out, their marriage became more rewarding to both of them, and they were able to work out or accept more of their differences without wildly escalating quarrels.

It sometimes happens that the couple focuses so much energy on the children that the marriage suffers. When two sets of children are combined into one family, with the clash of two different family value systems about childrearing, there are many problems. When the children are adolescent, the renewed Oedipal conflicts can be especially problematic. Sometimes the presenting family member may be a child who is doing poorly in school, becoming delinquent, using alcohol or drugs, running away, or misbehaving sexually. A family approach is important in treating such problems. Emotional cutoffs from the parent the child is not living with must be remedied as part of the treatment.

Constructive resolution depends on the love the spouses feel for each other despite the conflicts and their willingness to renegotiate issues of dominance, conflicting loyalties, conflicting role expectations, styles of expression of frustration, and tendencies to triangulate when dealing with ambivalence.

Books which can be recommended to couples considering remarriage, to those who are remarried, and to therapists working with stepfamilies are:

References

Maddox, B. *The Half-Parent.* New York: Evans, 1975.

Visher, E. B., and Visher, J. S. *Stepfamilies: A Guide to Working with Stepparents and Stepchildren.* New York: Brunner/Mazel, 1979.

Levinson, D. J., et al. *The Seasons of a Man's Life.* New York: Knopf, 1978.

Gould, R. L. *Transformations: Growth and Change in Adult Life.* New York: Simon and Schuster, 1978.

LEONARD J. FRIEDMAN, M.D.
Assistant Clinical Professor of Psychiatry
Harvard Medical School;
and Faculty, Cambridge Family Institute
Cambridge, MA

70. Common Issues in Recoupled
   Families and Therapy Interventions

Question:

We are a social work department in a day care center located in a large city. The staff consists of eight social workers whose main responsibility is counseling parents of the children enrolled in the day care program. As a result of the increasing number of recoupled families, through remarriage or live-in situations, we would like a better understanding of these families. Would you discuss 1) the common issues which the recoupled family must handle; 2) factors affecting the recoupled family, and 3) effective intervention with the new family system.

Discussion:

Let me preface my discussion by saying that there are many names applied to stepfamilies such as recoupled, remarried, blended, reconstituted, synergistic, etc. This reflects the confusion about these families which are proliferating but not yet realized as a norm in our present culture. Generally, I prefer the terms stepfamilies, recoupled or remarried families.

First I will touch on common issues and then discuss therapy interventions.

Common issues which recoupled families have to deal with are: money, discipline, bonding, new kin and old kin, former spouse, custodial children and visiting children, sexuality, sibling rivalry, and confusion over surnames. The two most troublesome areas are money and discipline.

Money. Money is a basic issue in all recoupled families, affluent or poor. Money is often used as a weapon and means of control. The mother may withhold visitation if the father does not send money; the father may withhold money to punish his ex-wife; the children get caught in the middle. There is less money for the old family as well as the new family.

Prenuptial agreements are often contracted in second marriages. Even though a formal agreement has been made, partners will often hide some money for emergency exit should the new relationship fail, giving rise to distrust.

Discipline. One of the most frequent sources of friction in stepfamilies is discipline. While the original hope is that each parent in the new relationship should discipline the children, difficulties arise when put into practice. The biological parent may consider the stepparent too harsh or quick. As an early intervention, a counselor might educate the stepparent in ways to ease into the new role, e.g., the stepparent might be more a friend at the beginning until the relationship has been strengthened. However, when the biological parent is absent, the other adult must act *in loco parentis*. (The live-in partner has an even more tenuous position as disciplinarian.)

Bonding. Bonding is a gradual process and second families often expect instant love. The children have trouble bonding because of the feeling of disloyalty to the original parent. The adults are surprised that the feeling for the stepchildren is not one of immediate love, or the same as for one's own children. The personality of the people involved also makes a considerable difference.

New Kin and Old Kin. Because of the extended kinship network that often comes with a remarriage, children may find more adults available to them. The kinship network of the present and former family becomes intertwined and the loyalties have to be rearranged. Remarriage affects all generations on both sides of the biological parents and stepparents.

Former Spouses. There is always at least one former spouse in remarriage. If there are children, the former partners usually have to continue to relate to each other. Often the new mate, if not married before, is threatened if there is no previous partner to relate to, especially if the former spouses have a fairly decent relationship. In some instances, the former spouse becomes depressed when the divorced mate remarries because that means they are *really* divorced and it is final. (For some people this is more threatening than the divorce itself.)

Sexuality. In stepfamilies there is heightened awareness of sexuality because it is a readymade family without the gradual acquisition of the incest taboo. The couple are in the honeymoon period but may find privacy difficult to obtain. The sexual atmosphere may be more intense if there are adolescents in the family. Sexual attraction between stepparent and stepchild and between stepsiblings is not uncommon.

Sibling Rivalry. In first families, sibling rivalry is common, but it is often exacerbated in stepfamilies. Occasionally a stepparent will allow a child to act out for him/her by not properly disciplining and allowing the child to scapegoat a stepchild.

Custody and Visiting Children. Custodial parents have the advantage of parenting on a daily basis and by their presence communicate to the children that they have not deserted them. This means that custodial parents are seen in the role of disciplinarian. Noncustodial parents, who show the children a good time and give presents, are viewed as the "good guys." However, the latter feel that they do not have the children long enough to impart their values to the children.

Visiting children may feel alien because there may not be space set aside for them. There are some stepfamilies, however, who are able to incorporate visiting children into the new system.

Surnames. Although surnames are a minor issue, it is one that needs to be mentioned. Children are often confused as to whose surname should be used under which circumstances. For example, when the child has a different name than the remarried mother problems may be created in school.

Therapy Interventions in Remarried Families

In practicing family therapy with remarried families, the techniques are the same but many of the goals are different.

One of the first issues to be dealt with is the mourning process for all involved, whether it is a loss through death, divorce or separation. Both children and adults need to be helped to express their grief. An early goal would be to strengthen the couple relationship, because if they have a fairly strong alliance, it will be easier to work out other problems in the family.

One needs to help recoupled families to clarify the roles and expectations, both spoken and unspoken. Because this is new territory for all involved, the members become aware that they are charting new ways of relating and have not been prepared for the unexpected problems which arise.

Still another goal is to keep the boundaries of the family system permeable so that children can enter and leave both sets of families with ease and without guilt. Older children need more freedom and independence to move in and out of the family easily. In some families the adolescent is literally extruded and goes off on his/her own. In a recoupled family, there is usually less cohesion than in a nuclear family. In a family with young children, there is more possibility for cohesion to take place.

If there is a problem with a child, the custodial parents, the children and the noncustodial parent should all be involved. The best approach is to ask permission of the custodial stepparent to include the biological parent in the therapy. This should occur fairly early in the process. When all are brought together, issues can be explored more fully. The positive feelings still existing between the former partners should be elicited in a way that is not threatening to the new partner. This technique helps the children feel that they do not have to split their loyalties, because the biological parents still have some caring feelings for each other.

Bringing the two sets of parents together facilitates negotiation between them. It is also an opportunity to be explicit about the importance of the continued contact between the noncustodial parent and the child. It is necessary for the child's self-esteem to know that the noncustodial parent cares enough to maintain the relationship.

When discipline is a recurring problem, it is often because one stepparent is seen as too strict, rigid and harsh. Often, it is the stepfather who has not been a parent before. These parents can be supported by commenting on how difficult it is to have instant parenthood thrust upon one; further, the caring and responsibility that this parent is trying to show should be underlined. Often parents find themselves in the position of defending their own children. There are even some cases where the parent seems to favor the stepchildren by having his/her own children give in for the sake of peace. Occasionally, because of the new roles and uncertainty, parents may have a child who becomes a tyrant. They need help in learning to work together in setting limits and maintaining them.

Sibling rivalry can become a serious problem in stepfamilies. The more children there are, the more the problems may multiply. Parents may have to learn to tune out some of the noise and to intervene only in extreme instances. It is interesting to observe that a new baby in the stepfamily may pull the children together and facilitate cohesion.

Sexuality is an issue which should be surfaced when seeing recoupled families, especially with latency and adolescent children. The children often find the demonstration of affection between the newlyweds discomforting because they still feel closely attached to the absent parent. It is important to introduce the topic of sexual attraction between people—sometimes between stepparent and stepchild and between stepsiblings—because if not discussed and aired, the attraction may take the form of rejection or unkindness toward the person in order to ward off any awareness. Skill is needed in dealing with this topic.

Treating recoupled families can be challenging. It is necessary to teach them to negotiate and renegotiate. One efficient way to get history and a detailed picture of the family, and also to flush out family secrets, is to do a genogram.

As preparation for recoupling, an educational program for those who are planning to remarry or are already living together is recommended.

MARY D. FRAMO, M.S.S.
Branch Supervisor
Family Service of Montgomery Co.
Ardmore, PA

71. Planning Conjoint Family Therapy with the Remarried Family

Question:

We work in a small community-based family counseling center. Over the last five years, we have seen an increase in the number of remarried families seeking treatment. These families are most commonly referred by either school personnel or juvenile court personnel. That is, the symptomatic person is usually a child between the ages of 5-17. Most frequently cited symptoms are lying, stealing, bedwetting, tantrum and fighting behaviors in children under 12, and truancy, running away, drug use, poor school performance and other acting-out behaviors in adolescents. Our center uses primarily a family systems theory, conjoint-family model of therapy with all families who request help. The questions we pose are: (a) how is this model of therapy used with a remarried family; (b) how does the therapist decide whom to include in the therapy, especially regarding the noncustodial parent; and (c) what special difficulties can be expected in employing this treatment model with the remarried family?

Discussion:

There has been an upsurge in literature on the treatment of families in the last 20 years. While many strategies and techniques have been developed and described, almost all of these therapeutic applications are either explicitly or implicitly meant for use with the nuclear, intact family. Statistics, however, show that one-third of American children do not live in an intact, nuclear family, and approximately 15 million children under the age of 18 live with a stepparent. The remarried family is the third most frequently encountered family configuration, following nuclear and single-parent. Literature on the clinical treatment of the remarried family is finally beginning to emerge. Currently, Visher and Visher (1979) provide one of the most complete guides for both stepparents and clinicians working with remarried families. We would like to share our methodology for working with this type of family.

Our center has long used conjoint family therapy based on a systems theory approach. Our assumption is that the presenting problems or identified patient represents a dysfunction within the family system rather than only within the individual. It seemed to us that not only can this assumption be generalized to the remarried family but is, perhaps, even more obvious than in the nuclear family. Therefore, the following procedure has been utilized.

When a call comes in to the center, an Intake is done over the phone by a counselor. The following information is gathered; names, sex, ages and marital status of everyone in the household. If this information elicits the fact that one or more of the adults was previously married, information is collected on names, ages, location and dates of the marriage with previous spouses, as well as the names, sex and ages of children who may not be living in this household. After all the necessary information has been collected, the Intake counselor makes an appointment for the family with a cotherapy team of two, and specifically requests that all members of the household be present. There is relatively little resistance to this as most of our referral sources indicate that is our policy when they make the referral, so the caller is expecting this request.

The first two sessions are considered to be an assessment period. In addition to the usual things a therapist looks for when making an initial evaluation of a family, in the case of the remarried family, the therapists are also looking for the answer to the question: Who should be included in the therapy? As is apparent, in a remarried family there are many more possibilities, e.g., not only all the members of this household or subgroups of it, but also noncustodial parent(s) plus, perhaps, their new spouses, and grandparents, to name a few of the possible configurations.

If the presenting problem seems to be related to conflict between the child and stepparent, lack of clarity of roles within the new family, rigidity of old family alliances and loyalties, and/or chaos in the logistics of family functioning, then the therapists would probably conclude that the family is having difficulty in blending and reorganizing two families into a new family. The therapy would then include all members of the present household. Subgroups might be seen for varying lengths of time and grandparents might be brought in for a one- or two-time "consultation" session. The bulk of the therapy, however, would be with all members of the household. With everyone present, work can proceed much more effectively on clarifying roles, understanding each other's differences, diminishing unrealistic expectations, and in general, educating the family on what to expect from their remarried family status.

In some cases, the presenting problems of the identified patient may be symptomatic of the hostility and tension—"the unfinished business"—between the child's divorced parents. Children become the most accessible avenue for divorced parents to gain revenge on each other. In these instances, the therapists encourage the family to bring the noncustodial parent into the therapy; if this parent has also remarried, his or her new spouse may also be included. A model for this specific aspect of therapy—i.e., the noncustodial parent in conjoint family therapy—has been written about previously (Baideme, Hill, and Serritella, 1978). As might be expected, there is often a great deal of reluctance and anxiety about bringing in an ex-spouse and many families do refuse. We have been very pleased to note, however, that when families agree to this, the success rate runs quite high. That is, tension and conflict between the divorced parents are significantly reduced, resulting in diminished symptoms in the child.

Another aspect of the family which the therapists are evaluating during the assessment phase is the family's capability to shift from an identified patient focus to a family systems orientation. It has been observed that when one or more members of the family have intrapsychic problems, the therapeutic group process may be seriously hampered or disrupted, and the chances for success with conjoint family therapy are greatly diminished. A second important contraindication is when there is a high level of blaming and scapegoating by the family. If family members continue to resist changing the perceptual focus of their problems from "out there" to "how am I responsible," despite modeling by and teaching of straightforward communication skills by the therapists, then it might be predicted that there will be difficulty in getting the family to understand and agree that the problem is a family problem and not one individual's. For these families, we then advocate utilizing a conjoint family modality with the goal of symptom relief. Within a symptom relief model of treatment, all family members continue to be seen on a conjoint basis. The symptoms, however, are never fully translated by the therapists to a systems view. Rather, the therapists will work with the family to find ways to relieve the problems with which they have specifically requested help.

It has been our experience that the transition from an individual/symptom approach to a family systems approach is a critical stage. It is at this point that many families withdraw from treatment prematurely. It is our belief that this happens even more frequently with remarried families than with nuclear families. With one or more failed marriages behind them, the adults may be especially fearful of looking at the problems in their present marriage, and may also be feeling guilty about the impact of the divorce on their children. Thus, it is suggested that therapists be especially thoughtful when making this therapeutic shift and that their decision to do so be based on a thorough assessment of the family's capability to make use of a systems therapy and the family's desire to achieve the goals consonant with that kind of therapy.

Therapists often have higher expectations for a family and its level of functioning than does the family. Thus, it may sometimes be a struggle for the therapist to keep the pace slow and within the family's goals. These families will probably feel ready to terminate when they have achieved some relief from their presenting problems. Although the therapists may not view this therapy as ideal or complete, the family's goals must also be taken into consideration. Often to the surprise of the therapists, these families report very positive results from the therapy.

In summary, then, we have learned through experience that even though theoretically and philosophically our allegiance is to a systems view of family therapy, pragmatically that strategy doesn't work with all families. The therapists need to consider that the goals for a well-functioning remarried family are not necessarily equal to the well-functioning nuclear family. We advocate that therapists be especially sensitive to the specific needs of the remarried family when selecting an intervention strategy. If the therapists accurately assess the family's potential to work within a systems model, and if the family is shifted slowly into this mode of treatment, there is an increased probability of success.

References

Baideme, S. M., Hill, H. A., and Serritella, D. A., Conjoint family therapy following divorce: An alternative strategy. *International Journal of Family Counseling,* 1978, *6,* 55-59.

Visher, E. B. and Visher, J. S. *Stepfamilies: A Guide to Working with Stepparents and Stepchildren.* New York: Brunner/Mazel, 1979.

SALLY M. BAIDEME, M.Ed.
Assistant Director

and

DANIEL A. SERRITELLA, Ed.S.
Director
The Odyssey Family Counseling Center
College Park, GA

SECTION VI

Special Areas and Issues

PART A

Multigenerational Issues

72. Helping Dysfunctional Family Members Reconnect with Sources of Strength in Their Family Network

Question:

As a family therapist in a mental health center and in private practice, I often deal with families whose members experience ongoing emotional crisis, e.g., severe depression, marital break-ups, attempted suicide, destructive enmeshments, and psychotic manifestations. I feel that when members of the nuclear family begin to feel desperate and unable to cope with such dysfunctional patterns, they can gain additional strength and support by re-connecting with their own family and social network. How do I initiate this process? Once the network is assembled, what is my role in it?

Discussion:

You are quite "on target": When relationships among family members have reached a desperate point, and when the feelings of helplessness prevail among members of the family, inclusion of the extended family and social system can help energize the members of the nuclear family and bring about new options and alternatives for crisis resolution. Family network, also called family network therapy or family network intervention, is a therapeutic process which allows mobilization of the social support system of the family, relatives, friends and neighbors in a collaborative effort to solve an emotional crisis. It is usually a time-limited, goal-oriented approach led by a small team of interventionists.

Professionals involved in networking efforts have found that mobilization of the family network results in the formation of productive changes in dysfunctional family systems, increased communication and the development of family connectedness, with its extended social systems leading towards crisis resolution (Garrison, 1974; Rueveni,

1979; Rueveni and Speck, 1969; Rueveni and Wiener, 1976; Speck and Attneave, 1973; Speck and Rueveni, 1977).

When you determine that a family can potentially benefit from mobilizing its extended network, you need to team up with at least one or two professional colleagues who have some experience with groups and family work. You will need to meet all members of the nuclear family, preferably at home (since it is their own turf, and since the network meeting will be held at home, if possible). If a meeting at home is an impossibility, a two-hour office visit can be considered. During this meeting, you and your team need to help family members discuss their feelings about sharing their concerns with 40-50 family members and friends whom they will have to invite to their home.

You explain that during such a meeting all the family concerns will be shared and discussed and that the goal is for the invited people to become familiar with the concerns and problems of the family, so that they can be of help and support. When you reach a decision with the family to mobilize the network, you may wish to instruct them to prepare lists of their family, friends, neighbors and others who they feel might be of help to them. During this pre-network "screening" meeting, you need to determine the date for the meeting. It is best to have such meetings in the evening for 3-4 hours, or during weekends. This allows for maximum participation. You also need to agree on the amount you will be reimbursed by the family for your services and, in the event you and your team plan to tape such a session, to secure written releases from both family and their invited network.

To begin such a session, your team and you (assuming you are now the leader) need to arrive at the family's home at least one half hour before the meeting begins to plan the last minute details of your strategy, to discuss the list of expected people, and to answer any last minute questions from members of the family. It is also advisable at this time to take a brief "house tour." At a recent network meeting, a note by the identified patient, left in her bedroom and found by a team member, provided additional stimulus for further exploration later in the session.

The network session should not start before the family can actually convene 40-50 people in the room. You will need that many people in order to insure a successful process leading towards the formation of temporary support groups of at least 10 members in each group.

Your role as a team during the sessions is to be able to help the assembled network of participants experience the various network phases described below, which lead towards crisis resolution and the formation of the temporary support groups for each member of the nuclear family.

The Network Phases

Initially, you will need to help the assembled network *retribalize*, by using unison singing, milling around, or any similar activity involving the participants in energizing the system (see Rueveni, 1979). This initial warm-up activity helps the network participants interconnect and reduces their feeling of isolation. Following this activity, you will need to have members of the nuclear family share their concerns and tell their invited guests how and in what way they might be of help to them. This activity will result in the disclosure of a variety of conflicting feelings about the nature of the problem, and you and your team members will need to encourage this process which is termed *polarization*, a phase where different viewpoints are shared. During this phase, you may want to suggest to the participants to sit behind the nuclear family member whom they wish to support, or encourage other people in the network who have not spoken, to share their views about the problem. An important component of the network process is the sharing of family secrets, and you may want to ask whether anybody in the family knows of any secrets that need to be shared. Since secrets are full of energy, they can speed up the process of engaging the network members with the specific family problems.

As the process continues, you will find that a number of network participants become quite active in taking the lead, suggesting specific solutions for consideration. The team members need to encourage this activity since this is a positive phase termed *mobilization*, which allows these network activists to identify specific family problems and offer their help and support for resolving them. This phase is usually followed by a lull from activity where both family and other network members begin to feel exhausted, unable to break the impasse, and that the problems may be too overwhelming. This *depression* phase is characterized by feelings of helplessness, boredom, irritability and lack of progress in achieving practical solutions. The team's role during this phase is to plan a strategy which can break this impasse.

A series of active choreographic (psychodramatic) strategies can be developed and implemented (Rueveni, 1980). For example, if a confrontation seems appropriate between mother and daughter, the daughter can be asked to step up on a chair, expressing her feelings towards her mother who sits down looking up at her daughter. If the father seems to be the target of many conflicting feelings by others in the family, the team may wish to temporarily "kill him off" by suggesting he close his eyes and pretend to be dead, then have others in the network express their feelings toward him. These intervention strategies need to be timed so that they result in a greater investment by both family and their social network and provide sufficient energies for moving away from the depression phase into the next final phases of *breakthrough* and *exhaustion-elation*. During these phases, positive and hopeful signs are experienced; members begin to feel that solutions can be formulated. It is best at this point for team members to suggest the formation of support groups, meeting around each of the nuclear family members in an attempt to consider alternative options for solving the problems. Support groups should have at least 10 members or more. They should meet for at least 30 minutes, reporting their progress or lack of it, to the entire network assembly at the end of the session.

You may want to determine whether there should be another network session at the end of the first one. If a sufficient number of solutions seem to come forth, it may be an indication that no further sessions are needed. In that case, the support groups can be scheduled to meet on a weekly basis, consulting with the team on a periodic basis. On the other hand, if the meeting ends in depression (which is frequently the case), it may be an indication of the need for further networking. In that case, the group may be asked to consider meeting for one or more sessions in future weeks.

To summarize, your team role is to be able to become affective strategists for change. You do it by working as a team in retribalizing and mobilizing the family system, by using choreographic moves and strategies which can enable the network members to reach out and experience the family pain, and by acting as resource consultants to the family and network members. Above all, do not take over the responsibility for changing the system, act in the periphery and encourage others in the system to take responsibility for reconnecting with the system. Hopefully this will create a networking process which should provide the ailing family members encouragement and support for solving their immediate crisis.

References

Garrison, J. Network techniques: case studies in the screening-linking-planning conference method. *Family Process*, 1974, *13*, 337-353.
Rueveni, U. *Networking Families in Crisis: Intervention Strategies with Families and*

Social Systems. New York: Human Sciences Press, 1979.

Rueveni, U. The family therapist as a strategist for change. *Interaction*, 1980, in press.

Rueveni, U. and Speck, R. V. Using encounter group techniques in the treatment of the social network of the schizophrenic. *International Journal of Group Psychotherapy*, 1969, *19*, 495-500.

Rueveni, U. and Wiener, M. Network intervention of disturbed families: The key role of network activists. *Psychotherapy: Theory, Research and Practice*, 1976, *13*, 173-176.

Speck, R. V. and Attneave, C. *Family Networks*. New York: Vintage Books, 1973.

Speck, R. V. and Rueveni, U. Treating the family in times of crisis. In J. Masserman (Ed.), *Current psychiatric therapies*, 1977, *17*, 135-142.

URI RUEVENI, Ph.D.
Acting Director
Division of Social & Community
Intervention
Eastern Pennsylvania
Psychiatric Institute
Philadelphia, PA

73. Problems With Family Genograms

Question:

I have just begun to use family genograms in a lot of my work with families, and especially with couples. The problem I'm having with using the genograms with some of these couples is that a few of my rather obsessive couples, mostly professional people, seem to get very wrapped up in the details of it all, and it's hard to elicit any feelings that might come up as we construct the genograms. I'm not sure how much doing genograms is *supposed* to get at unspoken feelings and how much it's really geared toward more intellectual understanding. Is there some way I can use family genograms productively with very "tight" couples, without them intellectualizing the whole experience?

Discussion:

The major use of gathering family history with the aid of a genogram is to organize the enormously complex material of the family patterns and background to allow the therapist and family to review the information to get a sense about the issues and relationships in a structured way. The genogram is designed for intellectual understanding which will help people begin to rethink their family relationships and perhaps motivate them to begin changing them. It is not a tool to elicit affect, although it frequently does. The actual work of dealing with unspoken feelings is more likely to occur outside the therapy setting, between the marital partners and their family members.

The following comments are oversimplified since the theoretical model of Bowen systems theory, on which the use of the genogram is based, is quite complex. The questions a therapist asks in constructing a genogram develop from that framework and would not have meaning as isolated questions.

My experience is that constructing genograms can be especially useful with somewhat obsessive couples because of the structure they offer for questioning about emotionally loaded issues in a family in a calm, nonthreatening way. The therapist may thus often get through barriers which might be insurmountable in a less structured context.

Guerin and Pendagast (1976) give a good example of this along with quite a few specific suggestions for conducting the session.

As the therapist asks about the membership of the family (who entered the family when and how, and who left it when and how) it is possible to ask all sorts of questions directed at the family relationship system: One can use Toman's (1976) profiles for sibling positions to ask whether family members have tended to fall into the typical sibling patterns or not. For example, is the oldest an overresponsible leader or the youngest a "little prince"? One can thus get a sense about how the family views different members. Asking how much an oldest has tended to fall into the typical problems of overresponsibility normalizes such characteristics. It describes issues in terms of patterns of functioning rather than individual pathology and may thus make it easier for people to respond. The labels families ascribe to members can give many clues about how to move therapeutically. For example, if the siblings are described in negative terms and the couple has come in for marital problems, resolving the sibling problems will probably be helpful in resolving the marital problem.

Another highly significant area the genogram opens up is that of cut-offs. Where do family members live, what is the extent of contact with living family members, who initiates it, and what reasons do people give for any lack of contact? This will tell much about how family members deal with conflict and closeness, and again will suggest therapeutic moves.

Closely related to the issue of cut-offs is the issue of deaths in the family. Asking about people's parents and grandparents leads into questions about how family members have died, who was there and how the deaths were handled, did the family members have a chance to resolve the issues between them before the deaths, etc. Has the person visited the grave since the relative's death, how is the dead person remembered and how often? This is a fruitful way to find out about other problematic relationships as well, since the question also arises, how did one's siblings respond? Differences here are often good indications about family triangles, etc.

In addition, factual questions about any family member can open up many emotional issues: when they were born, what they were like, what they did for a living or for recreation, what kind of marriage they had, where they lived, how they handled illness and death, etc. These questions often lead to reminiscences about significant moments in the relationship with that person. The memories people have about their grandparents, and what stories they have heard about how the grandparents treated their parents may be powerful clues to family patterns in the next generation.

Pursuing family patterns can lead to an understanding of how the family has typically responded to stress in the past (e.g., whether they tend to talk, somatize, work harder, drink or distance from each other), as well as much other information about the cultural and emotional context of the family. My experience is that frequently, when clients get interested in their genograms, they are able to relate a great deal of personal material which would be highly threatening if they were talking exclusively about themselves. In other words, it can greatly enrich the therapeutic context. Exploring the genogram often brings out unspoken feelings because those feelings are part of the system that becomes apparent as one explores the structure of entry and exit of family members and their ways of relating. As one asks a person about his grandfather's attitude toward women, children, or work, one learns a great deal about the family attitudes that have probably been operating for many generations.

I usually ask people to bring a family tree with them to the first session, including all children, siblings, parents, aunts, uncles and grandparents. I ask them to include dates for birth, death, marriage, separation, divorce and significant illness. I also ask them to list the cause of death of those members who have died and to make up, along with the family tree, a family chronology, listing all events they think have been significant in their past, including moves, job changes or other relevant events, in addition to the dates already asked for.

During the first session I go over the basic genogram information, reviewing the material they have brought after the session. I control the questioning, which goes into relationship patterns, emotionally significant nodal events, etc., in the family's history. If a person is greatly interested in details about his or her cousins I look over the written material but may not pursue it in the session.

References

Guerin, Philip J. and Pendagast, Eileen G., Evaluation of family systems and genograms. In P. Guerin (Ed.), *Family Therapy* New York: Gardner, 1976.
Toman, W. *Family Constellation, Its Effects on Personality and Social Behavior*, 3rd ed., New York: Springer, 1976.

MONICA McGOLDRICK, M.S.W.
Clinical Assistant Professor
Department of Psychiatry
Rutgers University
Medical School
Piscataway, NJ

74. Family of Origin Work
in Couple Group Therapy

Question:

My wife and I have been conducting couples group therapy for a little more than four years. Invariably, the majority of the couples get involved in family of origin work. However, each time that a couple has attempted to do this work simultaneously, it seems to slow the process down, to discourage either from getting very deeply into it, or to encourage the two of them to discontinue the work altogether. Can a couple do simultaneous family of origin work effectively, or is this something that one partner at a time must do?

Discussion:

Couple therapy, especially couples group therapy, provides a good format for family of origin work. And increasing numbers of therapists are facilitating work with their clients' families of origin, especially those therapists who have engaged in their own pilgrimages within their families of origin. Usually there are several individuals within a couples group who are working on family of origin issues and, as a result, they can facilitate and aid one another. Since there is no research to date on this particular subject, clinical experience must be relied on.

In my experience, there are several factors that contribute to effective family of origin work. First, the couple must have individuated enough to allow one another to do some things independent of the partner. They need to be invested in the mutual growth of each, and they must be able to look at each other with a reasonable degree of objectivity. Finally, they must have broken the cycle of blaming one another simultaneously or alternately for the marital difficulties, and have begun to see their mutual contributions to the areas of conflict. If family of origin work is attempted before some of these goals have been attained, it is likely to be ineffective.

Effective family of origin work also requires teamwork between the partners so that, as one goes about his/her archeological work, the other steadies the relationship. Most often the partner for whom family of origin work is easiest is the one who goes first, with the more reluctant partner following suit later on, if at all. This relationship is analogous to a couple sitting in a boat; as the one engaged in family of origin work reaches down with his/her net to pick up pieces of past relationships and interactions with the family of origin, the spouse helps by steadying the marital boat. Oftentimes this work stresses the marriage, and the spouse's ability and willingness to be a reliable resource is essential if his/her partner is to make progress. However, if the partner psychologically stands on the other end of the boat and raises a commotion, this can force the one involved in family of origin work to stop and turn his/her energies toward the marriage, lest they capsize. Both partners working intensely at the same time on family of origin issues tends to cause excessive motion for the marital boat so that neither is able to progress and both become discouraged with the endeavor.

Of course, family of origin work is not a neat step-by-step process where one spouse does work in this area and when finished hands the explorer's net over to his/her partner. Nor is it a precise process in which one partner moves along in a regular, steady pace before the other takes up the work. Most of the time it is a life-long process for individuals, so what we are discussing is the initial stage whereby the therapists help individuals to get started on their pilgrimage. Typically one partner will move ahead and do a substantial amount of work with his/her family and then take a break or reach a plateau, at which time the other partner will begin to do some concentrated work with his/her family, reach a point of temporarily stopping, allowing the first partner to resume work again.

One of the values of pursuing family of origin work in a couples group is that individuals can profit and learn from others' work in this area. Another way the group helps the individual involved in this work is by supporting him/her whenever the spouse becomes threatened or in some way becomes disruptive to the work. By having a support group, neither partner has to sacrifice the positive work they have achieved up to that point.

Therapists and group participants can facilitate members' progress in family of origin work in a variety of ways.

1) Start with the spouse who is most receptive to engaging in this work, and let his/her partner participate in a supportive role. The therapists need to keep a close watch on the more reluctant partner,

especially in the initial stages lest his/her anxiety interfere with or discourage the partner's efforts. Sabotage or distracting maneuvers by one partner can be quickly detected by other group members and dealt with on the spot.

2) A related issue is to help the couple look at how this extended family work is influencing their current relationship. Discussion of this influence helps them in particular and the group in general to recognize and understand how past family issues affect current marital and family functioning.

3) It is important to involve the total group in this enterprise at the beginning in order to be most effective in helping one another and aiding each person with his/her own work. Sculpting a current or typical family scene by using group members to roleplay family members is an excellent method for fostering understanding of a particular family and the individual's place in it. As various individuals identify with family or origin members, they become increasingly invested in helping fellow group members to experience constructive corrective change. In addition, they usually start thinking about their own families of origin and often gain motivation to go to work within their own families.

4) An individual can be prepared to deal with a particular emotional issue with a parent or sibling face to face by having the person write a letter to this person, tape the letter, and play it for the group. Such preparation highlights the readiness (or lack of it) to deal directly with the family member. Others in the group can easily recognize when more preparation is needed and comment upon it directly. In such instances, roleplaying of direct encounters with family members can be initiated.

5) Two other valuable resources for individuals engaged in family of origin work in couples group therapy are: a) tape of actual conversations with family members, which are later shared with the group, and b) videotapes of sessions by clients and their families with the therapist. Individuals are thus able to receive feedback from other group members about their interaction with members of their families, and group members can gain courage and some degree of assurance that their fearful fantasies about what might happen may not come true.

6) Finally, the group can offer the other spouse support and confirmation as the one pursues the work within the original family. The group is an appropriate place for the spouse to express hopes, fears, anger and pleasure without unduly influencing the work in progress. Also, the group can help a spouse determine realistically

whether the family of origin work is, in fact, important to the growth of the marital relationship or, as some spouses begin to suspect, an excuse for ignoring current marital concerns. Some spouses need assurance from time to time that the prolonged focus on the extended family is truly related to the marriage and that the waiting will probably be worth it.

MILO F. BENNINGFIELD, Ph.D.
Private Practice
Dallas, TX

75. Helping Couples to Differentiate from Their Families of Origin

Question:

When counseling married couples, the therapist is often challenged with how to help either or both spouses disentangle themselves from inappropriate and controlling behaviors and good intentions of the parents of either or both partners. The parents are eagerly casting votes about any and all details of the married children's lives. Or, the parents may be setting inappropriate expectations or conditions of the responsibility the children have to the parents. When the parents are unavailable or unwilling to participate in therapy, how can the therapist help the couple effectively manage the relationship in a productive way?

Discussion:

Interest and good intentions of parents of married children often become attempts to manage the children's lives, fostering continued dependency and leaving the children and the parents frustrated and bewildered as to what is happening. The challenge to the therapist is to help the couple resolve the frictions or misunderstandings without alienation or severence of the family bonds. The assumption is that grown married children need a continuing constructive interaction with parents, and parents of married children need a continuation of relationship with the children. The relationship is inappropriate and counterproductive when it is simply an extension of the patterns which existed when the married person lived at home. The potential exists for parents and their married children to evolve a productive, reciprocal, healthy relationship. Parents, however, at times foster their own neurotic or self-centered goals which derive from discomfort in letting go of the children; or they react from a sense of confusion about responsibility for the son or daughter and the additional in-law son or daughter.

The most effective impact on such a dysfunctional system would ordinarily be one which includes the parents in the therapy process, so all persons impacting dysfunctionally on the system could be involved in the needed shifts and alterations. When this is not possible, for whatever reason, the married couple must assume responsibility for instituting the conditions which will in effect formulate a new and more functional definition of how the relationships are to operate.

First, the therapist must relate to and understand the various dimensions of the problem and the feelings of each of the persons involved in the situation. The couple's strivings and the parental concerns must be understood. The parents' feelings are often obscure to the young therapist who may encourage severance of the family bond, seeing this as the only resolution for "meddling in-laws." The parents are usually behaving within a continuation of the parental responsibility and prerogatives exercised when the son or daughter was still in the home. They are working from old patterns which originated at the birth of the son or daughter, carried through childhood and adolescence, and still continue after the son's or daughter's marriage. This reaction is accentuated when the son or daughter is employed in a family business. Most parents feel justified in expecting children to comply with parental wishes, even in very personal matters, if the reward is rights to the family business. When employment or other family threads and bonds are continued after the young adults marry, the lines of demarcation between parental responsibility and son or daughter prerogatives and freedoms become clouded. For example, a sure fire way of confusion of the territories of jurisdiction results when a married child continues to live in the same household after marriage, even in a separate apartment, especially if the rent is free.

Both parents and married children are strongly ambivalent about the children's independence. The parents insist they want the married child to be independent, while their own inability to let go results in actual perpetuation of the dependency. The children, too, have a feeling of eagerness for economic and psychological independence, but the payoffs of continued dependence may weaken their resolve. The young married partners whose parents are supporting their education or their start in business have little inclination to bite the hand that feeds them. Conditional love thrives best when the rewards are monetary and tangible. Many a son or daughter has sold a portion of his/her freedom to grow for continued security of parental resources. Genuine independence, personal or economic, can be easily postponed to a more propitious time, in spite of protestations and constant complaints about parental control or manipulation. Or, on the other hand, the parental payoff is great when a dutiful son or daughter still tickles the parent's ego with compliance to parental wishes and with words of gratitude and appreciation.

Disentangling such potent forces and evolving a new definition of the relationship does not come easily. The therapist is expected to assist in a painful growth step, and to accomplish the task without disruption of client comfort. Autonomy, selfhood, marital happiness and success in life are the identified goals, while the forces countering growth are inertia, security, postponement of discomfort or effort, and various relationship payoffs which have been received for many years.

The therapeutic goal is to foster growth by shifting the reward systems to a new and better structure of the interpersonal system. Independence and selfhood for the individuals and for them as a married couple is achievable by redefining the interactional patterns. The parental hopes for the children are nearly always consonant with the married children's goals once the details and the process are therapeutically explicated.

Therapy helps the couple clearly establish a priority system, with the marriage and independence not to be compromised regardless of the rewards. Fidelity and consideration for the spouse must always take precedence over duty, obligation, courtesy or caring and love for the parent. Should this psychological and realistic goal be unacceptable for either spouse, there may be need to do individual therapy to unravel the unhealthy bond to parents. A useful therapeutic detail is to help the couple come to a unity of purpose and activity in achieving the goal. In-law and parental intrusions into the marriage are best resolved from a unified or couple effort. The couple must work together as a team, otherwise they can very easily be divided and conquered by parents committed to a perpetuation of old parent-child patterns.

Once the couple has settled the priority dilemma, they can move to redefining the relationship with the parents of in-laws. Since parents may not understand what is happening, or they may be caught up in problems of their own marriage, the burden of understanding and change will best be therapeutically focused on the available couple.

A series of helpful therapeutic steps can systematically move the couple into a more functional interaction system with the in-laws:

1) First, the couple must be helped through the process of coming together on their feelings and ideas of the goal they are after. At first they will feel from each other what they perceive to be an

intent to take over and demand change without understanding the issue. A husband who is thoughtful and considerate of his aging parents and wishes to be helpful to them, albeit spending too much time and energy on them, will be viewed by the wife as putting her second to his concern about the parents. The couple will need help exploring their feelings, expressing them in nonaccusatory ways, and mutually coming to the observation that the obstacle to their togetherness can be resolved. In other words, it is possible to be dutiful, courteous and helpful to parents and still retain the spouse as the number one person on the priority list. Once the husband sees how he can be responsive to his parents' needs and the wife can see her own needs being met, each can soften up his/her position and stand ready for negotiation on how to remove the obstacles to their flow of good feelings and understanding. A key to this step is practiced empathic understanding, coupled with self-disclosure and self-expression. Effective listening and open expression (e.g., Miller, Nunnally, and Wackman, 1975) invite understanding and set the stage for review of patterns and ways to resolve the issue.

2) From the understanding evolved, the couple is helped to acknowledge the priority of the marriage with all other issues moving to a secondary place. Each partner must feel the spouse's commitment to him/her and, emotionally as well as pragmatically, know he or she is the primary interest and concern, and not the parents.

3) Parental behavior and attitudes often convey the idea to married children that their continued dependency is the preferred status. Usually this perception is a distortion arising from garbled communication and failure of parental specification of intentions. Thus, to identify the common goal of parents and children as one of suitable independence for the son or daughter and his/her marriage is a helpful therapeutic step.

4) Another step in the process is outlining the procedures to be used by the couple on some specific issue where the parent has obviously inappropriate expectations or behavior. For example, if the parents, when in the couple's home, decide the couple should rearrange the furniture in the front room to suit their tastes and preferences, the couple can be instructed how to manage the situation. Frequently, the couple, not wishing to offend the parents, acquiesce to parental wishes, then feel anger and frustration at the parents, at themselves and often at each other.

5) Resolution of the dilemma may require greater understanding of the couple's feelings and instruction through behavioral rehearsal.

Feelings about confrontation and fear of outcomes need discussion and preparation. The couple may need help in determining who will be spokesperson and detailed instruction as to how they can meet the challenge. The first step could be for the couple to say to the parents. "We like it the way it is." If this doesn't register adequately, the next step in the sequence could be, "We prefer our arrangement and do not intend to alter it." A still more direct statement may be needed: "We want it this way and we think it inappropriate for you to suggest change." An ultimate position may be necessary: "We like our arrangement, and unless you stop trying to tell us how our furniture should be arranged we will ask you to leave." One of these steps will most likely bring the situation into focus to alter the problem area.

6) The next logical step is anticipation of both parental and couple reactions. The therapist needs to address the fears and discomfort of the couple and the astonishment and bewilderment of the parents. The couple must be prepared for a possible dramatic reaction by parents, even including a challenge to their position, expressed incredulity that a child of theirs would say such things, or even threats of disinheritance.

7) At this point encouragement must be given to the couple to hold their ground and persist in maintaining their position.

8) The final step is to reassure the couple that, as the parents register the new way the couple are defining the relationship, they will comply with the couple's expectations. As I have gone through these steps with couples in therapy, some parents have reacted to dampen or thwart efforts of the adult children; some have tried to dissuade the couple from continued therapy; others have tried to lay a heavy guilt load on the adult children; and some have sought therapy to resolve their own hangups. In most instances the parents have brought themselves into compliance with their children's preferences and definitions of the relationship. Usually the parents feel better when they can relinquish responsibility for any details of the married children's lives. The relationship can then be more productive, with the married children assuming personal responsibility and full jurisdiction over their lives; and the parents can retreat to a position of support and encouragement for their children, with a focus on their own relationship growth.

These steps restructure the parents' outmoded definition of the parent-child patterns and make possible a new, higher quality love interchange between the married children and their parents, and, in addition, significantly extinguish the pattern of stifling conditional love.

Reference

Miller, S., Nunnally, E. W., and Wackman, D. B. *Alive and Aware*. Minneapolis: Interpersonal Communication Programs, Inc., 1975.

VEON G. SMITH, M.S.S.A.
Professor
Graduate School of Social Work
University of Utah
Salt Lake City, UT

76. Involving the Family in Premarital Counseling

Question:

I once heard Carl Whitaker say at a workshop that one of the greatest myths about marriage is the idea that "I didn't marry your family, I married you." This makes me wonder when it would be appropriate to involve the families of the two people planning to get married, when the couple goes for premarital counseling.

Discussion:

Marriage is the union of two families. Or, to offer another quote from Carl Whitaker, "Marriage is the effort of two families to recreate themselves by sending out their scapegoats." The usefulness of involving the family in premarital counseling, then, is to make the mission of the scapegoats clearer, partially saving them from the complications of operating as undercover agents in the marriage.

When the premarital counselor thinks and works in terms of whole families, the addition of the families of origin to the counseling is an enriching experience. A healthy family has a sense of itself as a three to four generation integrated whole. The family and the subgroups and the individuals relate to an intrapsychic family of three or more generations (Whitaker and Keith, 1981). The goal of the counseling is to facilitate the integration of the multigenerational family. I cannot think of times when it would not be appropriate. The only danger is that someone might become upset and call off the marriage. But the homeostatic mechanisms in the families are usually heavily reinforced around the marriage. It has been my experience that people in the routine premarital "psychosis" have massive protection against upset. While they may be able to make use of counseling and discussion, they are never good candidates for psychotherapy.

If there are high voltage tensions about the marriage, they are much better exposed and diffused in the context of the expanded family than allowed to amplify covertly in the family triangulation system.

There are some standard operating procedures for organizing and conducting extended family conferences which might be useful to know. The counselor only need offer a conference with the families. The romantic leads have veto power, of course. If they are afraid of a conference, then it should not occur. Be certain that the marital pair takes responsibility for getting their families to come. The counselors can offer to accept phone calls from anyone who has questions about the purpose of the meeting. Make it clear that the family members are being invited in to help with the counseling, not to be counseled.

I think it best to use cotherapists for the multifamily, multigenerational conference. The counselor's primary job is to provide a place and a time for the meeting. The families' curiosity and anxiety should be allowed to take them wherever they want to go. The main goal is to get each family to tell its own story. Ask the fathers to describe their families and how they work. What was the groom like when he was a little boy? Ask each set of parents to describe their courtship and to reminisce about their wedding. What was each marriage like before the children arrived? What role did the in-laws play in their marriage? How did the fights about divorce begin?

The best arrangement would be for the two families to meet together, although there are some options. One would be for one family to come in at a time. Where it is not possible for families to come in, the counselor might suggest that the couple visit the families of origin as a way to find out more about the family's functioning and background. They could take a tape recorder home and ask some of the above questions.

Several years ago, an expatient called and asked if I would see her, her husband-to-be and their families for a premarital conference. We met for two hours on the afternoon of the wedding rehearsal. This conference had a lot of potential stress built into it as the new marriage was to be a mixing of religion; he was Presbyterian and she was Jewish. And his parents had been divorced 15 years previously. The families of origin had not met previously. Although the pseudomutual homeostatic syrup ran a little heavy for my family therapist's taste, the meeting was a warming human experience and I was delighted to be a part of it.

For most families, involvement in the premarital counseling would be a rewarding adventure, accomplishing in an organized way what is otherwise done informally and in fragments—getting to know one another. The usual pattern is for the families to become partially acquainted, then never to see each other again after the wedding. Perhaps activating the two-family whole before the wedding will enable the group to respond in a coordinated way to future change in the new family; births, changes in job or residence, support for child rearing. The extended family is almost always a factor in divorce. If the two families are a group at the start, they may provide a more adequate background for the couple to struggle with the crises which lead to divorce.

Anyone who extends premarital counseling to the whole family ought to write about it.

Reference

Whitaker, C. A. and Keith, D. V., Symbolic-experiential family therapy. In A. S. Gurman, and D. P. Kniskern (Eds.), *Handbook of Family Therapy*. New York: Brunner/Mazel, 1981.

DAVID V. KEITH, M.D.
Assistant Professor
Department of Psychiatry
University of Wisconsin Medical School
Madison, WI

77. Dynamics of Relationship Between Career Mothers and Young Adult Daughters

Question:

In the past decade, an increasing number of married women with children embarked on careers and became successful in business or in a profession. This new trend has had many ramifications in regard to modifying the dynamics of family interaction. Daughters of career mothers seem to be internalizing more multifaceted images of womanhood, as the role models their mothers present, combined with society's expectations and values regarding a "woman's place," continue to change. The various and often conflicting expectations are causing confusion leading to new presenting problem constellations in the therapists' office with the daughter as the identified patient.

What are the mother-daughter dynamics in a family in which the mother is a successful career woman and the daughter perceives her as a fine role model? What are the dynamics when the daughter believes her mother's involvement in her career represents a rejection of her role in and commitment to the family? What kind of therapeutic interventions can help the daughter find her separate identity within such a family context?

Discussion:

There are numerous problems daughters of successful career mothers present in therapy that seem to emanate from the special constellation and dynamics of the dual-career family (Rice, 1979). We will illuminate two of the major problems seen clinically with this population by way of illustration. The mothers being referred to are in the age range of 35-55 years and their daughters are 15-25. These comments apply to women's roles in the 1970s and 1980s; as society changes, so will the specific nature of the challenges which society's members face.

In families in which the mother is a successful career woman and the daughter perceives her as a fine role model, the daughter is faced with the dilemma of how she can be as good as, or better than, a "superwoman." These superwomen, who are successful in combining and juggling career and family, are by definition bright, competent, ambitious, tenacious and energetic. Many daughters of these women feel that their mothers have set standards for them which are very high or even unattainable. These daughters feel pressured to live up to their mothers' expectations. These expectations are not merely implicit, since mom is actively pursuing her own objectives, but rather comprise a compelling, if unspoken, message that it is taken for granted that the daughter will be extremely successful in both her personal and her professional life. For the most part, these daughters internalize these standards for themselves. Those daughters who would like to combine career and marriage but feel unsure about being able to do this well may become depressed, anxious and/or anorectic. Depression and anxiety may also be seen in those young adult women who are very close to their mothers and identify with their strength and exciting life style, but who are unable to separate enough from them to develop their own personal and professional identity. Furthermore, these young women are acutely aware of the conflicts and the many time and energy demands which confront a woman who desires to combine family and career. They may question whether the advantages of this stimulating family/career package outweigh the problems they associate with it.

At the other extreme are those families in which a daughter believes that her mother's involvement in her career is a rejection of her family. When this is the girl's perception, she may rebel against all which she believes her mother to represent. Many of these young women feel that their mothers were selfish in pursuing their careers and resent the fact that their mothers neglected them by not being available to bake, or shop, or to be "on call" as needed. Or, in less extreme cases, the daughter may be unhappy with playing "second fiddle" to her mother's career. Typically these young women are rebellious, angry and unhappy. They manifest their sense of abandonment and deprivation by acting out and they often do poorly in school. Acting-out and poor academic performance may be the daughter's way of expressing her feeling that she is not capable of being a successful career woman or that she would prefer to be a homemaker, remote from the demands of the work-a-day world. These young women may rebel in an attempt to get more attention from their mothers; getting into difficulty being a "cry for attention." At other times these young women may present as being critical, evasive and taciturn, alternately withdrawing to hide their longing for being more important in mother's life and attacking to demean her. Their resentment of and anger towards their mothers may become so consuming that their entire lives revolve around hurting and defeating mom.

It should be noted that the problems of all of these young women are similar to those faced by sons of successful fathers. However, in today's society there are many more and varied male role models and mentors for these young men to emulate, also it is expected that they will have a career and marry. By contrast, a young woman's mother may be one of the few females she encounters who is pursuing both simultaneously. Other adult women she knows may be fine wives and mothers or accomplished business or professional women whose career aspirations led them to chose to remain single or contributed to a divorce. Does she really have the option to be only one or the other, or will settling for only half of the gestalt make her feel like a failure?

When the daughter comes to therapy because of either depression, anxiety, suicidal ideation, anorexia or a general state of discontent and lack of direction, or because of difficulties caused from anger and rebelliousness, and talks a great deal about her mother, it is important to insist that the entire family be present at the next session (Napier and Whitaker, 1978). The father's attendance is also particularly critical as it is important that the daughter feels from the outset that both parents care enough about her to participate in the sessions. His being there is also imperative to help diffuse the intensity of the mother-daughter involvement, when the time is right to do so. His presence also provides the therapist with an opportunity to assess the dynamics and quality of the relationship of the parental dyad, the father's interaction with the daughter, whether daughter's perception of mother's role seems objectively realistic and is consensually validated by other members of the family, where other siblings fit, and why this youngster was vulnerable to becoming the identified patient. One intervention approach that seems to be efficacious is to ask everyone present to describe what they see as the reason for the session and what they view as the strengths and weaknesses in the family. Depending on how much is revealed that is pertinent to the presenting concern, the therapist might next ask each to comment on their perceptions of and feelings about mother's career. The father's responses should be attended carefully as they may provide clues as to whether: 1) he has been resentful but unwilling to express it and so the daughter has become the martyr in his stead; 2) he is delighted with his wife's accomplishments and pleased that she is bright and dynamic and contributes to the family income, easing the financial burden he would otherwise carry alone; 3) he welcomes his wife's independence and shares her high expectations for the daughter—who, in light of the strong parental coalition and mutually held goals for her, feels overwhelmed and helpless about carrying out a different destiny; 4) he is ambivalent and the daughter also vacillates between loving-identifying with and hating-rebelling against her mother; or 5) he is overshadowed by his wife and passive in his dealings with his daughter. The therapist also has to determine, by skillful probing, how the mother sees herself, what her priorities are in the present and what they were as her daughter was growing up, how much awareness she has of the impact of her choices and actions on others in her family, and her perception of her daughter's dilemma.

Once a solid understanding of the dynamics and structure of the family, past and present, is ascertained, treatment focuses on: 1) Helping the daughter really accept her desire to be a whole and separate individual, yet still connected with the family as a vital and loving member (Boszormenyi-Nagy and Spark, 1973); 2) Helping her not to engage in self-destructive behavior to punish her parents and, instead, to determine who she is and what she wants to do and be. It is important that she choose what is right for her and not simply to conform to or oppose her parent's wishes; 3) Helping her become assertive so that she can make her needs, desires and decisions known, and can insist on respect for her boundaries; 4) Facilitating the parents' ability to accept and communicate their willingness to let her be her own person and not a younger replica of her mother; 5) Intercepting and interrupting any efforts by her mother to keep her overly enmeshed or to push her beyond her level of capability and ambition; 6) Grappling with any desires the wife had for her husband that she had projected onto her daughter—so this pressure is alleviated and the underlying issue confronted; and 7) Helping mother to flaunt her achievements less and decenter her areas of concern to include her family more.

Where the syndrome includes acting-out in order to gain attention, it is crucial to see that the mother rearranges her schedule so as to have time, during her daughter's adolescence and early twenties, to spend with her when both are relaxed and interested in each other, and that mother be helped to show affection, support, acceptance and encouragement. This may necessitate redistributing finances to hire more household help to free up more of mother's time or to free the daughter from burdensome homemaking tasks, which have increased her resentment. Others in the family, including mother, may all have to pitch in to redistribute the tasks to be done.

If the young woman is living away from home and insists on working the problems out in individual therapy, at least one family session should be held and a family perspective should be used throughout her individual treatment.

Regardless of the treatment modality, the therapist should be mindful of his/her own biases about the attitudes toward dual-career marriages and how parenting roles are lived out. *Options for women* subsumes a whole repertoire of potent choices for mothers and daughters, and the important men in their lives.

References

Boszormenyi-Nagy, I. and Spark, G. *Invisible Loyalties*. New York: Harper & Row, 1973.
Napier, A. and Whitaker, C. *The Family Crucible*. New York: Harper & Row, 1978.
Rice, D. G. *Dual-Career Marriage: Conflict and Treatment*. New York: Free Press, 1979.

NADINE JOY KASLOW, M.A.
Ph.D. Candidate—Clinical Psychology
Department of Psychology
University of Houston
Houston, TX

and

FLORENCE W. KASLOW, Ph.D.
Professor
Department of Mental Health Sciences
Hahnemann Medical College
Philadelphia, PA

PART B

Communication, Imagery and Symbolism

78. Communication Training in Nonbehavioral Marital Therapy

Question:

Most of the research I've read about communication training with couples talks about a highly systematic, sequenced, modular approach. It's also clear that most marital therapists, even those who are more psychodynamically oriented, place a high priority on improving a couple's ability to communicate. Are there really any serious disadvantages in working on a couple's communication in a generally more unstructured type of treatment? Can't the same skills be taught as part of the natural "flow" of a more insight-oriented approach?

Discussion:

The advantages and disadvantages of working on a couple's communication within a relatively unstructured therapeutic approach have not been addressed in research investigations. As noted in your question, the majority of researchers have focused upon the efficacy of highly structured communication training programs in which couples are exposed to a preplanned sequence of exercises of roleplays. The data obtained generally indicate that these structured programs have a significant positive impact on communication. However, the results must be interpreted cautiously since much of the research involves young couples who are not experiencing severe marital distress. This may introduce a positive bias into the findings, since these couples are probably the ones most likely to accept and respond well to a highly structured program.

It is clear that certain research priorities, such as the need for a detailed and replicable treatment program, often contribute to the degree of structure in the programs studied. In fact, many researchers have noted that their programs provide clinicians with techniques that should be integrated with other treatment methods or that the "flow chart" of the component modules should be modified, depending upon the needs of each couple. On the basis of clinical experience, it could be argued not only that highly systematic preplanned modular approaches are not necessary, but that there could be serious disadvantages to routinely following such programs with most couples in marital therapy. Many couples may find the presequenced programs artificial and/or irrelevant to their problems. Additionally, there may be less generalization of communication skills from the session to the home if therapy is very highly structured and systematized. Of greatest importance is that a more unstructured approach has the clear advantage of allowing the therapist to be responsive to the particular needs and interactional pattern presented by each couple. In sum, it appears advisable, rather than disadvantageous, to be prepared to work on communication in a less structured therapy than that described in research reports on communication training.

A more difficult question involves the degree of structure necessary within any particular therapy session. Structure in a session for the purpose of communication enhancement is here defined as a direct focus on current communication patterns, achieved through therapist control of the content and/or form of the in-session discussions. For example, one can be reasonably unstructured and work directly on communication patterns by giving feedback on a particularly problematic or helpful communication as it occurs naturally over the course of the sessions. This feedback could occur during problem-solving discussions, or during explorations of the spouses' defenses or their patterns of interaction in their families of origin. Alternatively, even within the context of a more unstructured therapy, one can impose a high degree of structure through a roleplay or training exercise, for all or part of any session or series of sessions.

Although there are no data-based guidelines to follow, it may prove helpful to consider the following variables when making decisions regarding the degree of structure necessary within a session (or across several sessions) to work on successfully improving a couple's communication skills.

The level of communication skills displayed by the couple can affect the degree of structure necessary, in that couples who are extremely hostile and deficient in skills may at times require a more structured approach. This suggestion may appear to be in contradiction to the statement made earlier regarding the appropriateness of systematic, modular programs for young couples who are not in serious distress. To clarify, the present recommendation for highly distressed couples is for occasional within-session structure. That is, although these couples may not respond well to a preplanned, sequenced program, it may be advisable to impose a structured approach at various times over the course of the therapy, when attempting directly to teach particular skills. For example, in unstructured discussions, couples with very problematic interaction patterns would be continually breaking certain "rules" of communication, so that corrective feedback on their difficulties would become extremely intrusive to the point of being the focus of the sessions. Additionally, if the spouses are extremely hostile toward each other, structuring the discussion can be an effective method of (a) increasing their ability to receive (hear) feedback in a helpful way, and (b) prompting them to shift from an exclusive focus on content (what they are arguing about) to a consideration of process (how they are arguing). Often, communication training with these couples involves structured exercises that shape basic skills.

If the therapist prefers not to impose a great deal of communication-oriented structure on the sessions, he/she may decide to give feedback only on a few communication difficulties that are (a) very basic and clear impediments to discussion, e.g., lack of eye contact, constant interruptions, and/or (b) fairly easy to identify and change, e.g., lack of "I" statements is often recognized more readily by the spouses than are counterattacks and cross-blaming statements, the latter being more difficult to change because of the spouses' need to defend themselves.

The therapist's assessment of the particular interactional skills the couple needs to learn can also indicate the degree of advisable structure. Examples of skills that might be most readily learned in a structured format include empathic listening and sharing of feelings. Empathy training exercises, designed to teach these skills, have been evaluated positively in a number of outcome studies. Interactional skills that could be more effectively shaped within an unstructured context involve a client's difficulty in communicating clearly at the time he/she is experiencing particular emotions. Providing feedback when this difficulty arises during the natural "flow" of a session can have much more impact than an exercise designed to induce the emotional reaction. For example, to develop congruence between verbal and nonverbal messages, the therapist could give feedback when he/she notes an incongruent communication, such as a spouse saying "I am not angry" in a loud voice.

In addition to being responsive to the degree of hostility and overall communication skills displayed and the particular skills a couple is lacking, a therapist should be sufficiently flexible so as to modify the degree of structured work on communication, depending upon the couple's progress in therapy. One can incorporate varying degrees of structure into a variety of therapeutic approaches. For example, a therapist may be working on perceptual distortions and projections that contribute to inaccurate messages and unempathic responses, but may also choose to do structured empathy training as either a preparation for or an adjunct to the insight-oriented discussions. Additionally, certain insights, such as an understanding of how a spouse is repeating his/her parents' patterns, can increase both receptivity to feedback and the motivation to learn new skills.

Thus, it seems clear that interactional skills can be taught as part of the natural "flow" of a more insight-oriented approach. The present discussion has raised issues to consider in deciding if and when it is necessary to interrupt that flow and provide a more direct, didactic focus on communication.

HILLARY TURKEWITZ, Ph.D.
Research Associate
Department of Psychology
State University of New York
Stony Brook, NY

79. Sensitive Communication: Making Impact Consistent with Intent

Question:

Couples frequently ask a counselor to help them improve their communication. The partners might report that they often begin discussions with good will, sincerely hoping to understand each other's viewpoints and feelings on a topic, or hoping to arrive at a mutually satisfactory approach to a problem. Unfortunately, the discussions become unproductive, marked by emotional responses of guilt, anxiety or anger, by defensive responses of denial, withdrawal, derailment of the discussion or attack, and by decreased esteem for the relationship, the spouse and the self. Here, in contrast to some communication problems, the channels of communication are at least partially open and the initial intentions are positive, but the ultimate impact is negative. How can counselors help couples learn to make the impact of these communications more consistent with the intent—positive and productive, not negative and destructive?

Discussion:

Regardless of the degree of disharmony within a marriage or the presence or absence of psychopathology in either partner, most partners can still communicate well on some topics. Their problems arise primarily on sensitive topics. Typically a topic is sensitive when it presents a perceived threat (physical or psychological) to a person who lacks experience in reducing such threats through calm, equalitarian deliberations.

Psychological threats often involve frustrations which stem from unmet expectations. Often, as Albert Ellis points out, these are instances where the negative outcome of some event is perceived to be far worse than it actually could be: catastrophic or terrible, rather than unfortunate or inconvenient. A partner feeling threatened tends to distort everything else going on and to attribute undesirable motives or incompetencies to the other spouse. If he or she lacks successful experiences with calm exchange and discussion, the partner is likely to try reducing the threat or stress by hurriedly escaping (perhaps through a guilt-eliciting power play or through a change of topic) and to avoid discussion of the topic in the future—unless really prepared to "win" next time.

Partners seeking improvement in their communications could perhaps extrapolate useful ideas from a course addressing the whole area of communication. Also, they might do well to spend some time analyzing how they interact and how they preceive each other as they discuss nonsensitive topics. However, their time with the counselor will be best spent if they focus attention on the specific problems which arise during their discussions of sensitive topics. Most importantly, they need to recognize when a communication is becoming threatening, to identify what sorts of issues and behaviors evoke perceptions of being threatened, and to know what actions each can take to reduce those threats more effectively or to prevent their occurrences in the first place.

Initial Meetings

Certainly, during initial sessions the counselor will devote more time to rapport building and information gathering, and in subsequent sessions spend more time on practice discussions in the office, on assigned discussions at home, and on drawing implications from these learning experiences. Nevertheless, an observer would probably find no clear-cut distinction between an assessment phase and a treatment phase. New concerns might be assessed—complete with questions covering the topic's general nature, its relevant historical background and its more specific current functioning—not only in the first session, but also in the tenth or twentieth session, should treatment last that long. On the other hand, some suggestions are quite frequently obvious and appropriately given before the end of the first session.

Regardless of likely diagnosis, communication-oriented marital therapy has a here-and-now emphasis on making use of each partner's "normal" processes, rather than on effecting personality changes. Furthermore, the main requirement is that each partner possess a strong motivation to communicate better with the other. If he or she has other motives which are in conflict—for example, if John wants to save the marriage at all costs and Mary feels uncommitted—all three must examine the discrepancies (together and individually) to determine whether the conflicts are likely to undermine the couple's common goal of improving their communication. Throughout treatment, the current motives of each partner will remain an important assessment concern.

Communication-oriented assessment has much in common with other types of marital assessment. However, the counselor especially looks for recurring patterns which might indicate the most relevant areas of threat. Relevant questions include: What sorts of topics seem to be sensitive? Do they fall into some sort of hierarchy, from least to most sensitive? What are the threats? What are the predominant ways each partner reduces these threats? Do discussions with negative impact progress along a predictable pattern? Are there any particular events or circumstances—coming before or during the discussions—which make either or both partners more vulnerable to threat when talking with each other? Answers to these questions do not always come by the end of the first or even the tenth session. Finding answers sometimes requires individual rather than conjoint interviews. Sometimes the answers only gradually emerge as clients and counselor analyze the circumstances surrounding any problems which recur between sessions or during in-session roleplays.

By the end of the first session, the counselor typically has some ideas of which topics are least and most sensitive, and why. Thus, the counselor can probably make several reasonable interim suggestions, both for communication per se and for keeping going whatever momentum got the couple to seek help. Frequently, the counselor may ask the couple to hold a moratorium on the discussion of all the sensitive topics except the one that falls lowest on their sensitivity hierarchy. For that topic, the counselor may ask them to have two "discussion dates," following such rules as: 1) do not stray on to other topics, 2) choose a time and place for the date which is most likely to lead to uninterrupted, emotionally controlled discussion, 3) avoid prediscussion activities which may cause either partner to be unduly emotionally vulnerable (e.g., involving drugs, fatigue or negative emotions generated from other parts of their separate or conjoint lives), and 4) set a time limit of 20 minutes for each of the dates.

Whether or not having discussion dates seems appropriate for a particular couple, the counselor will probably ask each partner to keep a diary which covers any sensitive interactions occurring before the next counseling session. The diaries increase each person's awareness and help the partners more accurately report what sorts of things were going on before and during discussions, what was being said, how it seemed to be said, how each person felt, and how each person reacted to the other.

In the second meeting, depending on the case's complexity, the counselor may devote additional time specifically for information-gathering purposes. Less formally, however, the partners' reports of the week's positive and negative interactions may provide clues on the types of habits (both cognitive and behavioral) each needs to develop. For further assessment and treatment purposes, the counselor may then ask the couple either to reenact part of a previous discussion date or to attempt a slightly more sensitive topic in his/her presence.

The counselor's very presence provides some sense of security, perhaps analogous to the referee in a boxing match who tries to prevent participants from seriously injuring each other. In contrast to the referee, however, the counselor must allow threats and maladaptive responses ("low blows" or "cheap shots") to occur so that partners can be made aware of their use and impact. Thus, while a counselor's presence must insure enough security to encourage some risk taking and genuine confrontation, providing too much security is a common pitfall.

Two other common pitfalls involve partners attempting to cast the counselor in the role of either Great Problem Solver or Judge. It is the partners' role both to solve their problems and to decide what is right for them, and the counselor's role only to aid them in various ways, most notably by helping them communicate more effectively. Undue expansion of the counselor's role simply fosters countertherapeutic dependencies.

Besides providing information and suggestions, the counselor increasingly shows partners how they might approach future communication problems on their own. Most notably, the counselor has the couple temporarily interrupt counterproductive interactions, to ask themselves what is going on—what did John hear or see Mary do, how did he feel, what thoughts came out . . . and what was Mary actually trying to do? Perceived references to something marginally relevant or to something they have tacitly agreed not to bring up—"forbidden topics"—can turn productive discussions into bitter arguments. The counselor's focus is on helping the partners learn to reduce such threats, both cognitively and behaviorally.

When threats are verbalized, the counselor helps both partners understand how a normal person could—with a given cognitive-perceptual "filter"—feel threatened. As their awareness increases, the partners begin to remind themselves and each other to use more helpful filters. Each partner is also shown how to replace his or her typical current behavioral methods of coping with threat (attacking, withdrawing, etc.) with more effective methods. Most important here, each is taught to "compare the impact with the intent"—to honestly, nonpunitively, noninterpretively report his/her own emotional reactions to a specific incident and to request a report of intentions from the other person.

Finally, the sender of the communication is shown alternative ways of sending messages which can help make the impact more consistent with a nonthreatening intent. A most important distinction here is between a communication's content message and relationship message. The content message would be the words taken literally. The relationship message is made up of all other aspects of the exchange. It suggests the speaker's evaluation of the listener and the speaker's view of the relationship with the listener—and it "tells" the listener how to interpret the words which were spoken. The relationship message, whether positive or negative, is conveyed not so much through words as through the ways they were said and the context in which they were said.

While relationship messages are obviously very important, most people have not consciously practiced sending them. A negative relationship message—often just a suggestion of a sneer or a hint at a known weakness or problem—can have a considerable impact on a discussion. Recognizing the effects of these small bits of aggression inserted into a discussion which is labelled as an honest attempt to resolve a problem can go far toward eliminating them, if both partners cooperate. Thus, one partner calmly pointing out the negative relationship message as soon as it occurs can help restore balance and objectivity needed to resolve the issue directly under discussion.

Not only may the partners inappropriately send negative relationship messages, but also they frequently miss opportunities to send positive ones. Especially with sensitive topics, it is important to pair a positive relationship message (e.g., a touch on the arm which conveys, "I have commitment to you, John") with whatever content is needing to be said (e.g., "John, I would like to attend a two-day conference in Chicago next month") in order to reduce the chances of a perceived threat. The concepts and techniques here often draw from research in family communication systems and nonverbal behavior.

Occasionally, of course, the questions which follow the temporary interruption of a sensitive discussion reveal that (for the moment) the sender indeed had threatening intentions. In these cases, the focus shifts to whatever the sender was feeling. The sender probably felt threatened also or would not have resorted to the counterproductive tactics.

By the end of the session, whether or not the discussion's sensitive topic got fully aired, the counselor has the couple summarize the suggestions on how to cognitively and behaviorally restructure their communication patterns. Before next session, they will have more discussion dates, either on the same topic or on more sensitive ones, continuing to record their interactions in their diaries.

Subsequent Meetings and Termination; Fostering Generalization

A similar format typically occurs on subsequent sessions, all the way to treatment termination. Probably the most consistent themes throughout are that the partners need to give feedback for positive and negative impact and that they need to check out intentions when the impact is negative. For at least several sessions (and sometimes over many sessions) certain problems persist or new ones arise, requiring new approaches as well as refinements of old ones. But even before the frequency of needed refinements and new approaches starts to drop off, the counselor begins working toward termination by systematically turning more of the responsibility for good communication over to the couple. This is essential if the partners are to generalize and apply what they have learned. More and more they should decide which topics to handle, and when, where and how; they become responsible for analyzing the successes and failures of attempted discussions, for drawing implications and for rehearsing how to handle future situations.

As the counselor gives more responsibility in-session and between sessions, he/she may also increase the couple's responsibility by increasing the intervals between sessions. Typically, early sessions would be one week apart. As intervals increase, couples are assured that they can schedule an emergency appointment if they encounter a crisis, though they are told to first try resolving the problem themselves. For their own long-range security, they need to be as self-reliant as possible before termination; relatively speaking the counselor's availability represents only a short-range security.

While there is no set rule of thumb, terminations generally seem appropriate after one or two one-month intervals between sessions. The main criterion, however, is that the partners show a high degree of self-reliance in constructively approaching potentially sensitive issues. Being human, the partners will never reduce their percentages of bad impact to zero, but they can learn to recover from instances where the impact was negative, analyzing for themselves what went wrong and more effectively preventing similar problems in the future.

RALPH W. TRIMBLE, Ph.D.
Clinical Psychologist
Psychological and Counseling Center
University of Illinois
Urbana-Champaign, IL

80. Identifying Hidden Expectations
   in Marital Therapy

Question:

Sometimes I feel almost overwhelmed by the complexity of marital relationships I treat in therapy. But I know that there are a lot of hidden expectations in marriage and "double binds" that are quite common. Could you identify these for me?

Discussion:

Discord and unhappiness in marital conflict are often experienced by marital partners as unclear feelings—ambiguous and ambivalent—with the partners themselves uncertain as to the rationale for the negative reactions they are experiencing.

These feelings often stem from misprogrammed and fallacious attitudes and beliefs rooted in their historic past or "childhood consciousness" which are largely unknown or outside of the awareness of the individuals concerned. Family systems theory, in using genograms (three-generation family maps), attempts to trace early learnings that have been handed down in the form of current emotions, behavior and attitudes in the marital relationship.

The list of marital mishaps that follows is designed to focus immediately on those underlying attitudes and beliefs that are most commonly involved in marital discord and disillusion. It is written in simple, easily understood, every-day language, with some humor, as learning takes place more easily and defenses are more quickly dropped in a nonthreatening, laughter-inducing atmosphere. In using the list as a checklist (in individual, conjoint and couples group sessions), marital partners have been able to recognize and acknowledge with little defensiveness those sources of discomfort that have led to bitterness, pain, fear, anger and/or withdrawal. A more cooperative climate of openness, curiosity, humor and understanding begins to take place. The simply-worded, illustrated checklist surfaces those very attitudes and beliefs that are creating marital problems and opens up for discussion the different reactions spouses have to what each has deemed "reasonable" expectations, the "knots" in their intimate relationships.

Although certain key items in the list repeat with high frequency (i.e., #1 for both sexes, #13 for men), the list ventures to cover the range of reactions in intimate conflict while acknowledging the futility of attempting a complete list. At a didactic level, the list is designed to surface differences in five areas: closeness/distance expectations, separateness/togetherness, strength (power)/weakness, independence/dependence and sex-role expectations. The author has found that an initial reading of the list evokes both humor and sober reflection by the partners of the *range of misconceptions* each is capable of in their relationship. Fruitful discussion of areas in which they differ and a more focused, nondefensive exploration of the origins of their expectations then becomes possible. In addition, reeducation of what are reasonable or logical expectations can begin immediately, as each opens to exploring the previously concealed facets of self and other.

In summary, the list has been found to be a useful tool for rapidly creating a nonthreatening, nondefensive climate, characterized by openness and humor. In this climate, work can proceed to explore and discuss those responses which lead to marital pain, disillusion and breakdown. Relearning and reeducation can begin immediately.

Marital Knots (Nots)

1) If you loved me you would know . . . what I think, feel, want . . . and you would give it to me. Since you don't, you obviously don't care. So why should I care what you think, feel, say, want or do . . . So when you tell me what you want, *I* will be withholding . . .
   i.e., if you loved me, you would . . .
   talk to me (or listen to me)
   always agree with me, want what I want and like what I like
   want to take care of me
   want to do things for me
   bring new excitement into my life, plan it and make it happen
   you would . . .
   You don't. You don't love me.
2) If you tell me your feelings, I must do what you want. That would interfere with what I want . . . think . . . feel . . . so I don't want to hear (know) your feelings.
3) If you tell me what you want, I feel controlled. If I feel controlled, I feel weak, inadequate. I cannot give you what you ask for, without my feeling bad.

4) If I try to tell you my feelings you interrupt, correct, judge or ignore me. I am angry, frustrated. I won't tell you my feelings. (I distance.)

5) If I give to (do for) you and *you* don't acknowledge it, I feel unappreciated, empty. Since what I give you is unappreciated, I will give you nothing.

6) If I acknowledge *how much* you do for me, I feel beholden, burdened and obligated to do for you. I don't want to. I cannot acknowledge what you do.

7) If we don't agree, one of us must be wrong. If it is me, that implies that I am bad, stupid, ignorant or inadequate, so it can't be me. I must *prove* it is you, to protect me from feeling like a failure.

8) If I acknowledge that I see your pain, I must be able to fix it. I don't know how to fix it. So I won't acknowledge that I see it.

9) If you are in pain, I should be able to fix it. I don't know how to fix it. I feel inadequate. I am angry at you for making me feel inadequate. I withdraw from you, blame you, when you are in pain.

10) If you are in pain, I see you as blaming me. So I withdraw, leave or get angry. If it is my fault, I am bad. I am angry at you for making me feel inadequate, bad.

11) If I tell you how I feel, you will be angry. You will attack me. I am afraid of your anger. I can't tell you.

12) If I tell you how I feel, you will be upset. I can't stand how I feel when you are upset. I can't tell you. I live a lie.

13) If I were what *I* should be, *you* would be happy. I would be able to solve (fix) everything. Since I can't, your unhappiness makes me feel inadequate, guilty, angry. I distance from you.

14) If I were what *I* should be, *I* would never be: weak, tired, inadequate, distant, impotent, afraid . . . (I am.) I feel inadequate. I must *hide* what I feel so you won't find out how inadequate I really am.

15) If you were what *you* should be, *you* would never be: sad, angry, unloving, worried, suspicious, tired, loud, sick, selfish, weak, disagreeable, clumsy, controlling, flirtatious, demanding . . . (You are.)

16) If you were what *you* should be, *I* would be: happy, successful, popular, attractive, virile, potent, sexy . . . (I am not.) It's your fault.

17) I have a belief that:
   A MAN is never . . .

     A WOMAN is never . . .

If *I* am these things, *I* am bad, stupid, inadequate, sick, crazy. *I* am defective. I must hide.

If *you* are these things, *you* are defective. I am betrayed. You broke the contract.

18) I have a belief that:

     A MAN is always . . .

     A WOMAN is always . . .

If *I* am not, I am bad, stupid, inadequate, sick, crazy. *I* am defective. I must hide.

If *you* are not, you are defective. I am betrayed. (You broke the contract.)

19) If I let you get close to me, I fear I will be trapped, engulfed or smothered. You will control me. I must keep my distance from you and not allow you to get close.

20) If I let you get close, you will find out my secrets, my fears, how inadequate I really am, and then you couldn't love (respect) me. I must keep you at a distance.

21) If I let myself get close to you, I will need you. I will lose the ability to be alone, to function on my own. I will become weak. I am afraid. I must avoid closeness.

22) If I am too close, too dependent, need (love) you too much, I will not be able to survive without you. I must distance from you, care less, to be sure I won't miss (need) you too much, when you are gone (die, leave me).

23) If I love you, I will need you. I cannot trust you to be there. Therefore, I cannot (will not) love you.

24) If you are distant from me, you could not love me. Therefore, why should I love you?

Marital Knots (Nots) and Double Binds

1) If you criticize me, I feel inadequate. If you compliment me, you are placating me, by only saying what you think I want to hear.

2) If I tell you what I want and you do what I want, it doesn't count because I had to tell you. If you do what I want, but not *the way* I wanted you to, it still doesn't count. If I don't tell you what I want, you don't do what I want. I feel unloved.

3) If I do what you want, you love me. You only love what I do . . . not me. I feel like nothing. Therefore, I will do nothing.

4) If I am what you want me to be, I dislike myself. I resent you for

wanting me to be what I don't like. If I am myself, you won't like me. I resent you for not letting me be myself. I resent you for controlling me.

5) If you want to be alone, it means you don't want me with you. If you loved me, you would always want me with you. If you always want me with you, I feel smothered. . . .

6) If you comfort (give to) me, and I am comforted, you are more powerful than I am. I will not accept your comfort. If I comfort you, you *are* comforted. I resent you for being comfort-able when I can never be.

7) If I work hard for you to love me, you are happy. The harder I work, the more tired I get. The harder I work, the wearier I am, the happier you are. I can't be happy when I am so weary. I hate you for being happy when I can't be.

8) If you give to me, I feel beholden, obligated, burdened, and I distance. If you don't give to me, I feel unloved, uncared for, unwanted and I distance.

9) If you need me, I feel obligated, pressured, burdened, responsible. If you don't need me, I think you don't care.

10) If I am angry, I cannot tell you, for you would . . . leave, withhold from me, retaliate, abandon me. I am afraid to be without you. I am a coward. I hate you for making me a coward.

11) If I distance from you, I miss what I have with you. I draw closer. If I need you, I am weak. I hate myself for being weak. I hate you for making me weak.

12) If you don't love me, stay with me. I will die. I must cling to you no matter what the price. The more I cling, the more you distance. The more you distance, the more I cling.

13) My commitment to you is too restrictive.
     I wish to change it.
     I cannot tell you.
     You would be upset.
     To see you is to experience my guilt.
     I will find reasons to be angry with you, so I need *not* feel guilty.
     I will provoke you, anger you, drive you away, to give me a *reason* to be angry with you.
     So I can feel justified in my behavior, in breaking my commitment.
     And not feel guilty.

14) I am weak.
     You are a witness to my weakness.
     You are the cause of my weakness.

I must punish you for seeing, causing this in me.
I will use power to make you suffer, so I will feel stronger.
I must find a way to make the punishment seem reasonable.
I will look for things to blame you for, so I may punish you, so
    I may feel more powerful, stronger and forget that I feel so
    weak.
I will feel stronger by making you feel weak.
        And yet,
       I love,
        need,
          want you. . . .

False Beliefs

If you loved me, you could read my mind.
Difference means one must be bad, wrong.
Closeness is dangerous.
If I need you that means I am weak.
A loving partner must always do what the other wants.
A man should know everything, be able to do everything, fix
    everything.
Strong feelings are dangerous—pain, fear, anger, love,
    pleasure, need.

LORI EISENBERG, M.S.W., A.C.S.W.
Director
The Family Relations Institute
Falls Church, VA

81. "Unsharable" Secrets in Sex and Marital Therapy

Question:

In my practice of sex and marital therapy, I frequently find myself the recipient of confidential material, particularly some sexual "transgression" which one partner wishes to keep hidden from the other. I feel a professional responsibility to honor the confidentiality, but often find myself in a bind in the therapy when I observe the consequences of the secret played out in the couple's interaction. Being constrained from interpreting its meaning hampers my effectiveness. In the reading I've done I haven't found a systematic discussion which could provide me with a rationale for deciding when such secrets are a contraindication for conjoint (sex) therapy, or when, if ever, therapy can proceed despite them. I'd also like some advice on how to handle the situation with the individual or couple once it is presented to me.

Discussion:

The presence of unsharable material is a problem which frequently arises in the course of sex and marital therapy, and for which no satisfactory solution has been proffered. In scanning the literature and conversing with colleagues, I have collected a variety of approaches, ranging from a belief that therapy is not possible without full disclosure of all secrets, to the caution that therapists are too often insistent on disclosure of secrets best left for the individual to struggle with on his or her own. In my practice, which consists primarily of sex therapy, I take an intermediate stance—preferring disclosure, but considering in each case what secrets could be tolerated without undermining the goals or procedures of the therapy. To explicate the bases for making these judgments, it may be helpful to define those goals and examine the consequences for both couple and therapist of the kinds of secrets most frequently encountered.

In contrast to marital therapy, the primary goal of sex therapy is more narrowly focused: to reverse the sexual dysfunction by modifying the specific factors in the sexual system which impair adequacy. The prescription of graded sexual tasks, providing an "in vivo" desensitization and opportunity for new learning, further differentiates the two therapeutic modes. However, in order to function effectively sexually, one must be able to abandon oneself to the erotic experience. Fears of performance, intimacy, vulnerability, and issues of power serve as effective barriers to that abandonment. Thus, to carry out sex therapy without attention to the couple's interpersonal transactions is a hollow and futile exercise. For couples seeking help with a sexual difficulty, the role of sex as the "physical language of the primary emotional bond" (Scharff, 1978) has been elevated in significance. Whether as cause or effect, those issues of mutuality, trust, intimacy, vulnerability and fears of rejection have become channeled in the sexual exchange. It comes as no surprise, then, that various sexual behaviors or fantasies, past as well as present, constitute the bulk of the secrets encountered by the therapist. Some of the most frequent confidences shared with me have been: extramarital affairs; homosexual activity or desires; pretenses within the relationship (never been "turned on" to partner, never enjoyed sex, never had orgasm); and sexual trauma, such as incest or rape.

There are some general consequences for the couple when this material cannot be talked about. Any significant secret represents a withholding of a part of the self, and, to varying degrees, requires erecting a protective barrier around the secret and the affect attached to it. The degree of insistence that the secret remain hidden is often a mirror of its potency. As such, it continues to operate in the intimacy of the sexual relationship through the secret-bearer's guardedness, need to deny, project, behave in overly submissive or apologetic ways, or otherwise deal with whatever guilt and shame accompanies the secret. The partner often senses the constraint, and, being denied access to the explanation, elaborates reasons in accord with his/her own fears of inadequacy and rejection.

Further, as argued by Scharff (1978), protection of the partner, the reason often given for maintaining the secret, is demeaning and self-serving. While there may be circumstances in which the revelation of a secret could precipitate a severe psychological disturbance in the spouse, more often the secret-bearer's "protection" is a self-protection against the anger and disaffection of the partner and against facing his/her own shame and guilt. Such "protection" of the partner prevents a choice based on all the facts and contributes to a situation of inequality in which one member of the couple is experienced as having all the power in the relationship.

Corresponding consequences may be experienced by the therapist. Being the recipient of just one partner's secret can create an ambivalent alliance, upsetting the always precarious balance the therapist must maintain—equidistant from each member of the couple. Also, the maintenance of the secret makes what may be a major source of anxiety unavailable to therapeutic attention and, where the specific content of the secret is pertinent to the problematic sexual interaction, prevents the therapist from providing facilitating understanding.

Do these concerns imply a requirement for complete disclosure or no therapy? I don't think so. Depending upon the nature of the secret and the degree of interference, I have found it possible to proceed with therapy without disclosure. Some examples may help clarify the circumstances.

Extramarital affairs. My experience has been that the presence of an ongoing sexual liaison (whether secret or not) is a contraindication to sex therapy. In addition to the questionable marital commitment, the availability of another partner provides too easy an escape from the anxiety and discomfort brought out by the prescribed sexual tasks. The motivation to struggle with that anxiety is markedly diminished. On the other hand, I have been able to ignore a past affair, particularly if it appears that it occurred in response to circumstances which are not centrally operating in the couple's current relationship.

Not infrequently a dysfunctional partner will "test" him/herself with others, hoping for reassurance of sexual adequacy. The nondysfunctional partner may also have sought outside liaisons, in frustration, anger, or as an attempt to prove that it is not he/she who is "causing" the partner's problem. While the success or failure of such attempts is important data for the therapist, it is not the primary issue in a therapy which views the couple's sexual interaction as the "patient." However, a significant problem arises when the outcome of such encounters leads to a covertly communicated ascription of fault and responsibility (to self or partner). It may then be necessary to explicitly discuss these secret encounters, unless the therapist's direct focus on the joint responsibility is sufficient to alter the underlying message. The request for disclosure in this situation should aim towards enhancing each partner's empathy for the other's predicament—the attempt to feel adequate and repair damaged self-esteem.

Homosexual behavior and fantasies. It is possible to maintain secrecy about homosexual behavior if it does not play a central role in the couple's dysfunction. However, confidential material about significant homosexual desires, acted upon or in fantasy, which intrude into the couple's sexual interaction cannot be bypassed if a therapeutic process is to ensue. While the "homosexual" partner's fear that the information will be greeted with shocked intolerance is understandable, in my, albeit limited, experience there is often sufficient underlying congruence in the couple's values to mitigate against the feared loss of respect and rejection. Understanding the self-esteem issues for the spouse may be helpful. While there is usually a painful sense of rejection of that person's sexual identity (as woman/man), it may be counteracted by some relief that it is not his/her personal qualities to which the other is unresponsive. Further reparation to self-esteem may be achieved by the feeling "I am so important and loved, he/she wants me despite his/her homosexual desires."

Sexual pretenses within the relationship. Many couples have kept from each other years of frustration and disappointment in their sexual relationship. Having pretended for so long, they fear that disillusionment and untrustworthiness would be engendered should past pretenses now be revealed. Women, more frequently than men, have masked an absence of desire, enjoyment, orgasm—in part because women can more easily simulate sexual responsiveness. But the pretense began, also, because of cultural influences regarding male and female sex roles. Many couples still harbor the notion that the woman's sexual pleasure is the man's responsibility. One can see then that this would lead to the fear that exposure would be devastating to the male sexual ego. It is precisely because these "myths" represent barriers to the direct communication necessary for enjoyable sexual interaction that they must be brought into the therapeutic arena.

Sexual trauma. An assumption of guilt for having "participated" in an incestuous relationship is often the underlying reason for an individual's wish to maintain secrecy. It may be possible to talk about guilt and its effects in the therapy without having to specify its source. When the woman has been a victim of rape, the consequences of secrecy are more problematic. In addition to guilt ("Did I invite the attack?"), fear and anger towards the partner, who represents the male aggressor, leaves him with a sense of wrong-doing whose source he can't identify. He may then react defensively to this unacknowledged ascription of blame.

Given these considerations, what can you use to guide your decisions? The initial evaluation in the sex therapy model includes both conjoint and individual sessions. The individual sexual history session provides the opportunity for, even elicits, information the individual may wish to keep confidential. I inform the person that this is a confidential interview, and ask that I be apprised of what information cannot be shared. I also indicate, however, that I may feel that therapy would not be possible without the client's disclosure of certain material at some point. When such material is presented, I explore the imagined consequences of disclosure and the degree of anxiety mobilized. The individual interviews also allow the exploration of each partner's fantasies about the other; what might not be known, but could be imagined. On this basis some clinical judgment is possible regarding how facilitating or damaging a particular secret might be. However, I am willing to accept that the individual's longer association with the partner may make him/her more knowledgeable than me. If I decide to proceed with therapy despite an insistence on secrecy, later individual sessions can be used to urge disclosure if an impasse has been reached.

It is never the therapist's prerogative to divulge a secret. It is the therapist's responsibility to try to provide an atmosphere which would allow each partner to take the other into his/her confidence. When that does not seem likely, exit as gracefully as possible, offering whatever rationale is appropriate and believable. It clearly would accomplish no useful purpose to tell the couple that sex therapy is not indicated because there are unsharable secrets!

Reference

Scharff, D. Truth and consequences in sex and marital therapy: The revelation of secrets in the therapeutic setting. *Journal of Sex and Marital Therapy*, 1978, *4*, 35-49.

KAYLA J. SPRINGER, Ph.D.
Associate Professor of Psychology
Department of Psychiatry
University of Cincinnati
College of Medicine
Cincinnati, OH

82. Treatment of Extramarital Sexual Affairs

Question:

I perform marital and family therapy in a community mental health center and also have my own part-time private practice. I've heard that extramarital sexual affairs are quite common and yet I hear very little about them from my patients. It makes me wonder if I serve a biased sample or if my treatment approaches keep these issues from being revealed. When the subject of affairs does come up in sessions, I'm never quite sure what to expect or how to handle these issues. At times I hear a lot of accusations being made but only rarely are affairs actually discussed in therapy. Are extramarital affairs widespread? If so, what are their consequences for the marriage? How are they best treated?

Discussion:

Extramarital sexual affairs have been around since the beginning of humankind and promise to always be with us. Kinsey, Pomeroy, and Martin (1948) and Kinsey, Pomeroy, Martin, and Gebhard (1953) declared that by middle age half of American husbands had engaged in one or more affairs and a little over one-quarter of American wives had done the same. In the 1970s, Hunt (1974) stated that the rate of affairs for wives under the age of 25 had increased 300 percent since the Kinsey studies. A more recent study of *Redbook Magazine* readers (Levin, 1975), drawing from a sample of well-educated, young woman, concluded that up to 40 percent of American wives may now engage in affairs. A study performed by myself and Leslie Strong (1976) revealed that approximately half of the cases treated by members of the American Association for Marriage and Family Therapy involved the complaint of infidelity by one or both spouses. From these various studies it would appear that marital and family therapists who only occasionally hear about such complaints need to reexamine their therapeutic approaches to couples. Somehow, these therapists are blocking patients from sharing these emotionally loaded issues.

To help insure that therapists have access to all facets of every couple's difficulties, it is imperative that at some point in the initial evaluation sessions each marital partner be interviewed alone by the therapist. Complete confidentiality and neutrality must be granted to the person regarding the contents of individual sessions. Therapists who refuse to utilize any interviewing modalities except conjoint or family sessions are failing to offer patients with extramarital sexual (EMS) partners the opportunities they need to share, discuss and evaluate their affairs in a more neutral therapeutic environment. When these individual sessions are made a routine part of the evaluation process, they will facilitate the candid revelation and discussion of EMS relationships and their perceived meaning to the patients.

When therapists know that affairs are going on, or have gone on before, treatment plans should be followed which will include routine individual sessions for both marital partners along with conjoint or family sessions. During these individual sessions, individuals participating in EMS relationships are offered opportunities to clarify their feelings towards their spouses and towards their extramarital partners, to evaluate the probable impact of the affairs on their marriages and family units, and to make decisions regarding the continuance or discontinuance of these outside relationships. These tasks are handled more readily when patients do not have to deal defensively with hurt and angry marital partners sitting next to them. Individual sessions with the spouses who are not participating in EMS allow these partners to vent their feelings of hurt and anger, or of suspicion, or of puzzlement about their partners' behaviors or attitudes. Conjoint or family sessions can be utilized to deal with issues concerning the affairs if they are nonsecretive, as well as dealing with other general issues in the marriages.

Regardless of the alleged openness of marital partners to alternative lifestyles or of their emancipation from old moralities, the impact of knowing that one's partner is having an extramarital sexual affair almost invariably constitutes a serious threat to a marriage. Marital partners invariably feel hurt, deceived and angry when they learn of their partners' infidelities. Husbands often feel more threatened when wives have affairs than wives do when husband have affairs. Men do not experience sexist socialization patterns the way women do. The women are repeatedly told "men will be men"—meaning they will occasionally "stray" and women should put up with these male "imperfections." In addition, male egos may feel extremely threatened because "real men ought to be able to take care of their wives"—meaning satisfy all their sexual needs—a male myth that implies sex is everything in a relationship.

It is essential in the therapy sessions to examine the implications that the EMS relationships have for the marriages and for the family units. How will their wives/husbands and children feel if they find out? Are the affairs love affairs or are they primarily sexual diversions? What are the feelings of the other persons? Only rarely are the other persons interviewed by therapists but their attitudes, behaviors and levels of commitment to the affairs need to be explored. Frequently, partners participating in extramarital affairs report high levels of ambivalence towards their spouses. They "like" them; they "respect" them, "*but . . .*".

This ambivalence must be resolved one way or the other before valid decisions about the continuance of the marriage can be made. If those having the EMS relationships decide to terminate their affairs and concentrate on strengthening their marriages, the focus of therapists' work will shift to those goals—for both the husbands and the wives. If the EMS persons decide to divorce, therapists then deal with the issues concerning that process—including the preparation of the marital partners for such a course of action.

If EMS relationships are out in the open from the beginning of therapy, more of the therapeutic work on issues of hurt, anger, ambivalence and marital continuance may be addressed in the conjoint sessions than would otherwise occur. Even in these instances, however, it is important to allow both partners periodic but regular individual sessions to work on their own individual feelings. A recurring theme among couples in which EMS has occurred is that of broken trust. Both partners in these marriages need to closely examine and attempt to resolve their own individual feelings about these issues. Throughout all sessions therapeutic strategies are similar to those performed in all marital and family therapy; therapists facilitate communications, help develop understandings, clarify feelings, make the couples aware of both their intrapsychic and their interpersonal needs, strengths and behaviors, and assist them in facing reality. Therapists must grant confidentiality to all marital partners *and must deliver* on these promises.

It is not the prerogative of therapists to decide when, or if, affairs need to be "confessed." It is a myth that there are no such things as secrets within families. A large percentage of EMS affairs are conducted without marital partners' or the children's knowledge. Modern living styles, especially occupations that require much travel and irregular working hours, make keeping secrets relatively easy. Revealing EMS affairs to marital partners virtually guarantees the creation of major voids between husbands and wives. Individuals in secretive EMS affairs should be cautioned to weigh fully their own reactions to their affairs (from guilt to deep love) and the reactions that their marital partners might be expected to have. Those who choose to keep their marriages, to terminate their affairs and to keep knowledge of the affairs restricted to themselves and their therapists, stand an excellent chance of maintaining or rebuilding satisfactory marriages—all other things being equal. Once these secrets are known to the marital partners, however, even when the nonparticipating marital partners appear ready to "forget and forgive," couples face months and years before complete trust can ordinarily be regained.

Some therapists find it very difficult or even morally unacceptable to treat EMS problems without imposing the therapists' own moral codes upon these allegedly "guilty" partners. In these cases the therapists—unless they clearly identify themselves to couples as sectarian or pastoral counselors—should refer couples to different therapists. Couples are quick to pick up cues about therapists' values. When individuals engaged in EMS activities perceive that certain therapists completely disapprove of EMS relationships, they will attempt to avoid going to these therapists for help or will discontinue their interviews. Therapists' vocabularies are one tip-off to patients. Asking if either partner has "committed adultery," for example, is far more value-laden than posing the question, "Have either one of you ever been involved sexually with someone outside of your marriage?" Waiting rooms may alert patients to therapists' values. What magazines are to be found there? Are there strong profidelity slogans hung on the walls? Are patients required to fill out questionnaires that are blatantly blaming or guilt-producing? If therapists are careful to convey both an image and a reality of neutrality in respect to these emotionally laden subjects, they will find patients responding in constructive attempts to resolve these difficult issues. Frequently, these resolutions will not be to the satisfaction of all parties involved, but this fact is equally true in a significant number of other marital and family problems.

References

Humphrey, F. and Strong L. *Treatment of Extramarital Sexual Relationships As Reported By Clinical Members of the AAMFC*. Paper presented at the meeting of the American Association of Marriage and Family Counselors, Hartford, May, 1976.

Hunt, M. *Sexual Behavior in the 1970's*. Chicago: Playboy Press, 1974.

Kinsey, A., Pomeroy, W., and Martin, C. *Sexual Behavior in the Human Male.* Philadelphia: W. B. Saunders, 1948.

Kinsey, A., Pomeroy, W., Martin, C., and Gebhard, P. *Sexual Behavior in the Human Female.* Philadelphia: W. B. Saunders, 1953.

Levin, R. The End of the Double Standard. *Redbook, 144* (October, 1975): 38-44, 190, 192.

FREDERICK G. HUMPHREY, Ed.D.
*Associate Professor of Family
Relations
University of Connecticut
Storrs, CT*

83. Use of "Language of Awareness" in Teaching Partnering

Question:

Thought forms have the power to create reality. Words can affect thought processes and thus change one's vision of reality, which in turn alters the way one relates to the world. How can I make most effective use of this principle in teaching couples to improve their relationship as partners?

Discussion:

We give the name "language of awareness" to a series of simple rules of basic communication that we model and teach. We hear repeatedly from couples and families that they apply their new learning with one another, value it, and often make radical life changes within a relatively brief space of time. They report their changes appear to have a ripple effect among their friends and associates.

The pain that brings a couple or family to us motivates them to seek change. Characteristically each is losing a sense of mastery over his/her own life circumstance. We want to capitalize on the motivation for change as soon as possible, even in the first session, by offering each partner ways of relating effectively with the other.

We create an atmosphere of trust as soon as possible, without which constructive change cannot occur (for the defended person is a closed person). We define the experience as a collaboration between us as outsiders to their system and them as experts who will teach us about themselves operating within their own system.

The therapist or therapist team (which we prefer) carefully models the language of awareness tools. Learning to use these tools, each partner may emerge with a sense of being able to take back into self parts given away to the other. Often unwittingly each has given to the partner critical life decision-making power. New-found ways of expressing verbally one's real meaning significantly reveal to both partners a true intent. We repeatedly encourage both to share our consistent bias that each statement the partner is making in his/her own behalf reveals, often with deep feeling, his/her own unique point of view. We frequently encounter a strong tendency for living partners to hook emotionally into the other's expression rather than simply acknowledge what they have heard.

Offering gentle, firm boundaries as we enter the initial session, we slow down the communication process and lay a new, clean communication base.

As a therapy team we prefer to sit in a square formation, with the spouses at opposite corners facing one another and the therapists in the other corners. We explain that this will make it possible for them to be in direct eye contact and to communicate directly with one another. From almost the very beginning we conduct the session as a dialogue between the two partners. As we take each succeeding step, we check with the partners whether the structure we are offering is acceptable to both. In this way we model one principle of the language of awareness, i.e., that I do not assume that I know what your feelings are. If they prefer not to contract for a structured procedure, this, too, is perfectly acceptable. From the start we want them to know that they will be encouraged to take an active part in the process of what happens during the consultation and that nothing will be imposed upon them without their willing acceptance and active collaboration.

Building upon this foundation, we gradually offer a number of communication tools. They may include, as appropriate:

- Make "I" statements rather than "we" statements. ("We" statements assume I know what you feel without checking it out.)
- Make "I" statements rather than ask questions. (Questions tend to put the other on the defensive.)
- Make "I" statements rather than "you" statements. ("You" statements tend to invade your territory.)
- Check out any and all assumptions. (When I "assume," I make an "ass" out of "u" and "me.")
- Speak directly *to* the other rather than *about* the other in his/her presence.
- Stay in eye contact.
- Be specific rather than general.
- Make positive rather than negative statements.
- Acknowledge having heard the other before moving on.
- Experiment with substituting "I don't" for "I can't."
- Try using "and" instead of "but."
- Take responsibility for your own attitude and expression.
- Allow for equivalent air time.

We may proceed by asking each person to tell the other what his or her hopes are for this opening session (which typically lasts for two hours). We encourage each in turn to make such a statement to the partner. We deliberately refrain from focusing on "problems."

One of us may then suggest that each partner take five minutes to tell the other what his or her life is like at this moment in time. The other is asked simply to maintain eye contact and listen to the partner without response. When one partner has taken five minutes we reverse the process, asking the new speaker to start afresh, saying what his/her life is like without reacting to what s/he has heard from the partner. We monitor this interchange very carefully so that the partners stay within structured guidelines.

We then ask each to feed back to the partner simply what s/he has heard in the original statement, without reacting or editorializing. After the initial feedback each has an opportunity to add anything of importance the partner may have not fed back so as to be sure that the partner captured the meaning of the original statement. To encourage more complete and accurate communication (sending and receiving skills), the therapists may then add anything further that they may have heard in the original statement (always waiting for the partner to feed back first). We do this both ways so that both partners have an opportunity to learn how to ensure that their respective messages are received.

In addition to practicing improved communication skills, each member of the couple will also by now have laid a careful foundation for further exchange by clarifying for the self and hearing clearly from the other where each finds him/herself to be in his/her life at that point in time. To be truly heard by one's partner is a rare luxury. The gentle and careful boundaries that are laid around their beginning communication exchange serve to set the tone for ultimate respect for self and other from the very outset of the interview.

As they proceed with the interview, the therapist team, always with consent of both clients, may monitor their dialogue in such a manner as to ensure their improved utilization of the language of awareness. Thus, each partner may be gently reminded when tending to make a "you" statement, such as, "You make me angry when . . .", that s/he might experiment with changing that to an "I" statement. They will usually come up with something like, "I get angry when . . .", which allows the initiator to take more responsibility for his/her own emotional expression rather than project an emotional response upon the partner.

Couples and families habitually use "we"—often to the point where the individuality of the particular member becomes submerged in the whole group. If one partner says to the other, "We never do anything together," the therapist may suggest that s/he try an "I" statement, which will come out something like, "I never do anything with you." This is a first step toward awareness that I have within myself the power to do something with you if I so choose, and can take an active role in making that happen. As long as the expression is "we" rather than "I," I may feel powerless since I have given away my freedom of action. By my assumption I may have denied myself the opportunity to discover afresh your desire (complaining at the same time that you never speak up or I never hear from you).

Thus, we are actually structuring a careful training session in basic communication based on nonjudgmental respect for self and other. It is easier to listen when not talking. When I acknowledge that I have heard you, somehow I gain your respect.

Our objective is to mobilize quickly the positive growth force within each person. We want gently yet firmly to rock each person into assuming responsibility for self. We want to give each within the session the experience of space and selfhood, and tools that can help each to recontact the ability to be the creator of his/her own reality.

JANE DONNER SWEENEY, Ph.D.
VINCENT C. SWEENEY, M.D.
Founders and Directors
Center for Study of Human Systems
Chevy Chase, MD

84. Utilizing Myth/Game Systems With Couples in Conflict

Question:

Knowing there is a great deal of emphasis placed these days on the role of the myth and the game in marital therapy, I would appreciate your addressing yourself to several aspects of the subject. First, would you define what you mean by "myth" and "game." Then, please answer the following questions: 1) How do you employ the concept of myth and game in differing techniques of marital therapy? 2) How do you acquaint your patients with the fact that you are attempting to involve their myths and games in your treatment process? 3) What conditions auger for the least and most favorable prognosis when you utilize the myth/game system concept in conflict resolution? I would hope, incidentally, that when you deal with these questions you will provide your reader with some rather explicit examples of what the myth is, the game is, and the language you and your patients use in contending with these elusive phenomena.

Discussion:

Let me answer the third question first. If patients can recognize and understand the myths and the games by which they are motivated, the influences adverse to their conflict resolution stand a good chance of being eliminated. On the other hand, prognosis for resolution of marital conflict is very poor if either party cannot or will not relinquish their myth/game systems.

Even before I try defining the myth and the game it should be remembered that myths have something of the paradox in them. Hence, paradoxical statements made to patients in conflict often have the same kind of effect that whispered commands do to children who are accustomed to being yelled at—paradoxical statements attract attention. I never cease to enjoy watching the behavior of a couple who are confronted with the plausibility of the myths they may be living. Each mate will register their attention with startled, perplexed, quizzical and thoughtful looks, denial, etc. This results from the fact that statements representing their myths seem contradictory, unbelievable and even absurd upon first hearing. Later in the therapy each mate may have discovered that they have indeed been harboring beliefs which have been fanning the flames of their conflict such as the following: "If I let you near me you will destroy me; but if you don't try to come near me I will hate you," or "I want an unfettered adventure; when I married you I let myself get trapped; to be safe from you and entrapment, I must keep an emotional distance from you." Their behaviors which express these beliefs range from stormy verbal battles, to petulance and sulking, to vastly different demeanors when they are together in public than when they are alone together at home. When these discoveries are made, the myth statements cease to seem paradoxical.

The subject of myths and games plays such a prominent position in today's psychological and psychiatric literature (Lederer and Jackson, 1968; Paolino and McCrady, 1978; Sager, 1976; Steiner, 1974) that it seems superfluous to me to discuss the various definitions. This, however, in no way negates the importance to marriage therapists for knowing precisely what they hope to communicate to patients when using terms such as myth (legend, fiction, superstition, and mirage) and game (ritual, scheme, manipulation, maladaption, and acting out). Incidentally, I am using the words in the two sets of parentheses as synonyms. There exists among these similar words and terms subtle but important differences, which I do not intend to address in this paper, but which can affect the nature and quality of the communication between therapist and patient, and thus affect also the character of the therapeutic process itself.

To me, a myth is an unconscious, unfounded, hence, false, belief to which one clings because that belief does something the individual feels to be salutory. I see this unfounded or false belief serving in a covert manner to evoke self-indulgent and, more often than not, destructive behaviors which cause their host to function in less than an optimally efficient manner. In short, the myth produces behaviors which tend to supply the actors with an insufficiency of rewarding, gratifying feelings.

To me, the game is the *overt* manifestation of the unfounded, unconscious and *covert* myth. Berne's (1967) definition of game is acceptable for my purposes here. He sees the game as a series of complementary ulterior transactions which tend to progress to well-defined outcomes. The behaviors of the game players have undisclosed, ulterior and dishonest qualities, all of which tend to lead to "no-win" pay-offs to self and other. The ulterior qualities referred to by Berne are, to me, the *myths*; the behaviors are the *games* in which the players, more often than not, lose, because one cannot win (feel gratified) with false beliefs.

Conflict arises out of unconsciously motivated attempts on the part of one marital partner to manipulate (game) the other. Hence, it is my tendency in practice to assist patients to identify and to expose to one another their myths and, through verbal and nonverbal social inter-actions with each other, with me, and with others, to eliminate their myth/game systems.

I explain my premises about myth/game systems and conflict reso-lution to patients as early in their therapy as their ability to attend and comprehend this philosophy warrants. Obviously, if either or both partners enter my offices in such emotional deficit that rational ex-planations are likely to go unheeded, I postpone straightforward ex-planations. Under such circumstances, I have to approach them with whatever supportive measures may be called for. But it is rarely the case that within the first three sessions I have not been able to express my viewpoint and to enlist cooperation in the "search and destroy myth/game" mission.

The examples are plentiful: the husband tells me clearly that he loves his wife and has no desire to leave her. His behavior: he bullies her; he criticizes her grammar, her mode of expression, her style of food preparation. How does he account for the discrepancy between his affirmed belief and his critical behavior? He answers, "I know, I know. If I were in her place, I wouldn't live with me for one more minute. I don't know why I do this to her."

A wife tells me, "I love him, but if I open myself up to him he will explode on me." Her behavior: she nags him, recriminates, dwells upon past conflicts and their outcomes. How does she account for the dif-ference between her assertion of love and her fear of him, her recri-minations and ruminations and her desire to bring about a compatibility? She answers, "I don't know; I guess I don't have any options open to me, so I live with this and my headaches."

It doesn't seem to matter what type of therapy one practices in so far as the employment of myth detection, exposure and elimination are concerned. I am an eclectic therapist and practice all three psy-chotherapeutic approaches—supportive, reeducative, and reconstruc-tive (Wolberg, 1954)—simultaneously and separately. I have no reason to assume that any of the marriage and family therapy theories employ any other than these three techniques. The major difference in the application of myth/game usage arises in where, in the therapeutic process, I and/or the patients devote the time and energies to myth/game detection, exposure and/or destruction. During *supportive therapy*, I am the most likely of the three of us to be in the best position to detect the myth/game systems at play, for at that time I am in the position of providing first aid, comfort, nurturance, succor, advice and counsel while the patients are in severe deficit. The patients' responses to me and to each other through their compliances, defiances, counteraggressions, withdrawals, etc., provide me with hypotheses about their myth/game systems. I may reveal my hypotheses to them or invite them to speculate themselves on their respective behaviors. I may invite feedback from other participants to them in group therapy sessions. But primarily, in this phase of therapy, the myth/game complexes are targets for my own detection, not so much that of the patients. They are engaging each other at this time with irrational behaviors, in the forms of fear and either internalized or externalized aggressions. My neutrality, therefore, affords the principal opportunity for objectivity; objectivity is not generally to be expected from them at this time.

In *reeducative therapy*, I can and do utilize every opportunity for enlisting the patients to join me in the identification and exposure of their myths and games. I do this by inviting them to substitute acceptable behaviors for those which are noxious to themselves and to the other. They may even have been asked to record and graph the frequency, intensity and duration of the aforementioned acceptable and noxious behaviors. In this modality of treatment we can now talk about the facts and conjecture regarding the causes of their behaviors. "I guess I am acting like I want what I want when I want it, aren't I?" she says. "I guess I do give you orders like a parent to a child, don't I?" he says. The objectified behaviors in this phase of treatment can be used to formulate strategies for less damaging interactions—for the elimination of a pout or a sulk or an inappropriate lip quiver or snide remark, in short, for the eliminations of myth/game systems.

Obviously, as I move from behavior modification methods (e.g., Thomas, 1974) to those involving *reconstructive therapy*, much more interpretation and dialogue is entailed. The patients in this treatment modality, either alone in sessions with me, in couples groups, in individual singles groups, or together with me, are engaged both in exploration and conjecture as to the derivation of their destructive behaviors, the developmental history of these and the manner in which they have come to be represented in the here-and-now. Hypotheses are formulated regarding possible myths to see if these ring true and tend to lend credibility to the observed behaviors. "If I do this, I will be rejected," "I am afraid to do this because he/she will not love me," and, "If I let her get too close to me she will control me," are among the hypotheses formulated to explain datachment, attack, withdrawal, etc.

It is not enough simply to expose myth/game formulations. Because of the attention-getting qualities of what seem to be absurdities, I urge my patients to discuss their newly formulated myths and to portray them in as many ways as possible. I also urge patients to repeat their findings over and over, for with reiteration, paradoxes become plausible, then acceptable, then, hopefully, rejectable.

I ask the patients constantly to review the goals they set for themselves upon entering therapy and to not be reluctant to revise, reject, alter and reconsider these goals in light of confirmation of their hypotheses regarding existing myth/game systems. I, and they, can see their progress in resolving their conflicts in the fluency with which they exchange views on what formerly were "touchy" topics. It usually becomes apparent to all of us that a reduction in conflict is occurring when the strong affect prevailing at earlier stages of therapy has begun to dissipate.

To utilize this concept of the myth/game efficiently, the therapeutic process must be interlaced innovatively with varieties of techniques and tactics (i.e., sculpting, simulating, employment of "alter egos" to represent each mate, etc.). As I introduce this concept to my patients, I do so with a request that they strive 1) to look for ways to like each other, 2) to communicate with one another, both verbally and non-verbally, with the greatest possible efficiency, 3) to establish where the other is coming from on every topic, and 4) to find every way to give themselves incentives to work together. I have found that these four guidelines to behavior provide patients with a structure for exploring the myth/game systems as these may be affecting their dyadic relationship.

Out of all of the above, I have come to appreciate that the search for and the exposure of myth/game systems is one of my most useful therapeutic techniques for alleviating marital strife.

References

Berne, E. *Games People Play*. New York: Grove Press, 1967.
Lederer, W. J. and Jackson, D. D. *The Mirages of Marriage*. New York: W. W. Norton & Company, 1978.
Paolino, T. J., Jr., and McCrady, B. S. *Marriage and Marital Therapy*. New York: Brunner/Mazel, 1978.
Sager, C. J. *Marriage Contracts and Couple Therapy*. New York: Brunner/Mazel, 1976.

Steiner, C. *Scripts People Live*. New York: Grove Press, 1974.
Thomas, E., Jr. *Behavior Modification Procedure: A Source Book*. Chicago: Aldine, 1974.
Wolberg, L. R. *The Technique of Psychotherapy*. New York: Grune & Stratton, 1954.

SYLVAN J. KAPLAN, Ph.D.
*Clinical Psychologist in
Private Practice
Chevy Chase, MD*

85. Uncovering Spouses'
Future-Oriented Fantasies

Question:

Over the years in my practice of family therapy, I have encountered a potent phenomenon in marriages for which the terms,
"time bomb," "divergent lifestyles," "future marital vacuum,"
"interest gap" and "violated marriage contract" would all be appropriate descriptions. This phenomenon highlights a need in the
practice of family therapy for greater attention to the pull of the
future on the marital pair. Concern for conflicting tendencies in
the future orientation of the marriage partners has been overshadowed by the attention accorded to the relative importance
of past vs. contemporaneous events in the formulation of theory
and treatment approaches. A survey of current publications in
the family therapy literature and review of intervention techniques readily confirms that bias. It is appropriate, in service to
our client families, that we direct our attention to the future and
explore the role that future-oriented forces play in problem marriages. What are these forces? How can the family therapist identify these problems? And what intervention techniques are
available to enhance treatment effectiveness?

Discussion:

After working with a marital pair for about six months, I came to
question for myself as well as for them whether marital therapy was
beneficial or even necessary. The husband and wife were both in their
early thirties. The husband had a part-time job and attended graduate
school in dentistry. They had two small children, a boy and a girl. The
wife was the sole caretaker of the children. The husband used the only
automobile they owned. The wife's major complaint was that she was
isolated. The husband's predominant concern was his wife's seeming
inability or unwillingness to control and quiet the children in the
evenings when he had to study. He frequently took tranquilizers to
cope with the situation. The couple enjoyed pleasant and helpful re-

lationships with both sets of in-laws who were devoted to the children. They also had a close and active network of friends.

The couple offered, as the reason for marital therapy, the need to improve their marriage. They wanted to strengthen their relationship and improve communication. Both partners were bright, verbal, likeable and good-natured. They expressed their caring for each other but avoided any reference to love.

Each time that I questioned the benefits of the therapy, I was beset by compliments and gratitude. They spoke kindly of the benefits of the sessions in giving them the chance to talk things out. After asking where *we* were going, it occurred to me to ask where the couple were going with their lives. Probably because of my training in projective testing, I gave the couple an unstructured task by asking them what they would like their lives to be in 10 years. After questioning, "How do you expect your lives to be?" or, "How would you wish your lives to be?" I opted for the wish. The task became a fantasy projection of the future. I asked both partners to think about their fantasies, and then, without changing them, to share their thoughts.

The husband began by saying that he wanted to live in the country but teach and practice dentistry in the city. Keeping the flow of thoughts, values and interests free, I reduced the obstacles by suggesting that in 10 years there would be new highways from the countryside to the city, and computer controlled cars that traveled at high speeds. He proceeded to say that he wanted to teach at a dental school, and to have a small but lucrative practice. He would want to earn enough money to afford a nice home, an apartment in town and fine clothes. I arbitrarily set his earnings at $150,000 per year by the economic circumstances of the early 1970s. We went through his fantasy production hour by hour, day by day and week by week. He would teach and be impressive to his students. He would take liberal time for casual lunches with friends. Four nights of the week, after seeing patients in his private practice, he would go to his apartment, shower and then take in some cultural, musical or theatrical event, perhaps with a colleague or friend. On these occasions, he would sleep in town. No mention was made of his wife or the children.

I asked the wife to tell her fantasy the way she had thought of it before hearing her husband's story. She understood that she could wish for anything she desired whether it was realistic or not. Her future fantasy production was strikingly different from her husband's. She imagined living in a small, convenient suburban home, close to friends and family and within a short walk or drive to shopping facilities. She emphasized spending time with her children, perhaps adding another to the family in a year or two. She looked forward to annual vacations. On weekends, she would enjoy going to local movies. Evenings, she imagined staying at home, snuggling up with a good book or watching television. Her involvement with her husband would be routine attention to meals, preparation of his clothing and visits to parents on holidays.

The husband and wife were both impressed with the dramatic differences in their future fantasy projections. During the next two sessions, they talked more openly and frankly about their underlying feelings. Three months later, they decided to get divorced. The future-oriented fantasy uncapped deep and unspoken dissatisfactions that both partners had about their marriage. Their values, interests, goals and social preferences contrasted sharply. They wanted different things out of life. The wife's reason for marriage was wanting children and a family. The husband did what was "expected" of him. The partners liked each other. They were considerate of each other's feelings. Both were willing to stand by their marital vows and commitments even though they were unhappy in their relationship. Despite their self-doubts and dissatisfactions, they attempted to keep the marriage viable by negotiating and cooperating. Their revelation of future-oriented wishes in a safe and accepting atmosphere gave them the courage to express their deeper concerns and regrets, and to dissolve the marriage.

This illustrative case is, of course, grossly oversimplified. I have omitted references to underlying dynamics, contributions from the families of origin and issues concerning the children. I have likewise telescoped events to describe one salient aspect of the case, namely, the impact of the future-oriented projection. Opening up issues of diverging life interests and goals within a marriage is not a procedure for the amateur. When unresolvable conflicts and goals are uncovered, the ensuing sessions are emotionally heavy.

The procedure, even when there are differences, does not uniformly lead to marital break-up. Affectional bonds, willingness to compromise and the resolve of each party to let the other grow and become usually outweigh the decision to terminate the marriage. Partners in schismatic marriages who battle continuously do not react to comparable conflicts in their projections of the future. Sometimes, the partners come to understand their unique life interests more clearly and to be more accepting of one another. The technique gains its potency in those cases wherein the parties choose to end their relationship by helping them to face their true feelings about themselves and about each other, and to discuss them openly and honestly. Although there is pain, the process is basically humane. The choice to work on the differences or separate is always left to the participants, who are urged to take their time and make sure of the way they feel about and perceive their relationship.

By exploring the future step-by-step in fantasy, I have encountered other phenomena that exert profound influence on the marital pair and family in the here-and-now, but which are not elicited by discussions of past or present. One such group of events has in common the anticipated, unalterable movement toward some tragic or catastrophic outcome: death of a spouse or self, insanity, suicide, financial ruin, separation or divorce, incapacitating illness, etc. The expectation and fear of such events in the future can exert a powerful influence on relationships in the here-and-now. Usually, they replace discussion of desirable, wish-fulfilling future fantasy. For example, a wife is worried that her spouse, as her father, will die young and leave her dependent and alone. A man is certain he will become senile prematurely as his grandfather and father did, and, by the time he is 55, will be dysfunctional. A husband worries that his wife will be unfaithful to him after 15 years of marriage, as was his mother to his father and so reacts suspiciously toward her. Some wives worry about destroying their husbands by making excessive and unrealistic demands, but are unable to disengage from their controlling behavior. Laying bare these fears, and sharing them with the spouse, if he or she is not already aware of them, is a first step in the treatment. Determining the extent to which such fears are unfounded and acting constructively to gain control over one's destiny, or planning how to act in the event of the anticipated tragedy, and having done so, returning to constructive living are also helpful in therapy.

Another form of future-oriented fantasy, which reveals yet another type of stress that lies in the future, is the tendency for one partner to impose a series of objectives and goals on the spouse. The game plan of the moving partner has the quality of a test in which achievement or compliance by the spouse is tantamount to proof of love. A wife, for example, may pressure her husband to become wealthy. In some cases, this will be to match the economic level of her father; in other instances, it will be to erase her memories of poverty and prevent the occurrence of conflict which she hated in her parents' relationship. The need to keep a spouse dependent, impoverished and isolated as a means of preventing the partner from leaving are motives frequently encountered by probing the future.

When confronted and dealt with in a therapeutic setting, the emergent frustration and lack of gratification within the marriage can clarify the validity of the marital relationship, elucidate the legitimacy of expectations of one partner for the other, provide the basis for a new marital contract or encourage exposure of underlying needs and feelings. The technique offers the opportunity to restrict the adverse impact of unrealistic fears or unfair demands stemming from one's own inadequacy as well as the choice of terminating the marital relationship. Thus, "future orientation therapy" is equally useful in helping the partners resolve their divergences as in helping those who wish to escape from painful entrapment and emotional suffocation.

The idea that the future exerts considerable influence on the here-and-now behavior of individuals and families is not new, indeed. Gordon Allport illustrated the fact in his book, *Becoming* (1955). In the early 1960s, Lyman Wynne demonstrated repetitive family dysfunctional interactions in certain cases by having the family members plan a vacation trip. His technique came close to tapping future-oriented divergences, but was not as revealing as the open-ended projective future fantasy production, which permits greater latitude in selection of the fantasized areas of divergence and conflict. The present procedure opens new vistas for the futures of families as well as for the future of family therapy and should be at least as fruitful as the focus on contemporaneous and past sources of family conflict and dysfunction.

References

Allport, G. S. *Becoming: Basic Considerations for a Psychology of Personality.* New Haven: Yale University Press, 1955.

C. JACK FRIEDMAN, Ph.D.
*Clinical Psychologist in
Private Practice
Ardmore, PA*

86. Gestalt Therapy Strategies
   To Reduce Projection
   in Families

Question:

In my work with couples and families I often see projection and
scapegoating. Couples make negative attributions about each
other and their children that reflect denied aspects of themselves.
In working with couples or families where projection is a central
dynamic, I find myself limited to two strategies. I make structural
interventions that enhance differentiation between the confluent
members, thereby lessening the impact of projection. This approach works especially well when the use of projection onto a
child reflects unresolved and unnegotiated spouse conflict. I find
structural strategies are less efficient when the utilization of projection reflects internal conflict and internal splitting in one or
both spouses. This is especially true in the case of parents of
borderline children who are themselves borderline. The other
strategy I utilize is the direct interpretation of the projective
dynamic. I find making the direct interpretation often builds resistance and has little affective or behavioral import. Could you
suggest a technique or strategy that deals directly and experientially with projective phenomena?

Discussion:

The gestalt technique of the "empty chair" or "dialogue" is a useful
strategy for working with projection. In order to use the technique
effectively, it is helpful to understand the nature of projection from a
developmental object relations perspective.
   Couples' internal object relational difficulties often result in boundary and contact problems for family members, such as enmeshment,
scapegoating and projective identification. Both gestalt psychotherapy
and developmental object relations theory conceptualize marriage as
a relationship in which introjection and projection are central. To the

extent that the organization of the self is built around pathogenic introjects, the personality will be susceptible to extensive utilization of projection. Pathogenic introjections are organized in a polar manner (aggressor versus victim, grandiose versus inferior self). To the extent that introjects form the core of the self, there will be positive and negative projections onto significant others, be it spouse or child. If the child and/or spouse is poorly differentiated, then the child or spouse will internalize and identify with the projected role. This phenomena is known as projective identification.

A major focus of the object relations viewpoint is that our relations with real people reflect our internal representations of others, and our own internalized dialogues (Bauer, 1977). This implies that, just as there is an encounter-like quality between ourselves and others, there is a relational and dialogue-like drama within ourselves.

A person seeks modes of relating to others that reflect his/her earlier internalizations. We relate to significant others in terms of these internalizations, seeking to replicate in real life the drama of inner life. We do not simply internalize a person or attribution, but rather a mode of relating—a dramatic and relational polarity. We identify consciously with one dimension of the polarity, but both sides are inherent in the imagery. For example, if a child experiences a sadomasochistic relationship, internalizations would reflect the polarity of victim and victimizer. To internalize being punished is to internalize the punisher. We consciously identify with one side of the dialogue, disowning or splitting off the other side—the "not me" part. The cut-off, disowned and, hence, unconscious aspects of the internal dialogue may either be acted out on one's self, acted out directly on others or, often within a family system, projected onto a spouse or child.

Moreover, people shift their identifications within the polarity of the internal dialogues. Again, to use our example, the person who internalized the victim-victimizer relationship may shift from victim to victimizer. The nature of the shifting will depend, in part, on how split off the disowned role is and, in part, if there is a partner available to shift and play the corresponding role. As a person's internal relationships shift, this shifting will be reflected in his/her real relationships with spouse and children. This shifting is characteristic of many sadomasochistic marriages. For one period of time, one spouse is in the victim role and one is the victimizer. Then, under the influence of guilt and/or separation anxiety, there is a mutual shifting in which the victim becomes victimizer and the former victimizer becomes the victim.

The goal of the dialogue technique is to assist a person in reowning and reexperiencing the split-off part of the internalization. This is achieved by having the patient express experientially both sides of the internalized polarity. This practice assists the patient in assimilating the disowned part. The reowning allows for the decrease of unconscious acting out, the lessening of internal conflict and splitting, and a decrease in the utilization of projection. The basic technique is for the patient to role play both poles of the split while sitting in chairs which face each other. In role playing that which is projected out of awareness, the patient may rapidly become aware of what was formerly disowned.

In those clinical situations in which a parent projects onto a child or spouse, the therapist may interrupt the process of projection by having the parent use the dialogue technique. For instance, if the focus is on a child, the therapist may have the parent enter into dialogue with the imagined child in the empty chair. By having the parent give a voice to the imagined child, the parent begins to reown some of the projected parts; eventually, the focus will shift from the parent and child dialogue to parts within the parent himself or possibly between the parent and his or her own parent, hence locating the experience historically (Bauer, 1979). The empty chair technique is not a role-playing technique to help the parent get along better with the child (although it may be presented that way), but aims specifically at shifting the focus from between parent and child to within the parent.

For example, as a child Mary experienced a sadistic-masochistic relationship with her father. She internalized the drama of victim and victimizer and now plays out the drama in the family life. Her own male child, upon reaching adolescence is perceived by her as particularly vindictive and fearfully aggressive, while she experiences and identifies herself as all good and placating. By entering into a dialogue with her aggressive adolescent via the empty chair, Mary begins to reown her own aggression, and when the dialogue shifts to one between her aggressive self and passive weak self, she further assimilates her aggression. Then in another shift to the historical past, Mary recounts her experience of powerlessness with her father. The dialogue is again amplified between Mary and her parent, enhancing the reowning. It is by reowning her own agression that Mary can deal forthrightly and directly with her aggressive adolescent.

The technique is relatively simple to utilize. If the situation is one in which a child is involved in the projection, then the parent should work on his/her projections separate from the children. The reason is that the intensity and intimacy of such work would weaken generational boundaries. However, it is important and helpful for the spouse to be present. Seeing one's husband or wife work on his/her internal dialogues that are projected on to one's self supports differentiation and lessening of projective identification. Such an experience often provides for a direct and vivid understanding of one's spouse as a psychological individual.

I personally find that gestalt work is accentuated when the patient is in hypnotic trance. Gestalt work in trance facilitates not only the immediacy of experiencing the internal dialogues but facilitates maintaining the results of such work.

References

Bauer, R. Gestalt approach to internal objects. *Psychotherapy: Theory, Research and Practice*, 1977, *13*, 232-235.
Bauer, R. Gestalt approach to family therapy. *American Journal of Family Therapy*, 1979, 7, 41-43.

RUDOLPH BAUER, Ph.D.
Director of Clinical Training
Gestalt Therapy Training Center
Washington, DC

87. The Use of Photographs and Family Albums in Family Therapy

Question:

Can photographs and family albums be useful in family psychotherapy?

Discussion:

In the process of helping individuals attain some of the goals of Bowen family systems psychotherapy (1971, 1972), which include understanding the family and the parts they play in the operation of the family system, the establishment of personal relationships with family members, and getting to know people in the extended family as far back as possible, I frequently find the use of photographs invaluable. In contrast to other approaches that utilize photographs in psychotherapy (Akeret, 1973; Anderson and Malloy, 1976; Kaslow, 1978; Kaslow and Friedman, 1977; Zakem, 1978), I do not think it is always necessary to bring photographs to the therapy session or to relive and reexperience the feelings and memories in a cathartic manner during the psychotherapy session. My goal is to help the individuals obtain and/or maintain contact with their family of origin, and the photographs serve as an entrée to facilitate the process. What is necessary is for the individuals to understand the language and concepts of systems theory, which will aid in their interpretation of their family photo albums as they embark on the search for self and family history.

Photographs can function to address the question: What does it mean to be a person, a man, a woman, a child, in this family? They are of a prime importance not only for the individuals depicted in the photographs, but for their relevance for the family as a whole. They are signals of family life cycle ceremonies, rituals and traditions which are important for the development of the "identity" of the person involved, as well as for indicating the relevance of the event for the development of the whole family, for the "family identity." What is chosen to be photographed, recorded and documented for the family album reflects the ideals, traditions and values of the family. The activities surrounding the photographing of the events become as integral a part of family life as the events they commemorate.

As a family therapist, I am interested in who, what, where, when and how the family chooses to document their existence as a family. Given that the camera can capture and preserve a mini-slice of family history, important questions can be raised as to the meaning surrounding those activities, relationships and events that are selected to be rendered into permanent photographic images. The records form the history of the family and present a collective image of the family.

Typical picture-taking behavior in families occurs at important events in the family's life cycle, such as births, birthday parties, weddings, holidays, vacations and family reunions. Conversely, there is a sharp decrease in the number of pictures taken during periods of family stress, crisis or conflict. Firstborn children are generally photographed more than later children, and most pictures are taken while the children are relatively young and changing. People from all socioeconomic classes own cameras and take, keep and treasure their photographs. The size and prominence of pictures and portraits of family members hung in the home also reflect attitudes about the family. Families also tend to take pictures when events or changes represent progress, such as moving to a larger home, when a positive change is anticipated, such as cosmetic plastic surgery on a nose, or to recapture developmental change, such as loss of a child's baby teeth. Knowledge of these patterns of picture taking behavior is important because departures from these patterns may provide important clues for the therapist and the family about the emotional processes operating in the family. For example, if a second child is photographed significantly more than the firstborn, hypotheses can be raised regarding the second child's meeting the expectations of the family in regard to such issues as its sex or attractiveness, or some family secret regarding the first child, such as illegitimacy, handicap or disfigurement. Issues such as equality and favoritism are also raised when family members become adamant about trying to keep the amount of photographs of the first and second child about the same (Entin, 1979).

Favorite pictures of one's self, spouse, children and parents are significant in helping to understand their view of the emotional processes operating at the time within the self and family. Other leads for investigation involve speculating about what is happening in the picture at the time (the people, relationships, events, clothing and other items in the pictures), what the people may have been thinking and feeling about the events, and what happened just prior to and following the picture. Also, significant information is provided by charting a relationship process through viewing the same people or events in a series of photographs over time, noting changes in who is included and absent, and observing who stands next to whom and what they are wearing. What events are documented, and how and when the photographs change, are also informative. The dimensions of time and space, passages and transitions of the family as an expanding and contracting system through births, marriages, separations, deaths and divorces are all available for observation within the family photo album. It is especially interesting to see the same life cycle event, such as a wedding, pictured over several generations. The study of generational themes is further enhanced by observing parents and grandparents when they were both younger and at similar ages and/or life cycle stages. These photographs may illuminate the emotional processes of the family that have been operating for years, often subliminally, and give the younger generation a different perspective on their parents and grandparents. As stated by a photographer, "When I saw this photograph of my daughter, I felt as if I were looking at myself in the mirror, but in another time and place" (Frederick, 1980).

In my clinical practice, I find that photographs can have their greatest impact in the context of getting to know oneself within the context of the family of origin. When individuals are trying to get to know their family, to find out about the family myths, stories, events or history, many times family members either cannot or will not talk about their past. As an aid to memory or possibly to revive feelings which they are unable to otherwise verbalize, I suggest that they review photographs with their family to augment the verbal discussions and to get clues as to the themes, issues, goals, traditions and values of the family. This activity has powerful effects, both as a process of reminiscing and talking about previous memories and relationships, as well as developing renewed relationships in the present. During the course of therapy, I teach the concepts of family systems theory by discussion of clinical examples from their own family experiences. It is then suggested that they may learn more about the family processes by looking at their family albums to see if and how the same relationship patterns are operating. Usually individuals do this with their parents, although occasionally they may bring their albums to a therapy session. The "reading" of the photographs are open to multiple interpretations. The use of family systems concepts provide a new framework for viewing family albums. The clients' examinations, interpretations and experiences of looking at the photographs with their family become, in turn, the basis for further discussion in therapy in the facilitation of insight and understanding for changing themselves.

I suggested one family bring in some photos when I learned that this was the second marriage for each partner and they had been college sweethearts before either married. They were an attractive young couple in their late twenties who had been married about a year and were experiencing severe marital conflicts resulting in distance and a lack of intimacy. The consistent theme had been their lack of emotional involvement with each other. While one photograph may be an accurate mini-slice, characteristic of the relationship, or just happenstance, the accumulation of pictures begins to reveal the threads of consistent themes and patterns; they tell a story, the story of the family. At their wedding, this couple appear to relate to each other through her daughter by her previous marriage, a triangle.

While generally corny and staged, the wedding album photographs can, however, be revealing. On the way to the honeymoon, the bedroom upstairs at her parents' previous residence, the couple smiles gaily and eagerly on the bottom step. But, as the destination was approaching, the relationship pattern emerged immediately: She wants closeness and intimacy, and he is distancing and pulling away from her. This pattern was to persist in their relationship and culminated in their divorce. The verbal interpretation was consistent with the visual communication. Interestingly, in his memory of the wedding photographs, the husband was positive there was a picture of him pulling her up the stairs, with her resisting. That picture, if it exists, however, is not included in the "official wedding album." It is often significant as to which pictures are selected for inclusion in the documentation of events, which are left in the yellow Kodak envelopes, and which are discarded completely. What these choices reveal about the family system is important, as are investigations of an individual's "favorite pictures" which reveal their view of the family system.

My emphasis, as a family therapist, is on the study of photographs to aid in the understanding of family emotional systems. Photographs and family albums function as icons of the family, visually articulating the meanings and relationships of the family, while serving as landmarks for a history of continuity and change within the multigenerational family portrait.

References

Akeret, R. V. *Photoanalysis.* New York: Wyden, 1973.
Anderson, C. M. and Malloy, E. S. Family photographs in treatment and training. *Family*

Process, 1976, *15*, 259-264.

Bowen, M. Family and family group therapy. In H. Kaplan and B. Sadock (Eds.), *Comprehensive Group Psychotherapy*. Baltimore: Williams and Wilkins, 1971.

Bowen, M. Toward the differentiation of a self in one's own family. In J. Framo (Ed.), *Family Interaction—A Dialogue Between Family Researchers and Family Therapists*. New York: Springer, 1972.

Entin, A. D. Understanding yourself and your family better through family albums and multigenerational family portraits. Paper presented at the symposium—Photography and Psychotherapy: Toward a Psychology of Photography. May 5, 1979, Newark, Delaware. *Camera Lucida*, 1980, *Vol. 1 No. 2*, Milwaukee, Wisconsin.

Frederick, A., *Photographic Announcement*, Richmond, VA, Feb. 3, 1980.

Kaslow, F. The use of photographs, scrapbooks and diaries in marital and family therapy. Paper presented at the 1978 APA Convention, Toronto, Canada.

Kaslow, F. W. and Friedman, J. Utilization of family photos and movies in family therapy. *Journal of Marriage and Family Counseling*, 1977, *3*, 19-25.

Zakem, B., *Photo Therapy: A Developing Therapeutic Approach*. Submitted for publication, 1978.

ALAN D. ENTIN, Ph.D.
Independent Practice
Richmond, VA

88. Visual Imagery and Behavior Prescription in the Treatment of Parent-Child Conflict

Question:

In my practice, I work with many families with child behavior disorders as the presenting problem. These problems include aggressiveness, destructiveness, lying, stealing and noncompliance with parental rules and requests. The child's behavior is frequently associated with reciprocal hostility on the part of one or both parents (e.g., yelling, hitting, excessive punishment, threatening and generally attributing "badness" to the child).

In treating these families, I use an eclectic approach involving: 1) conventional family therapy techniques—exploration of feelings, clarification of interactional patterns, and encouraging clear communication; 2) parent education around methods of discipline; and 3) behavioral methods such as time out, changing reinforcement contingencies and contracting. While often effective, these methods sometimes fail with the more severe, long-standing behavior problems and in cases where a parent's hostility obstructs participation in the behavioral assignments. Why do these methods sometimes fail, and what other techniques can be used?

Discussion:

The methods you describe may fail if they do not create a more basic restructuring of generational power alignments, or if the parents do not fully internalize a new model for parent-child relating. In particular, child behavior disorders are frequently embedded in the father-mother-child triad in one of two ways: 1) the child is triangulated, with both parents competing to form a cross-generational coalition with the child against the other parent and undermining one anothers' attempts to set limits; or 2) the child is in a stable coalition with one parent ("the protector") against the other parent ("the harsh disciplinarian") so that the latter's attempts to exert control are undermined. The main treatment problem here is how to design behavioral or other interventions so that the parents will operate as a unified team in relation to the child's misbehavior.

In addition, a parent who is overly aggressive and attributes "badness" to the child frequently experienced this same kind of parenting during his/her own childhood. He or she lacks an internalized model of adequate parenting and empathy with the child so that behavioral suggestions and parent education techniques are not heeded or do not generalize beyond a concrete situation. The main treatment problem here is how to influence the parent to adopt new concrete disciplinary techniques and, more important, to internalize or generalize a new *prototype* of empathic parent-child relating.

Thus, when conventional methods fail in the treatment of child behavior disorders, the therapist must reconsider his/her techniques to see if in some way the interventions themselves are supporting the blurring of generational boundaries or are simply not restructuring the alignments in the family. Secondly, the overly punitive parent must not only learn new techniques of discipline but must also enter into some positive empathy-building experiences with the child. Below, I will describe an intervention with a specific case, designed to restructure a stable mother-son protective cross-generational coalition and simultaneously accelerate the "punitive" father's internalization of an appropriate parental model.

This family consisted of father, mother, I.P. son (age 11), and two younger daughters. The presenting problems were the son's misbehavior (aggressiveness toward siblings, noncompliance with parental requests, yelling at his mother, messiness, swearing and poor school performance) and the father's "violent temper" in response to the son's misbehavior. Father had been physically abused and medically neglected during his childhood by his own father.

Closer examination revealed that the problem behaviors occurred most often in a highly specific context. Typically, upon returning home from school, the son would misbehave in any one of a variety of ways, and mother would make an ineffectual-inconsistent attempt to set limits. For example, she would send him to his room and invariably go in to comfort him or otherwise not enforce the limit. Or she would instruct him to clean up his mess and then clean it up herself. Typically, the son would continue to misbehave until mother was at "her wits end" and threatening to tell father about son's misdeeds. When father returned from his long day's work, he was met by mother and her long list of complaints about son's behavior. Father typically flew into a "rage" and yelled at or spanked son, who by now was cowering in tears.

At this point, mother interceded as son's protector, criticizing father for being too harsh and "violent." Father would storm out of the house for a couple of hours, and mother would subsequently "give him the silent treatment" for two or three days. Then the cycle would begin all over again.

After four months of trying the conventional methods described in the question section above, a two-part intervention was designed. In order to help father internalize a new, empathic prototype of father-son relating, he was instructed in an individual session to choose someone from his past who played the role of a "good father figure." He immediately came up with Bill, who was a close older friend during father's childhood. Bill had protected him from neighborhood gangs and older boys who were threatening, and Bill had helped father with his preadolescent problems. The father contrasted Bill's helpfulness with his own father's hypercritical behavior. For 35 minutes, I instructed father to close his eyes and visualize scenes in which Bill played the role of a nurturing, protecting and strong father figure. Father was deeply involved and emotionally moved during this imagery session.

After this session, I felt it was necessary to arrange for this newly-revived internalized parent image to be reactivated directly in the family setting at the time when conflict usually occurred. I also wanted to build a more positive nurturing alliance between father and son and have the mother support the new father-son alliance. Furthermore, I wanted to put mother and son in a state of heightened anticipation during the period between the son's return from school and father's return from work, so that their usual pattern of misbehaving son/ineffectual mother would be interrupted. Lastly, I wanted son to greet father at the door in a positive way, rather than have mother greet father with the usual list of son's misbehaviors.

I therefore called the mother on the phone and instructed her without explanation to tell her son to greet his father by the name of "Bill" when he returned from work that evening. I previously had an agreement with the family that information from individual sessions or telephone contacts would be shared with all family members if I deemed it relevant. Thus this intervention left mother and son in a state of intense curiosity, anticipating some kind of surprise in father's reaction when son called him by the name of "Bill."

This intervention had a dramatic and long-lasting impact in breaking the original homeostatic cycle of the triad. Father responded to being greeted with the name of "Bill" by hugging his son for the first time since the son's infancy, and this new greeting ritual was repeated by everyone in the family for the next 12 workdays on their own initiative. Subsequently, in times of stressful family contact, the name of Bill was reinvoked and broke the escalating tensions. Also, father decided to reveal to son the secret of who Bill was, and this knowledge became a positive bond between them. Along with the new greeting ritual and reactivation of the new internalized parental prototype came a willingness on father's part to utilize the more benevolent techniques of discipline discussed in the earlier sessions. He also started a father-son athletic program without criticism for poor performance. The intervention, by creating a positive and empathic bond between father and son, induced mother to discard her overly protective stance as no longer necessary. She too began applying the disciplinary techniques she had been taught in earlier sessions and became more consistent.

Treatment terminated five weeks after the intervention. Son's behavior had improved to within normal developmental limits and his school performance also improved. At a preplanned six-month follow-up, these gains had been maintained within the family, and the son's school performance continued to match his potential.

Similar techniques in the treatment of parent-child conflict have been utilized with other cases reported in the literature. Erickson and Rossi (1979) report the use of hypnotic imagery in the February Man case. Basic concepts of restructuring can be found in Minuchin (1974). The use of behavior prescription has been pioneered by Watzlawick, Weakland and Fisch (1974) and Selvini-Palazzoli, Boscolo, Cecchin and Prata (1978).

Like each family in treatment, the case reported here is unique, and techniques should always be designed in accord with the family's unique construction of reality and involvement in therapy. However, two general goals seem essential in the treatment of all child behavior disorders: the parents must operate as a unified team in discipline and they must internalize new models of empathic parenting. All specific techniques such as the exploration of feelings or contingency contracting or visual imagery must be in the service of these goals in order to succeed.

References

Erickson, M. H. and Rossi, E. L. *Hypnotherapy: An Exploratory Casebook.* New York: Irvington, 1979.

Minuchin, S. *Families and Family Therapy.* Cambridge, MA: Harvard University Press, 1974.

Selvini-Palazzoli, M. S., Boscolo, L., Cecchin, G., and Prata, G. *Paradox and Counterparadox*. New York: Jason Aronson, 1978.
Watzlawick, P., Weakland, J. and Fisch, R. *Change*. New York: W. W. Norton, 1974.

ROBERT JAY GREEN, Ph.D.
*Private Practice and
Faculty, California Graduate School
of Marital and Family Therapy
Berkeley, CA*

89. De-escalating Couples'
   Power Struggles

Question:

Therapists routinely encounter numerous presenting problems
expressed by couples as the basis of their marital dissatisfaction.
These disagreements and complaints can often be reduced to a
single common denominator, the power struggle. The struggles
may be overt or covert, and usually constitute a vital aspect of
the marital system. Since therapists frequently encounter marital systems with escalated power struggles which are difficult
to resolve, what strategies provide useful results? How can the
couple resolve these power issues, and will the resolution endure?

Discussion:

Couples who complain about continuous fighting and unresolved conflicts in their relationship are locked in an escalated power struggle.
They may argue, fight and feud about money, in-laws, sex, social activities and other issues without realizing that the basis of these issues
is really power. The conflicts are often an on-going, long-standing
series of disputes which may culminate in serious verbal and/or physical abuse.

The therapist should begin the intervention by helping the couple
to understand that the issues are not the issue, explaining how these
recurring disagreements are struggles for power in their relationship.
S/he should concentrate on providing the awareness that the power
struggle is manifested in their confrontations about the other issues
in the marriage. Detailed examples taken from the couple's relationship history should be cited and emphasized to openly identify the
problem and provide support for the analysis.

Metaphors are valuable tools in inducing change. In animated and
vivid form, the therapist can depict the couples as two bald eagles who
are trying to act like parakeets perched in the same cage. They were
hatched, nurtured, trained and helped to become bald eagles in their
preparation for marriage. Illustrations of this shaping process are

taken from their family of origin, if available. The metaphor continues with the explanation that, in their attempts to move together toward intimacy, the bald eagle within them emerges. In marriage they are sharing the same perch; and their attempts to get close by cuddling like parakeets often result in bringing out the bald eagle in the other. First one lifts his/her massive wings and knocks the other off the perch. The attached eagle responds by swooping down and attacking with a flutter of its wings and a peck aimed at a strategic spot. Now the skirmish has begun and each eagle must preserve its dignity by responding to this call to battle. The pecking, pushing and clawing continues and escalates until one of the eagles is either too damaged or too tired to continue the struggle.

The therapist must vividly portray the flapping of wings, swoops and pecks to convey the message of the metaphor. It must be as pungent as possible. Again, the couple are labeled as bald eagles who think they are parakeets and many examples of their conflicts and fighting styles should be introduced into the metaphor to create greater identification. A cuttlebone can be used as a symbol of their strife. By pecking on the cuttlebone birds experience contact and involvement. These couples are described as experiencing a peculiar kind of involvement through their fighting and seem to need to peck each other when they are together. The therapist may act puzzled at this point and state, "I don't quite understand it but you two seem to peck each other and fight to be close. When you move together one reaches over and pecks the other on the head because without the pecking there can be no closeness." They may be told that they seem to need to behave like this with each peck being a peculiar kind of love message given to the other as a kind of closeness. Their basic problem is that they believe that love in marriage means to behave like parakeets instead of bald eagles.

Another metaphor conceptualizes them as gunfighters who frequently engage in violent shoot-outs attempting to hit the other in some vulnerable spot with their verbal bullets. They polish their guns with great pride, waiting for the right opportunity to prove their skill. In each gunfight they shoot down their spouse, then put another notch on their gunhandle to signify their success. When they promise to put down their weapons, they coyly sneak their gun out of the holster and place it under their pillow, anticipating another opportunity to shoot down their mate. The other does the same, secretly concealing his or her gun under the pillow until the right moment. When one goes for the gun, the other does also. With guns blazing, bullets zooming and barrels smoking, the shoot-out continues with the gunfighters pausing only to reload. These battles seem never-ending and the issues are not resolved. They will emerge again as an excuse for a future shooting match.

After describing the planning and preparation involved in their frequent shoot-outs, the therapist insists that their absence of fighting merely signifies that each has become more coy or sneaky about his/her use of weapons by hiding the gun under the pillow. It is not as visible, but remains readily available for use. When one displeases the other s/he reaches under the pillow for the concealed weapon and fires at the other point blank. When a spouse is severely wounded, the fighting temporarily stops, or nonfatal rubber bullets are substituted for the next confrontation. Vividly portraying their overt and covert shoot-outs, the therapist holds out his/her hands and asks for them to give up their guns. This dramatic gesture is the climax to the metaphor, with the outstretched hands representing his/her invitation for the spouses to give up their weapons by surrendering them to the therapist.

If they are dirty fighters who elevate their self-esteem by trampling the other's, the therapist can point out that their fights are dirty fights with each engaging in verbal crotch-kicking. These hits below the belt can immobilize and severely damage the other. They kick in the crotch because their intention is to do the most damage to the other, incapacitating them with their verbal barbs. By labeling them as "dirty fighters who are crotch-kickers," the therapist may be planting ego-alien ideas in their minds which will result in their desiring to change. Again, the therapist should dramatize and illustrate the metaphor in persuasive fashion by using their words and phrases each time as s/he demonstrates a kick.

Following the presentation of these metaphors, the therapist prescribes the symptom, assigning each spouse the responsibility of carefully planning and executing a good fight before the next session. They are instructed to carefully prepare for it, to decide on the best technique and to execute the plan, going through all the verbal bald eagle/gunfighter behavior they can muster. They must carry out this assignment by carefully devoting their attention to the planning of the details of what they will say and do to the other in this calculated confrontation.

The future sessions must reiterate the theme of power by briefly reintroducing the metaphors. Couples can again be told that they are bald eagles and not parakeets, the essence of the metaphorical message being emphasized again. If the therapist can succeed in catching the couple in the process of their behavior and can help them see the humor in it, the fighting will lose its sting in the relationship and they will be moving toward therapeutic change.

If the previous intervention does not provide the desired change, a two-stage strategy may be used.

Stage One—The Set-Up. As the therapist deals with various issues in therapy, spouses are instructed that they will not agree. The therapist states, "I know, Mary, you will see it differently." When the therapist speaks to John he adds, "I know, John, you'll see it differently, too." When they appear to agree on an issue, the therapist mentions, "You cannot possibly see it the same way."

Stage Two—Intervention. 1) The therapist labels each as strong and teases them about their bull-headedness. 2) The therapist slowly turns the issue toward sensitivity, explaining how easily upset each spouse is if anything is just a little different from what s/he expects or wants. 3) The therapist relabels anger as crying, discussing how through attitude and actions each spouse is saying to the other, "If you don't see it my way, I fall apart." They appear frightening to each other, but deep inside they are softies. 4) The therapist includes a description of how each experiences intimacy through these encounters (e.g., by engaging in these confrontations Mary keeps her husband feeling strong.) She may actually be baiting him to help him feel important and powerful. Instead of responding in her usual way to this set-up she might go up and put her arms around him and say, "Dear, if it happened this way, you are right. You're always right." 5) The therapist comments about how each lures the other by setting the other up. One sets it up, the other accepts it. During therapy, when this process occurs, the therapist may whisper to the spouse, "John, she's setting you up; you're walking right into it." Then s/he says to the other, "You sneak, you've set him up again." The therapist needs to demonstrate how each walks into the confrontations.

The task of the therapist is to catch them at their game and get them to focus on process, not content. Therapists should alter their confrontation agenda with demonstrative comments (i.e., "You walked into it again, John," or, "You got her again.") The success of this intervention is predicated upon the therapist's having established an adequate therapeutic relationship with the couple to permit this type of exchange.

WILLIAM J. HIEBERT, S.T.M.
Director of Educational Services
Marriage and Family Counseling Service
Rock Island, IL

90. Techniques for Treating Marital Impasses

Question:

The families who come to our clinical setting are often stuck in a marital impasse where the wife and husband have opposing views on how a certain child is to be handled, how the grandmother is to be dealt with, or whether the wife should be allowed to go to work, etc. In many cases the difficulties become critical when the wife, stirred by the women's movement, begins to be more assertive and the husband hardens his position in response. We are looking for some concrete ideas for helping these clients to break through such impasses.

Discussion:

Many family therapists consider the "marital impasse" the underlying source of any family trouble or any family member's problem. There is no doubt it ranks high in the list of critical issues faced in family therapy. There also is no doubt that many of these difficulties are intergenerational in nature, for example, the current spouse is enacting in this generation behaviors that his or her parent failed to enact in the last generation.

Developing detailed genograms that search for such leftover themes can provide the family with understandings that prepare them to approach conflict resolution with new energy, but learning "how to do it" is crucial for success in replacing impasse-producing behavior with creative problem-solving behavior.

It is necessary, at the outset, to discover if each spouse is committed to achieving solutions which are mutually satisfying. For many, this means letting go of the fear of losing and/or the need to win. It is readily apparent that if one wins and the other loses, the marriage and family is stalled in its growth.

An exercise I have found to be very useful at this point involves having the couple collaborate in writing a script of a typical fight. The following is an actual example of such a script, written by Jerry and Eileen:

Jerry: I invited my father over to spend a couple of days.

Eileen: You what?!

J.: I invited my father to sleep in the playroom downstairs. He has nowhere else to go.

E.: Tell him to go to Hell.

J.: Eileen, this is my home as well as yours and I can and will invite my father if I choose.

E.: You will have to choose—either I stay here or he can.

J.: You are not being fair. It is only a temporary setup. Not for more than a week.

E.: I do not want that slob in my house under any conditions.

J.: What would you have me do—throw him out in the street?

E.: Yes!

J.: Well, I won't—my offer to him still stands.

E.: You're still a Potz.

J.: What does that mean?

E.: You're still looking for parent approval.

J.: That doesn't change anything . . .

E.: It's his problem, and he doesn't deserve consideration from me and he is not going to get it.

J.: It's not entirely up to you. I made this decision and expect you to go along with it.

E.: You have no right to make any decision involving me without consulting me. I am a person!!!!

J.: All I ask is some concern for a serious problem. Not only that. I made this decision and you are stuck with it.

E.: F--- Y--!

(Curtain closes. Orchestra plays impasse music.)

The script writing places the couple outside the action. They learn to cooperate and jointly witness their own struggling. I have found this exercise extremely effective in producing a profound change in the couples. They generally become more optimistic and can laugh at themselves.

They are now ready to write in various endings—he wins, she wins and both win. This is how Jerry and Eileen worked out their endings:

He wins:

E.: I will move out right away—he can move in.

J.: Fine, I'll call him up—he will be so happy.

She wins:

E.: If he comes it is the end of our marriage.

J.: Well, I don't want that. I'll let my brother take him in.

Both win:

E.: He cannot stay here—we have no room and I want my privacy.

J.: Let's at least put him up for a couple of days, until he can find a room somewhere.

E.: O.K. As long as you tell him it's only for a couple of days.

Once it has been agreed that the only real victory is one that both spouses can share, the matter of how to do it can proceed.

The therapist needs now to function as a drama coach, teaching each spouse to speak clearly, hold their body in a position that communicates firmness and calm strength, and to use the voice, the eyes and the hands to convey the message, "This is important; I'm serious; I'm intent on having my ideas heard." Working with body language with each spouse as an individual and with the couple together is essential to the process and too often overlooked. The therapist can have the couple act out a sequence without using words and, if video is available, have them critique their own performance, looking for evidence of strengths and weaknesses.

The final ingredient is rules and procedures. Each person has a sense of what is fair and foul when it comes to fighting. They should be taught that it is their obligation to keep the process working by calling "foul" when a foul has been committed. The therapist can help them discover their rules and practice enforcing them.

Throughout, the couple should be learning what procedures to follow, what should happen first, second, etc. Problem solving begins when one person announces the presence of the problem. Here the problem is defined, and a time set for working on the problem. When the partners meet, each has considered the problem and brings proposals for its solution. The proposals are considered alternately until a mutually satisfying solution is found. No other issue is allowed to interrupt the work. Each person has the right to call for an intermission to do some further thinking, and both spouses are obliged to monitor the process.

Marital struggles which take place in the context of a family with children will inevitably involve the children in roles which regulate the process, maintaining the family in its familiar patterns. The functions of the various children can be observed and attended to when the work is done with them present. The work cannot be considered successful until all family members have made adaptations, come to see its worth and support the new learning. Once the children see that what is happening is going to work, they will be happy to join the team and begin using the procedures to gain justice for themselves.

PETER A. KINNEY, Ed.D.
Co-Director
Cape and Islands Family Istitute
Hyannis, MA

PART C

Aging and Death

91. Being a Therapist with One's Parents' Generation

Question:

In doing marital therapy with the geriatric population, it is easy to get caught into believing that "you can't teach an old dog new tricks." With increased homogeneity in living situations, we tend to live and work in age-segregated circles and this is especially true for professionals who work in urban areas. Thus, our daily contact with the elderly population is increasingly limited and our personal experience is primarily relegated to our relatives, if that. Those limited experiences may serve to strengthen the transference and countertransference in the therapy experience. I would like to see some discussion of the potential snags in doing marital therapy with elderly couples, as well as some of the relevant therapeutic issues for this group of people.

Discussion:

This question raises many issues in providing any mental health services for the elderly population, but some of these issues are heightened in marital therapy where parental and child transferences and countertransferences are easily evoked. This discussion addresses these transferences as well as some general issues that arise in therapy with this generation.

A common problem is the transference of the patients to the therapist. Although a parental transference is usually evoked in the therapeutic process, the situation gets more complicated with the presence of child transferences when the therapist is similar in age to the couple's children. A child transference is problematic in its lack of perceived authority, which is important for the therapeutic process. This results in a fear of surrendering control of their lives to "their children" with attendant loss of self-esteem. Resistance is then likely to be exhibited by discrediting the therapist because of his/her age. This is likely to emerge in establishing the therapeutic alliance and its (at least) partial resolution is essential before therapy can proceed.

If this transference is matched in the countertransference of the therapist the problem is compounded.

The common idealization of the therapist as a dutiful son/daughter is not likely to be problematic early in therapy, but will need to be faced at a later stage. The expectation is that the therapists will be everything the children were not, which results in pressure on the therapists to prove their caring, be overly nourishing, and accepting of the parents' denial. It may become a countertransference issue if the therapist is still seeking approval from his/her own parents. The parental is the most common transference and need not be problematic unless the therapist is not comfortable being in a parental role to patients who are the age of his/her own parents. Because the therapist is likely to be facing the caretaker role with his/her own parents, unresolved issues around dependency may be difficult. The issue of dependency needs is likely to be a primary one and needs to be addressed directly and realistically.

This group frequently has distorted views of the process of therapy. The expectations range from those of extreme suspicion of all "intellectuals" to belief of quasi-magical powers in the therapist. Either extreme will interfere with the therapy but the latter issue will impair the initial therapeutic alliance whereas the former issue is likely to be a problem after the alliance has been established.

The therapist's countertransference has great potential for being problematic especially for the novice therapist. Numerous unresolved parental issues can potentially emerge in the therapy process. As mentioned earlier, the lack of regular contact with this population heightens the potential transferences of parental or grandparental issues. Omnipotence fantasies of the therapist may emerge as overdetermined responses to problems seen in his/her parents' marriage. Although any idiosyncratic issues may emerge, a few issues are especially common. The therapist may view the patients as helpless and fragile and protect the couple from dealing with difficult issues or the therapist may view them as all powerful and approach them with fear. Either option prevents a realistic assessment of the patients' responsibility and power in the situation. Overidentification with the patients may result in side-taking over intergenerational issues with a blind spot to the patients' role in setting up interpersonal conflict. It is not uncommon for the therapist to overprotect the couple because of concern about "fragility" or viewing them as being "too old to change." Fear of parental disapproval or desire to please them may result in avoidance of areas of conflict. Some common areas of avoidance include illness, death and dying, and sexuality. Issues of dependency are likely to be prominent, and dependency demands may evoke anger in the therapist.

There are also more general issues that arise in marital therapy with the preceding generation. Although one can expect that some peace has been made with some marital issues, it is not uncommon for issues of individuation again to be heightened in the relationship. As Erikson suggests, each new stage allows opportunities to rework old issues. It is safe to assume that almost any early unresolved issue may present itself as a potential therapeutic problem as well as current developmental issues (i.e., generativity vs. stagnation; integrity vs. despair). Issues of dying, illness, loss of partner, retirement, relationships with children, loneliness, etc., are likely to be relevant even if not explicitly stated as a presenting complaint. If the partners are at different stages of development in regard to such issues, distance and lack of empathy and support may result. Attention will then need to be directed to developing their abilities to deal with differences and to support each other's needs.

The issue of dependency is paramount for this population and a good share of the therapy process is likely to involve working on present and anticipated dependency needs. Increasing age, decreasing physical capacity and illness may disrupt the old patterns of caretaking and dependency and increase the stress on the marriage. It is especially important to bring out fears and fantasies about dependency needs of the future. Widow- or widowerhood needs to be addressed in a realistic way with consideration of other social supports beyond the immediate couple relationship. Financial and estate issues may also be relevant and relationship dynamics are likely to be played out through them. This can be dealt with constructively if these events are dealt with as potential areas of growth for the patients and increased flexibility for the relationship.

The depth of therapy must be considered by the therapist in terms of how much turmoil will be opened up in order for successful resolution. Usually, the patients give you clues as to how much they are willing to reveal and how much relationship difficulty they are willing to tolerate. This can also be explored directly with them so as to avoid overprotection on the part of the therapist. Uncovering of issues needs to be carefully balanced with support.

Although the examination and resolution of transferences is central to the therapeutic task, some additional suggestions may be useful. Bringing in the children and grandchildren (if relevant) may be helpful in focusing the energy within the family to deal with existing problems.

It may also loosen some of the transference and countertransferences that may have distorted the therapeutic relationship. A cotherapist may be especially useful to the therapist who is a novice in working with this population.

In summary, the most common problems in working with patients of one's parents' generation are transference and countertransference issues. It is important for the therapist to be aware of this potential and continue to examine the mutual projections in the therapy relationship.

DOROTHEA TORSTENSON, Ph.D.
Clinical Assistant Professor
Department of Psychiatry
University of Wisconsin Medical School
Madison, WI

92. Marital Psychotherapy and Terminal Illness

Question:

It was Freud (1915) who said, "If you want to endure life prepare yourself for death" (p. 300). He was referring to one's own death, not that of others. However, I have seen that if you would live you must also prepare for the death of loved ones, and if not, the results can be disastrous. I have come across a number of cases of acute marital discord between a medically ill person and his or her spouse, where the ill partner died shortly after. A retrospective review of the cases, in both my own practice and the supervision of others, suggested that deterioration in the marital relationship was related to the medical and behavioral changes prodromal to death. In such cases, the proper therapeutic intervention can be very remedial.

Erickson (1963) in his description of the "eight ages of man," speculated that the last stage was characterized by ego integrity or alternatively, despair. The person with integrity has been able to deal with death without fear and with a sense of completion, while those in despair are filled with dissatisfaction, disgust and a sense of incompletion.

However, in most studies based upon this concept (e.g., Nehrke, Belluci and Gabriel, 1977-1978), the situational context has been relatively neglected. They overlook what happens in the immediate experiential confrontation with death in the seriously or terminally ill, not only in the patient but also in their relatives. However, dealing with illness and death is not only an individual task but a family one, especially for the surviving spouse.

Robert Browning's, "Rabbi Ben Ezra":

> Grow old along with me;
> The Best is yet to be;
> The last for which the first was made

presents an idyllic picture of marriage during old age. This peaceful image of a couple enjoying the culmination of a rich, rewarding

445

life together might strike an ironic note to a wife facing the serious and perhaps terminal illness of her husband; and the irony is compounded if that couple has grown old in a conflicted and discordant marriage. Can there possibly be an ending with dignity and ego integrity, without bitterness and despair in such cases?

Discussion:

Examples of efforts to achieve the goal you describe through marital therapy will be presented in this discussion, including the changes in my usual procedures that were necessitated by the nature of the task.

Case I

Mr. and Mrs. C., both in their early 70s, had entered a couples group, initially because of escalating marital problems precipitated by the wife's serious heart ailment, increasing physical feebleness, and growing dependence upon a resentful husband. At this time, the marital conflict was quickly resolved, and the tensions between them diminished considerably.

Some years later, however, Mrs. C. fell and broke her hip. She did poorly in the hospital, and went progressively downhill medically. Her husband reacted with a growing and implacable rage at his wife, and with persistent accusations that her condition was based solely upon her noncooperation in the treatment regimen.

I saw the couple at the wife's bedside two times and spoke to the husband individually, with no improvement in their relationship. Then Mrs. C. died suddenly of a heart attack. Mr. C. continued his insistent complaint that she had brought the death on herself through lack of cooperation.

Case II

Mr. R. was a 68-year-old man who was treated individually in the geriatric clinic for an acute manic episode, and then entered a therapy group with his wife. He presented with a long-standing history of heart disease which had necessitated an early retirement. While in couples therapy, his physical problems worsened. A pacemaker was implanted, but he also developed prostate and kidney problems. Concomitant with these medical conditions, marital discord escalated and the relationship deteriorated. Mrs. R. insisted that her husband was not really ill. She advised the extended family to phone or visit Mr. R. and admonish him. He, meanwhile, dredged up old complaints about her. When he said he went out to buy tylenol, she accused him of having a sexual assignation with his secretary, whom he had not seen for 25 years. The marital relationship was striking this discordant note when Mr. Robbins suddenly died.

The above reactions can be viewed as means taken by the couples to avoid coming to terms with medical illness and the implications of mortality. On the basis of such experiences, I now believe it is best to work to a greater degree with spouses individually, especially with the medically well spouse. The method involves individual work with the well spouse, coaching him or her in concrete measures for dealing with the medically ill partner. It entails the therapist becoming active and confronting in dealing with three major dynamic issues: 1) the re-arousal of old, unfinished marital and family conflicts; 2) the use of anger by both partners as a smoke screen to conceal the true situation; and 3) blaming the other partner for the illness. The results have been considerably more successful, as seen in the two examples that follow.

Case III

Mrs. B. was a 60-year-old woman, married 36 years to a husband 10 years older. She had a 35-year history of recurrent depressive episodes with frequent hospitalizations, dating from the first year of marriage. Recently, Mr. B. developed a serious and terminal malignancy. Obviously, he expected his wife to fall apart, because he immediately ordered her to be hospitalized. She was admitted to one of the psychiatric wards where she was assigned to me. Mr. B. had been admitted to another hospital, where plans were being made to send him to a nursing home. (He never got there.)

I arranged a family visit at his hospital bedside with Mrs. B. and their two sons. At the meeting his wife cried, quite appropriately, and was immediately labeled as sick by the three stoic members of the family.

"What will become of you?" asked her worried husband; "When I was alive [!] I was able to take care of you."

"That's right," echoed her sons.

Another family meeting was arranged for the following week. Meanwhile, Mrs. B. and I discussed her situation, and she received much coaching on how to deal with her husband; for example, to straighten his pillow, bring him juice and in other ways to demonstrate that she is capable, efficient and not helpless. She did so at the next visit and performed extremely well. Her husband was amazed and ecstatic. "She's all right!" he exclaimed, "She doesn't need to be in the hospital!" He then added, "Maybe I'll get better."

Unfortunately, he was a poor prophet, for he died shortly thereafter. Mrs. B. tolerated the pressures of the funeral and subsequent widowhood well. She has received no psychotherapy since her discharge from the hospital five years ago, but attends the lithium clinic regularly. She appears sad but very friendly, has a social life, and has had no recurrence of a clinical depression.

Case IV

Mr. and Mrs. W. are another couple in their late 60s, with a complex history of individual and marital pathology. Mrs. W. is an epileptic who was hospitalized for over a year at a state mental hospital. Mr. W. is a physically impaired man who plays the role of the martyred spouse of a mentally ill woman. After she was discharged from the state hospital, they joined my couples therapy group where they did very well despite, or perhaps because of, the airing of some intense marital conflicts. At one point, however, Mr. W. underwent an emergency operation for bleeding ulcers. A year and a half later he suffered a recurrence of gastric distress. An operation disclosed a malignancy which had perforated the stomach wall and spread. From all indications, he had become terminally ill.

Shortly after his return home from the hospital, Mrs. W. phoned me in a huge panic, virtually incoherent, and unable to hear anything I said to her. There had been a massive upsurge of marital conflict, in which his extended family was centrally involved. Mrs. W. then left her husband in the care of his sisters, to live with her son in Philadelphia and then with her daughter in Los Angeles. She returned after six weeks and made an appointment to see me.

Seen in individual sessions, her anxiety continued to be massive, as was her denial. She knew the nature of his illness, but said that she did not know and expected him to get well. Primarily, she spoke of her resentment at Mr. W. and his family. I insisted she accept the reality of his illness rather than fall apart and indulge in an orgy of blaming. I assigned concrete procedures she could follow to deal with him. I also made a home visit, where Mr. W. appeared as irrational as his wife and five times as angry, presumably at her. Our meeting was a chaotic one, and my visit seemed to make no difference, or even made matters worse.

However, Mrs. W. continued to see me and be coached on dealing with Mr. W. Their relationship improved dramatically, so that they became closer and more affectionate than ever. "There is love between us," she reported gratefully. I arranged another house visit and found him, indeed, a changed man. He was relaxed, reasonably content under the circumstances. We engaged in a sad but cathartic discussion of his cancer and his reaction, and a few weeks later, I arranged for the couples group to meet at the W. home. The good feelings between the couple spread to the entire group; the meeting was a very moving one.

Conclusions

Escalating marital dissension as a reaction to a serious or terminal illness in one spouse is a pattern frequently encountered in older couples. This paper presented a method, combining individual and marital therapy, which has been effective in helping such couples deal with this most meaningful and basic situation.

All of these reactions cited above may be viewed as serving a defensive function, with both partners in collusion to act out in order to avoid dealing with the illness, as though ignoring it would make it disappear. Freud said somewhere, "One's own death is beyond imagining." In the cases I saw, the death of a significant other was also treated as though it were unimaginable. The therapy was essentially directed towards increasing the sense of security of the sick spouse, and decreasing the feeling of helplessness of the well spouse, thus decreasing the anxiety of both. The result is an emergence of ego integrity and interpersonal closeness rather than flight and a surrender to resentment, anger and despair. Paradoxically, facing death is an act on the side of life and love.

References

Erikson, E. H. *Childhood and society*. New York: Norton, 1963.

Freud, S. (1915) Thoughts for the times on war and death. *Standard Edition*, Vol. 14. London: Hogarth, 1957, 273-300.

Nehrke, M. F., Belluci, G. and Gabriel, S. J. Death anxiety locus of control and life satisfaction in the elderly: toward a definition of ego-integrity. *Omega*, 1977-1978, 8, 359-368.

JOSEPH RICHMAN, Ph.D.
Associate Professor
Department of Psychiatry
Albert Einstein College of Medicine
Bronx, NY

93. Brief Therapeutic Strategies to Deal with Severe Death Anxiety

Question:

Despite the general effectiveness of family and marital therapy in dealing with issues of death, separation and loss, I have noticed that there are some "survivors" who return to treatment several months later presenting moderate to severe anxiety attacks, phobias or somatic symptoms which appear to be death-related. Since the initial therapy was structural in nature and consisted of changing the marital/familial organization consistent with the realities engendered by the loss, the return to treatment raises several questions. First, does the new problem suggest that my treatment was merely superficial and based on symptom removal rather than *real* change? Are such loss issues possibly too complicated for structural therapy to address? Do these families need a more insight-oriented psychodynamic approach? Finally, should I see these people again, and if so, is there any way that I can treat them on a short-term basis without disrupting or compromising my basic theoretical tenets or clinical style?

Discussion:

It is certainly disillusioning when people return to therapy after what appeared to be successful treatment outcome. The question about whether human loss can be effectively resolved without long-term, insight-oriented therapy suggests that there may be some ambivalence in the therapist's own mind about the long-term results of structural family therapy. In my experience, the use of structural therapy followed by a more strategic method I dubbed "oblique exorcism" has shown excellent results in dealing with some of the residual effects of death and loss (Coleman, 1980). Before elaborating on technique, however, it is important to give an overview of related issues.

Initial Presenting Problem and Treatment Approach

These families initially enter therapy in a state of crisis. They have either experienced a recent death or loss of a spouse, parent or significant other, or are in the process of losing one. In addition, these families generally are in a transitional phase of the life cycle and were either at a point of making a commitment to marriage, starting a family, or moving toward the "empty nest" stage of life when the death or loss occurred. Although the major issue appears to be the loss of this person and the impact that the loss has on continuing family relationships, a closer look may reveal additional problems. Thus, the loss itself could be a secondary issue that is shaking the foundation of a more primary problem—the familial context within which this loss takes place. Clearly, not all families need or seek help during a traumatic situation.

Frequently the loss of a member is imbued with incredible power because it threatens to evoke change in the family's homeostatic system. Thus, the focus of therapy must be on the family's hierarchical structure, their existing transactional patterns and the system's repetitive behavioral sequences. This is not to say that the therapist will be unconcerned with the family's grief; but the mourning must be in the service of working toward attaining a family configuration that will function effectively without the missing member or his/her ghost (Coleman and Stanton, 1978). Once the family finds alternative relationship patterns, it can shift to accommodate to the loss, and therapy can terminate. The family is now ready to handle responsibly any further grieving vis-à-vis its own support system, as reinforced in the therapy sessions.

Second Presenting Problem and Treatment Approach

When a member(s) of a formerly treated family returns to the therapist with a "new" problem, the vicissitudes surrounding the current symptom must be carefully examined. There are several important considerations: (a) The degree of overlap between the initial presenting problem and the current one must be determined; (b) The family's present structure and functioning need to be evaluated to see if the therapeutically derived reorganization has been maintained; (c) The therapist must assess the extent to which s/he focused too much on the loss and overlooked some of the other family problems; (d) The family's present stage in the life cycle must be delineated and any concomitant elements of conflict must be discerned. As noted earlier, these families are often in a transitional phase at the time of the loss. Because of their extreme difficulty in meeting the loss-generated crisis they may require additional therapeutic time and effort in order to make the changes that facilitate the continuing flow of growth and development. It is thus legitimate to assume that these families may need multiple sequences of brief therapy with intervening "vacations" from treatment.

After careful assessment of these factors, the therapist can assume that the family's return for additional treatment is a signal of readiness for further growth. The obstacle to surmount, however, is that which keeps most families stuck at any stage of life—fear. Before their loss these folks were already struggling with the passage to the next stage. The death or loss did not cause the conflict, it merely reinforced it. Thus, the therapist must: 1) look at the current presenting problem, most often expressed as a severe anxiety state, phobic reaction or somatization; 2) view it as functional and adaptive in maintaining the system's present state of being "stuck" at the same stage it was struggling with at the time of the loss; 3) see the resistance as a way of coping with the fear of what the next stage will offer; 4) view the symptom as a metaphor of being stuck between "death" (the recent loss) and "life" (what might eventuate if further change takes place); and 5) design strategic tasks to encourage change.

Oblique Exorcism. This technique utilizes the theoretical concepts of systems theory and the ideas developed by those associated with strategic family therapy (e.g., Haley, 1976; Selvini-Palazzoli et al., 1978; and Watzlawick, Weakland, and Fisch, 1974). Essentially, the use of oblique exorcism is based on the notion that the symptom never needs to be discussed, nor the treatment methods interpreted or explained. The therapist assumes that the family "wants out" of its untenable situation, and the therapist's sole task is to create the most viable means of extricating them. Each strategy must be individually designed to create change, which is best achieved by giving "homework" to be done between sessions. As with most strategic tasks, the presenting problem provides a major guideline for developing effective assignments. The following clinical examples demonstrate the use of oblique exorcism.

Robert A. had initially come to therapy with his wife for a marital problem. They had been married for eight years, were childless, and were facing the life cycle dilemma of starting a family. Therapy revealed that the marriage was not substantial enough to salvage and the A.'s left therapy after a trial separation and subsequently divorced. Within the same period, Mr. A. also lost his mother from terminal cancer. Despite his own marital distress, he coped with his mother's death and dying process in a mature manner and avoided becoming entangled with his family of origin. Approximately six months after terminating therapy, Robert A. returned suffering from severe anxiety attacks, which overwhelmed him to the extent that he could not take clients out for meals or handle any confined situations without feeling as if he were going to choke to death. He developed severe chest pains which were without medical origin. At times the attacks were so bad that he would run from his apartment and drive to the nearest hospital, sitting in his car outside the emergency room until the pains subsided. A few times he was actually admitted to a hospital only to be checked and discharged. My hypothesis was that Robert was still struggling with his losses and was stuck at a stage of development where he was about to make another commitment to a woman. Because he was now in his mid-thirties, if they married he would soon have to deal with the issue of children—a recapitulation of his former stage of developmental "arrest."

Therapy using oblique exorcism included the following sequence of strategic tasks:

1) Robert was first instructed to have an anxiety attack in the office. I then gave him a paper bag, demonstrated how he could breathe into it and told him to practice having a morning and evening attack daily until his next session. He also was to put the bag in his briefcase and keep it with him at all times.

2) The next assignment was to visit a neonate nursery and a cancer ward.

3) He then had to visit restaurants of various sizes and styles, sit alone for very short periods and eat only ice cream and soft or pureed foods in order to avoid choking to death. The latter was stated very explicitly and I made it clear that I could not tolerate losing a patient when s/he was in treatment; before he could eat solid foods in restaurants he'd have to terminate treatment.

4) He was to continue seeing his girlfriend, but he was to take control of all social activities so that he always knew where the emergency exits were and could "bail out" whenever he anticipated an attack.

5) He was to spend an entire week concentrating on the word "power" which he posted on all his mirrors, refrigerator, etc. Also, at work he was to answer the phone with the word "power" flashing like a neon sign in his mind.

6) He was to spend the next week in a weakened condition, feeling
helpless and like a baby, letting his girlfriend nurture him and tend
to his every whim.

At this point Robert decided he didn't need to go on. He was not
willing to give up the feeling of power and refused to become weak.
He is currently eating out in social and business contexts and has not
fled from any situations. Therapy is focused on Robert and his girlfriend and the future of their dyadic relationship.

Family B. has been in family therapy for several months as a result
of the suicidal gestures of their 19-year-old daughter who recently
returned home after an unsuccessful year of sporadically attending
two different colleges. The daughter, Alyce, was the younger of two
children; her older brother was a senior in college, engaged and living
away from home. The family was obviously struggling with their impending empty nest, e.g., they had "lost" their only son to his fiancée
and might easily lose their daughter to suicide. Alyce's suicidal attempts always brought about the following repetitive behavior sequences: She would threaten to take her life; her mother would rush
to save her by bringing her home; and Mr. B. would become sullen,
depressed and withdrawn. Once Alyce left home again, Mr. B. would
attempt to get the marriage going, but Mrs. B. would get depressed
and start to worry about Alyce becoming suicidal. Finally, Alyce would
call on the phone, threaten to kill herself and then have to come home,
and the repetitive cycle would continue. Family therapy focused on
moving Alyce out of her parent's relationship and helping Mr. and
Mrs. B. to keep her out. When things became significantly improved,
therapy was discontinued.

A few months later I received an emergency call from Alyce who
told me that she called to say "goodbye." She wanted to thank me for
all that I had done and wanted me to know that I had really helped
but that she had made a conscious decision to end her life. She was
home for a holiday celebration, and her mother's entire family of origin
were there, yet unaware of her dilemma. Her suicidal motive was to
make her parents really understand how they had deserted her when
she needed them so desperately.

I asked her how she could be so certain that they would be upset by
her death. I suggested that they might be relieved and that her death
might help their marriage. I told her that she should check it out first
as it would be a shame to make such an error. I engaged her in planning
a mock funeral in my office with her whole family present, suggesting
that the outcome of the mock funeral would determine her course of

action. Of course, if she was correct, I'd have to accept her suicide. We discussed every element of the proposed session, including the black dress she would wear, the black candles she would light and the poetry she'd compose. At the appointed time of the mock funeral session, Alyce arrived alone and handed me a drawing of a hen laying eggs marked "life." Alyce said that the funeral was cancelled because she had decided to go on living. She asked if I'd work with her on an individual basis if she promised not to kill herself. That exorcism took place approximately five years ago and Alyce has been out of treatment for approximately four and a half years, is symptom-free and is working to support herself in her own apartment. Her relationship with her family appears to be excellent and the parents are reported to be busy with their own lives.

In both cases, death and loss were major issues and each, whether symbolic or real, took place at a critical juncture in the family life cycle. The use of oblique exorcism provided strategic techniques that quickly and directly resolve serious conflicts that traditional therapies would take longer to change. Although there are other ways of resolving death and loss, oblique exorcism is particularly helpful when one needs a brief therapeutic strategy to deal with severe death anxiety in families who prefer to remain in therapy forever rather than risk change.

References

Coleman, S. B. Incomplete mourning in substance abusing families: Theory, research and practice. In L. Wolberg and M. Aronson (Eds.), *Group and Family Therapy 1980*. New York: Brunner/Mazel, 1980.

Coleman, S. B. and Stanton, M. D. The role of death in the addict family. *Journal of Marriage and Family Counseling*, 1978, *4*, 79-91.

Haley, J. *Problem Solving Therapy*. San Francisco: Jossey-Bass, 1976.

Selvini-Palazzoli, M. L., Boscolo, L., Cecchin, G., and Prata, G. *Paradox and Counterparadox: A New Model in the Therapy of the Family in Schizophrenic Transaction*. New York: Aronson, 1978.

Watzlawick, P., Weakland, J., and Fisch, R. *Change: Principles of Problem Formation and Problem Resolution*. New York: Norton, 1974.

SANDRA B. COLEMAN, Ph.D.
Director, Research and Evaluation
A.C.T. (Achievement through Counseling
and Treatment);
Clinical Associate Professor
Department of Mental Health Sciences
Hahnemann Medical College and Hospital
Philadelphia, PA

94. Marital Stress During the Transition to Retirement

Question:

I have read that people are retiring from work at earlier and earlier ages, while living longer and longer lives. I wonder what problems married couples encounter as they approach retirement. It seems to me that there must be special stresses associated with this significant life transition. What is known about marriage during this period? How might couples be helped to prepare more effectively for retirement?

Discussion:

The marital relationship cannot help but be affected by the retirement experience. Although most people make the transition from worker to retiree satisfactorily on their own, some need assistance. Furthermore, and perhaps more important, there is a growing retirement preparation movement which maintains that almost everyone can be helped to experience a more successful retirement.

Although the legal mandatory retirement age was raised to 70 in 1978, the trend over the past few decades has been to earlier and earlier retirement. The majority of workers retire before age 65. In 1957, 38% of men age 65 and older were working. Today, only 20% of this age group is working. On the other hand, a 1979 Louis Harris poll found that more than half the Americans surveyed said they planned to continue working when they reached retirement age.

One study (Groen, 1978) assessed the marital satisfaction of couples around the time of the husband's retirement from full-time employment. A sample of teachers who would retire in three years was compared with a sample of teachers who were already three years into retirement. It was found that the retirees were significantly more satisfied than the preretirees in several measures of satisfaction. The lower satisfaction of the preretirees was related to anxiety about the future, especially in relation to financial adequacy. Retirees expressed satisfaction with increased contact with the spouse, less concern with financial adequacy, and an orientation to the present rather than the future. In other words, once people actually enter the retirement phase of life they can anticipate enhanced marital satisfaction.

There are several factors that can create stress in a marriage as retirement approaches. These very same factors, if approached creatively, can contribute to the enrichment of the relationship.

Two Retirements. Increasingly, it is the case that couples have to deal with two retirements—his and hers. It is likely that individual life cycles will not be synchronized. Very common is the situation of a wife who assumes or resumes a career after spending some years raising children. Especially if she is younger than her husband, she may be reaching the peak of career success and satisfaction as the husband begins to slow down and think of retirement.

Looked at from a different perspective, a woman may face a retirement-like crisis much earlier than her husband. While he is absorbed in his career, she experiences a progressive diminution of the maternal role. A husband may not be sensitive to the identity crisis being experienced by his wife or her struggle to reconstruct her life on a non-family-centered foundation.

It has been found, by the way, that women are as work oriented as men, and more likely than men to take a long time in adjusting to retirement (Atchley, 1976). In a study of semi-skilled factory workers, female subjects were less favorable to retirement than males. Work-based friendship ties were the chief correlate of the wish to continue working (Jacobson, 1974).

Role Reversal. It is not unusual for men to assume more expressive roles as they get older and for women to assume more instrumental roles. As men withdraw from the work world, they are more free to develop the more "feminine" side of themselves. They may become more attentive to grandchildren, bring in flowers from the garden to decorate the house, or show interest in cooking or baking. Women, for their part, freed from child-rearing responsibilities, are likely to undertake more of the business aspects of the family, making decisions and becoming more assertive. Especially if the husband's health is failing, or if she has developed a life outside the home, the balance of power within the marital dyad is likely to shift.

Life Review Process. Mental health and happiness are related to successfully passing through a series of developmental stages, each of which requires reflection, recapitulation and new decisions as to the shape one's life is to take. For men, critical life reviews typically occur at the termination of the occupational career; for women, they typically occur at the termination of the family cycle.

Four dimensions of the marital relationship need review: 1) *self-esteem*: a positive sense of self-worth is a natural starting point for a satisfying retirement; 2) *interpersonal commitment*: the meaning and implications of marriage for the later years of life must be explored; "until death do us part" becomes more real; 3) *availability of resources*: the couple must be realistic about what they can do with what they have; 4) *goal consensus*: the couple must see themselves as a team working for shared goals. Choices have to be made about such matters as living arrangements, medical care, and relations with children (Medley, 1977).

There are several modalities for working with preretirees, for guiding them through their two retirements, the disequilibrium of role reversal, and the life review process.

Individual and Couple Therapy. This includes two dimensions. On the one hand, personal counseling involves providing support and assistance so that they can understand the changes they are experiencing. On the other hand, activity counseling is directed at the identification of appropriate work opportunities—paid or voluntary—and leisure activities. Many of the "young olds" might be encouraged to explore second-career or part-time work possibilities. This could be advisable especially in cases where the husband retires before the wife.

Small Group Sessions. Several peer couples might be brought together to explore shared concerns about retirement. One theme that recurs in groups is the struggle to maintain or reestablish the meaningful identity conferred by years of paid work. Also, participants recognize that retiring coincides with aging and that this often brings increased physical limitations or disabilities. Such prospects lead to fear of protracted illness, loss of faculties and death. The group can provide a support network within which such delicate topics can be explored.

Preretirement Planning Seminars. There are several structured package programs available. They are not therapy, nor are they mainly educational. Rather, the seminars are motivational, designed to stimulate the participants to explore actively the options available to them in a number of areas. For example, the Action for Independent Maturity (AIM) seminar consists of eight two-hour sessions on the following topics: 1) the challenge of retirement; 2) health and safety; 3) housing and location; 4) legal affairs; 5) attitudes and role adjustments; 6) meaningful use of time; 7) sources of income; and 8) financial planning.

Obviously, all of these are topics which husbands and wives should explore together. The seminar, led by an AIM-trained discussion leader, provides a nonthreatening context within which couple communication can be focused and encouraged. (Note: Information about the AIM Seminar can be obtained from Action for Independent Maturity, 1909 K Street NW, Washington, DC 20049).

Marriage counselors might consider getting training as discussion leaders. At least they should be aware of seminars conducted in their area to which people might be referred. And, while the seminar might seem indicated for some couples encountered in therapy, conversely, attending a seminar might prompt some couples to move into therapy.

Working with couples in this mid-life enrichment context can also have the serendipitous benefit of helping the therapist attend to his or her own eventual retirement.

References

Atchley, R. C. Selected social and psychological differences between men and women in later life. *Journal of Gerontology,* 1976, *31,* 204-211.

Groen, N. K. *Marital Satisfaction and Retirement.* Doctoral dissertation, Syracuse University, 1978.

Jacobson, D. Rejection of the retiree role: A study of female industrial workers in their 50's. *Human Relations,* 1974, *27,* 477-492.

Medley, M. L. Marital adjustment in the post-retirement years. *The Family Coordinator,* 1977, *26,* 5-11.

WILLIAM F. POWERS, Ph.D.
Professor of Sociology
Suffolk Community College
Selden, NY

PART D

The Family Therapist

95. Preventing Burnout in Therapeutic Work with Severely Dysfunctional Families

Question:

With the need for therapeutic work with severely dysfunctional families increasing dramatically, the demands of the work too often result in therapists feeling overwhelmed, confused, powerless and hopeless—in short, burned out. There seems to be a contagion of burnout in our agency. How does burnout occur and how can it be prevented?

Discussion:

Burnout is an all too common experience of therapists treating severely dysfunctional families, particularly families of schizophrenics and multiproblem families. It is useful to understand how it can occur so that therapists can realistically define their roles and responsibilities in relation to both family and treatment systems.

As therapist, you can easily get caught up in a contagion of anxiety and fear of catastrophic expectations, especially when one or more family members are paranoid, talking crazy, acting bizarrely, abusing alcohol or drugs, or posing a threat of suicide, violence or incest. You are likely to lose your treatment focus, direction and sense of control with a disorganized family chronically on the brink of chaos or rebounding from crisis to crisis. You may lose sleep on late night phone calls from a family in crisis only to have the family fail to show for regularly scheduled sessions. You may despair at ever convening a fragmented family or ever terminating with an enmeshed family.

The pervasiveness and rigidity of destructive interactional patterns can make you pessimistic, or even fatalistic, about possibilities for change. A family's denial of problems or resistance to your most valiant change efforts can leave you feeling frustrated, incompetent and doomed to fail. Seemingly limitless, unrealistic and conflicting expectations by family members can make you feel depleted and trapped in a no-win situation. Moreover, communication ambiguity may baffle you to the point that you doubt your own perceptions and responses to a family and may even start to wonder if it's you who are crazy.

If many of these symptoms are familiar, then you may have been successfully inducted into a severely dysfunctional family system. Becoming so embroiled may seem like sinking in quicksand. In such a predicament, it is extremely helpful to have supportive resources on firm ground. Unfortunately, the treatment system may not be providing essential support. The problem of therapist burnout, therefore, may also be symptomatic of dysfunction in the treatment system.

Governmental and institutional policies are often unclear, unrealistic and inconsistent. Hampered by economic, legal and political constraints, they may be poorly administered or out of touch with reality-based service needs. The community mental health movement has brought about a dramatic increase in the demand for family work with the reentry of former mental patients into the community, and yet funding is inadequate to provide for professional staff, resources (such as halfway houses), and research necessary to solve basic problems of patient reintegration with families and communities.

Treatment programs are too often fragmented, with rules and boundaries confused and even conflicting with therapeutic imperatives. Therapists who begin work with families on an inpatient service may not be allowed to continue beyond discharge, a transition most critical to the real world readjustment of patient and family. Such a policy also gives a message that the "cure" took place in the hospital and, at discharge, the family can simply return to business as usual. Many families fall between the cracks in transfer from agency to agency to meet administrative requirements. Multiple therapists and agencies may be involved simultaneously, with poor communication and even cross purposes, with various members of a family. Some families are in chronic treatment, passed from one agency to the next over the years. Such complications contribute to therapist confusion, "triangulation," and powerlessness. Stresses are compounded when therapists are overburdened with large caseloads, paperwork and meetings. Time pressures force staff isolation, reduce communication and lower morale.

In most treatment systems, the bulk of responsibility for the most difficult treatment cases generally falls to those members of the system who have the least power and experience. Therapists who work with severely dysfunctional families are typically underpaid and undervalued. The more senior and seasoned clinicians, partially due to their own burnout concerns, tend to assign and refer more disturbed and disturbing cases to junior colleagues and to beginning trainees. At the same time, they give explicit and implicit messages that these cases are probably hopeless.

It is no wonder that so many therapists treating severely dysfunctional families suffer burnout. Ironically, the most likely candidates for burnout are the professionals who are most idealistic and committed (Cherniss, 1980). Responsible therapists who are energetic, hardworking and dedicated are most likely to overfunction in response to underfunctioning family and treatment systems. A vicious cycle can ensue: The more responsibility you, as therapist, assume for a system in distress, the more helpless and dependent on you that system can become. The more you do, the more is expected of you, and the less responsibility the system takes in solving its problems. You should also be aware of your own rescue needs, for the greater the plight, the greater the rescue fantasies. You may find yourself in the position of an identified patient who sacrifices himself in order to keep the system from collapsing.

To avoid burnout, it is important to understand the problem in systemic perspective—how dysfunction in both family and treatment systems may contribute to burnout symptoms in the therapist. It is imperative to reassess and clarify your roles and responsibilities in relation to both family and treatment systems. Be careful to set realistic goals and priorities that are based on a sound evaluation of: (a) each family system, (b) the available resources and constraints in the treatment system, and (c) your own abilities and limitations.

When working with families that have severe organizational problems, poor differentiation and boundaries (Walsh, 1979), and fuzzy communication, you need to be especially clear in defining yourself in relation to the family. It is important to differentiate your role and responsibilities as therapist from those of family members. While it is your responsibility to take charge of and structure the therapy, family members must be actively encouraged to take responsibility for their own behavior and for their own roles in the joint resolution of problems.

You define yourself as therapist concretely in the structure you establish for the therapeutic context and in the goals and terms you set for your involvement. Setting rules for the therapy communicates that you are in charge. It also makes clear what you expect of the family and what can be expected of you. Mueller and Orfanidis (1976) actually give a list of their rules of therapy to each family member at the start of treatment, thereby communicating directly to all members and furthering the process of differentiation of individuals and their responsibilities in the therapeutic process.

Set whatever rules you need to work effectively. Some general rules may apply to all families, such as a rule that treatment sessions will start and end on time. Other rules may be set to fit particular treatment needs. For example, if you believe that a family member's drinking problem impedes your work with the family, you might set a rule requiring weekly AA attendance in conjunction with your family therapy contract. In effect, you are stating: "These are the terms of my commitment to work with you; I set them because I believe them to be essential in order to reach our goals."

Whatever rules and limits you set, be prepared to enforce them. You should anticipate that they are likely to be tested. When a family waits until the last minute of a session to bring up a hot issue and pushes to extend the session overtime, it is important to hold firm to the structure of the meeting time. While frustrating to the family, it also reassures them that the therapist can set limits when they fear going out of bounds or fear losing control. You can acknowledge the concern raised and table it to the next session or to a more appropriate time. This also places responsibility on the family to bring up sensitive issues at a time they can be worked on.

Be clear about the extent and limits of your availability to a family. Families who approach relationships on all-or-none terms are likely to hold unrealistic expectations for your total commitment to them. If you find yourself repeatedly spending long hours on late night crisis calls only to have the family miss their next appointment, you might, for example, set a rule limiting phone calls to three minutes. Simply returning a call and making contact can allay some anxiety. Keeping the call brief, you can hear and acknowledge the concern and redirect solution of the problem to the next session where it can be dealt with more adequately. Another way to handle phone calls is to set a regular daily time when you are available to receive and return calls. While some flexibility in setting rules and limits is necessary, it is important not to overaccommodate to the extent that you become overburdened and resentful of both family and job. Set terms that you can live with. Moreover, it is valuable for the family to experience a solid relationship based on commitment with limits.

The setting of realistic goals and limitations is perhaps the most difficult task for therapists. With severe problems, you may feel that no matter how much you do, it will never be enough. That may be true and is important to acknowledge. Likewise, I must accept my limitations in addressing the serious and complex problem of burnout, given the constraints of a brief response. I wish (my rescue fantasy) that I might present a comprehensive approach to the treatment of severely dysfunctional families and the prevention of burnout. Realistically, I must limit myself to a few points, which I believe to be central to the problem and prevention of burnout. Hopefully, this discussion can serve as a stimulus to therapists and treatment staff to reconsider roles and responsibilities and to find ways of working together as a more mutually supportive and effectively functioning treatment system.

References

Cherniss, C. *Professional Burnout in Human Service Organizations*. New York: Praeger, 1980.

Mueller, P. and Orfanidis, M. A method of co-therapy for schizophrenic families. *Family Process*, 1976, *15*, 179-191.

Walsh, F. Breaching of family generation boundaries by schizophrenics, disturbed, and normals. *International Journal of Family Therapy*, 1979, *1*, 254-275.

FROMA WALSH, Ph.D.
Assistant Professor of Psychiatry &
Behavioral Sciences
Center for Family Studies
The Family Institute of Chicago
Northwestern University Medical School
Chicago, IL

96. Developing a Family Therapy Program in a Psychoanalytically Oriented Setting

Question:

> How is it possible to introduce, develop and enhance the growth of a program for marital and family therapy in a well-established, complex and prestigious psychoanalysis-oriented organization?

Discussion:

A family therapy program in a traditional mental health setting quickly encounters many conflicts. On the one hand, the institution wishes to be sensitive and responsive to new human problems; on the other, it wishes to continue along those traditional paths with which it is familiar and secure. Therefore, establishing a program uniquely designed to meet new needs requires a knowledge of how to work in a system which contains many contradictions, both in the new program with its different paradigm as well as in the well-established organization itself. If the person or persons who wish to establish such a program are part of the organization and have been with it for some time, they are in a dilemma. They know the organization to some extent and are part and parcel of it. At the same time, they wish to introduce changes requiring some distance and separation from the structure and those patterns set down with such care and thought over a long period of time. Judson (1978) has said, "It is extremely difficult when one has found something that makes a difference, to recapture the way one thought before" (p. 51).

Family therapists believe they have found a way of thinking that makes a difference, and therefore that means they live in and look at the setting in which they work as if through two customs, two educations and two environments. This is an uneasy position. Other staff come to look at family therapists with some uneasiness, doubts and suspicions, as if they are aliens speaking a strange language. Those who are not part of a major group are thought of as odd, and unworthy motives are ascribed to them. The pride of the group is wounded by these "aliens." Jokes are whispered about them, especially their strange ways. For example, their eyes are busy many hours of the day watching and analyzing videotapes from which they draw strange and esoteric conclusions.

It is my intention in this discussion to throw some light on the complexity of the problem, its negative and positive aspects, by presenting an actual case history from my experience.

Approximately 15 years ago, some of the first reverberations of the family therapy movement reached the Menninger Foundation and the Veterans Administration Hospital in Topeka, Kansas. Murray Bowen and Nathan Ackerman came to the Menninger Foundation to speak about and show their work, quite aware of the resistances they might encounter, but also aware that there were those who might sense the importance of their work. They were right on both scores. There was much unfavorable criticism and there was much interest. Shortly after, Virginia Satir was invited, and then came Salvador Minuchin, the latter on a number of occasions, to meet with a small group of interested staff members in the Department of Education of the Menninger Foundation. Premonitions about the difficulties of introducing the work into a psychoanalytically oriented setting were felt at that time, since only a very few staff members showed great interest. Warnings about the obstacles which might interfere had come from Framo (1976) and Haley (1975), the latter summing up succinctly and with penetrating intent the serious consequences which might occur. His summary is too valuable not to quote again and again:

> If a mental health clinic introduces family as a treatment procedure, the consequences are likely to be disorientation of the staff, radically changed administrative procedures, less harmony among the professions and confusion in the administrative hierarchy. Staff members will find themselves asked to think in terms of a theory in which they are not trained and to diagnose social rather than individual problems. The staff will also be expected to intervene actively in human dilemma, to work with poor people, to do therapy under observation where all errors are visible, and quite possibly to have the results of their therapy evaluated. In exchange for confusion in clinic administrative procedures and stress on staff members, the clinic receives a relatively small return. There will be service to larger numbers of people, less of a waiting list, more time devoted to therapy, and less to other activities, and possibly better treatment outcome. Obviously this is not a sufficient return for a mental health clinic to undertake this adventure irresponsibly (pp. 12-13).

In 1971, several staff, including the author, spent a week in the Berkshires, at a workshop sponsored by the Nathan Ackerman Institute. We were impressed by this experience, I so much so, that I resigned as Director of Social Work, a position I had held for 10 years. Several colleagues joined me in the endeavor to learn, practice and teach family therapy. I think it is impossible to practice family therapy alone, without the support of some peers who will expose their work to each other and who will risk the sense of isolation and exclusion that quickly follows in the wake of individuals who introduce new ideas and new procedures. But, in addition, it helps for the program to be led by someone who has held an important hierarchical position in the organization itself, who is not an outsider, and whose clinical judgement and skill has been respected. But a leadership position and support of peers who are on a grass roots level, so to speak, are insufficient. There must be support from the highest echelon, a support which can only go so far and which will have its limitations. In our case, the President of The Menninger Foundation agreed to our having a small amount of money for a period of some years in order to train and teach, in order to install essential videotape equipment. The importance of video recording the work, observing sessions over and over again, of supervising the data, of teaching from it, cannot be stressed enough. As Judson (1978) comments, "Science is helplessly opportunistic, it can pursue only the paths opened by technique" (p. 135).

Several things happened when this was done. The President shouldered some criticism for this unpopular move, with several departments feeling they had less of his support for the traditional treatment approaches. On the other hand, the President also had criticism from the family therapy staff (at this time consisting of three or four people), who felt that his approval and support should clear away all obstacles in their path. Thus, a series of triangulations occurred, until the family therapists realized the contradiction—that they desired support from the most important administrative staff and, at the same time, insisted on having autonomy over intake procedures and on the designation of the family as the identified patient, rather than singling out one individual in that family as being mentally ill. These three conditions are, nevertheless, most important for initiating a treatment approach based on the family as a system: 1) that the leader in the introduction of a program must be respected by his/her colleagues; 2) that the leader must have the support of his/her peers in this endeavor; and 3) that the leader have the tentative blessings of the topmost leader in that organization.

These three conditions are enhanced by the importance of the program being built on a sound financial base and not dependent on draining money from the overall budget. As our intake procedures became less complicated and free of cumbersome red tape, families were seen very soon, after a call to the Admission's Office, and treatment procedures were swiftly instituted. Several important reactions were noted. Delighted with some of our results, and having captured these results on videotape, our enthusiasm ran high. We wanted to show our work to anyone who would stop, look and listen, not realizing that such fervor not only turns people off, but arouses apprehension, suspicion and withdrawal. We could not understand these reactions. We felt rejected, the burden of being outsiders, and with some guilt and disloyalty because of the years of patient training we had been given by our colleagues.

In our enthusiasm, we had ignored a fundamental principle in our family therapy work. This is that we had to understand the matrix in which our work was being conducted; we had to understand how to join it, how to be in it and outside of it. We had to appreciate the fact that all innovative ideas are, with good cause, regarded with suspicion and disbelief. One has only to look back at the past decade to understand the validity of disbelief, as new ideas and fads, one after another, are introduced on the mental health scene, raising enthusiastic hopes and expectations, only to have these new developments disappear and vanish on the horizon. We, therefore, learned to be discreet, to draw a low profile, to let the work speak for itself, to allow staff access to our work only if they so desired, to present our work with modesty, to bear the burdens of silence and scepticism without developing bitterness and a wish to give up. In this matter we were, and still are, only partially successful.

We are highly vulnerable to the pull of enmeshment, the pull to be in the organizational structure, without a clear definition of ourselves and the essential differences of our work. We received much urging to seek ways of integrating family therapy with psychoanalysis, an appealing idea which struck at our ambivalence at wanting to be with the organization and at the same time being differentiated from it. We saw ourselves (at least some of us had this experience) as being disloyal, which made us sometimes vacillate between depression or rebelliousness. We were sometimes called "cliquish," or accused of robbing other departments of their brightest people, when they became attracted to our work. Our students (whether social workers, residents in psychiatry or fellows in child psychiatry) occasionally found us smug, haughty, manipulative, contemptuous, but came to understand the difficulty they were placed in by our emphasis on social context and family systems, while with other faculty they were being immersed in psychoanalytic theory and psychoanalytically oriented psychotherapy.

When they became enthusiastic enough to espouse the family approach, they risked being exploited by us, without our awareness; or, being turned off by senior staff, they joined those who were hostile towards our concepts. A middle ground position could not be easily maintained.

It has been necessary, therefore, to resist temptations toward rhetoric and dogma; not to encourage staff towards any easy entrée into our training programs; not to present papers in the traditional fashion, which simply confuses those without training in our ways of working. We have been careful to not expand our program into territorial waters, claimed and possessed by others in the organization. We have not been opposed to other staff members who wish to practice family therapy without being affiliated with our core group or without having been through the Menninger Foundation Staff Training Program in Family Therapy. The result of not attempting to control practice has been that many staff members have discovered for themselves the imperative need for training and have then come to us seeking help on their own accord. When we have been encouraged to expand our services in certain directions, or when we have wished to sharpen the definition of our boundaries, we have expressed our concern and misgivings that to do so might harm the unity of the organization and, on many occasions, have decided not to effect that particular change. This has caused the administration to examine and weigh the risks and then to facilitate change themselves on the side of growth. This is not an artifice, but a genuine concern for the safety of the structure of our professional family.

Lastly, our work has been enhanced and encouraged by distinguished members of the field who have come to Topeka to help educate and train us without fear of being roughly mistreated or criticized by one of the pioneer centers of psychoanalytic training, treatment and research. Encouraged by the generosity of the primary teachers in the field, we have been made welcome to their centers of practice and to have those important interchanges which create new knowledge. A few others, and only a very few, have not been willing to come to Topeka, viewing our organization as one fused mass, not understanding that, as in a family, some of our subsystems (and not just the family therapy program) may be more differentiated than others, giving life and vitality to the whole organization.

References

Judson, H. F. F. Annals of Science DNA-I, Part 1. *New Yorker*, November 27, 1978.
Framo, J. L. Chronicle of a struggle to establish a family therapy unit within a com-

munity mental health center. In P. Guerin (Ed.), *Family Therapy: Theory and Practice.* New York: Gardner Press, 1976.

Haley, J. Why a mental health clinic should avoid family therapy. *Journal of Marriage and Family Counseling*, 1975, *1*, 3-13.

ARTHUR MANDELBAUM, M.S.W.
Director
Marriage and Family Program
The Menninger Foundation
Topeka, KS

97. Married Therapists
   Working As Cotherapists

Question:

I am a psychiatrist in private practice and my wife is a psychiatric social worker who works half time in a mental health clinic where she does marital therapy, working conjointly with couples or with marital partners separately. I have had considerable experience working as a single therapist with couples, but, as yet, my wife and I have not tried working together as cotherapists seeing marital couples. Recently we've been thinking about doing this. What guidelines would you suggest for developing our skills together as cotherapists? Also, on a private practice basis, what kind of fee is charged with two therapists working together at the same time?

Discussion:

The skills required for a married cotherapy team to do marital psychotherapy are, in some ways, very different from skills a therapist employs working singly with couples. One of the major reasons for this is the existence of what we have come to call "the marriage personality." Briefly, the idea is that as soon as you bring a marriage into a room you bring a third entity or personality which strongly affects other personalities, most particularly the personalities of the marriage partners themselves. Marriage partners act differently when they are together than when they are separate, and this will be true for the therapists' marriage as well as the patients'. Consequently, the primary insights for the therapists involve their ability to attend to their own marriage and its personality. This personality becomes, in the conjoint session, a major therapeutic tool.

Just as children see themselves as a collective personality separate from their parents, who together are seen as making up a parental personality, the patient couple will see you, not just as two single therapists, but as a marriage. In the typical marital treatment, the therapist struggles to stay neutral between the two mates as the therapy unfolds, while a husband-wife, male-female therapist team balances the marital equation. The neutrality issue is deemphasized as another one takes its place—an issue perhaps unique to this type of therapy, which has great advantage over other therapies affecting marriages.

As you work with a marriage in crisis your own marriage will be constantly exposed to view, examined and consciously and unconsciously "modeled" by the patient-couple. Thus, one of the major skills you will employ will be your capacity for insights into your own marriage, particularly your capacity as individuals to "coliberate" with each other. We use the term "coliberate" to indicate a process very different from cooperative "giving in," compromising, and holding back strategies of survival that individuals learn in the parent-child paradigm and carry over into marriage in the form of unwritten marriage contracts. Coliberation is the ability of individuals in the marriage to attend to and care for each other's freedom to be individual and to grow together in exploring each other's separateness. Needless to say, marriages in crisis are generally cooperative marriages engaged in some struggle over their unwritten marriage contract (which part of the aim of the therapy is to uncover). Obviously, if the therapists are acting on hidden contracts in their marriage, it will adversely affect the therapy.

Conjoint therapy with husband and wife cotherapists requires new concepts of transference-countertransference phenomena, and these are only just being worked out by cotherapists. But it is already clear that the reality of helping a dysfunctional marriage lies in allowing and making manifest a free flow of transference and countertransference interpretation, as the patient-couple most often places the therapist-couple in the roles of parents or siblings model.

Real change takes place slowly with a marriage, just as it does in individual therapy. Coliberative effort can't be legislated. In the process the patient-couple will be alert to how you are in your marriage: how you listen to each other in the sessions, how you employ authority with each other, who defers to whom and when, who talks the most, how you regard each others' educational and training background—in short, they will quickly size up whether the cotherapists are truly cotherapists. To the extent that they are coliberative all these qualities are skills you bring to bear in the cotherapy session, and before you enter into this kind of therapy it is well to consider whether you have them or are willing to develop them.

We recommend that therapists looking toward doing cotherapy seek a therapeutic experience themselves, with male and female cotherapists if possible, so they can experience firsthand bringing their own marriage into new focus. It is crucial to be honest with yourself about whether you are willing to engage in a constant investigation of your own marriage and to expose your marital interaction to the scrutiny of others.

Though there are as yet no studies comparing the benefits derived from traditional marital therapists to the benefits derived from marital partners as cotherapists, our own experience suggests that the benefits are considerable. Developing skills with this method certainly enhances the therapists' marriage, and the patient-couple can hardly fail to be affected, at least this is what our own follow-up of couples we have had in the past 12 years indicated.

As to the fees for private practice, doing cotherapy with one's spouse, or, for that matter, any other cotherapist, is not terribly rewarding financially. The reason for this is that there are two therapists working at the same time with the same couple. It is difficult even with the most affluent of patient-couples to charge a fee twice that of the usual for a single therapist. We work only on a double-session basis, that is 1½ hours (two 45-minute sessions back to back) and charge at the per session rate, making no allowance for the fact that the two of us are working together at the same time. Many therapists are reluctant these days to get into cotherapy arrangements because of these financial limitations. It would be wise to take this issue carefully into consideration with each other, because it will serve as a source of unconscious hostility if you are not comfortable with the fee you are charging. Reimbursement for psychotherapy is still almost entirely tied to the old model which charges for time only. Other medical specialties have long since dropped this archaic concept in favor of a more realistic method of charging by procedure.

JOHN P. BRIGGS, M.D.
Assistant Professor of Psychiatry
Columbia University
New York, NY

and

MURIEL BRIGGS, M.A.
Tarrytown, NY

98. The Pros and Cons of Spouse Cotherapy

Question:

I hear more and more about husband-wife therapy teams working together with couples, families and groups. I am wondering about the consequences of such an arrangement for both clients and therapists. What are the pros and cons of spouse cotherapy? If my wife and I decide to try working together, how could we enhance our chances for a successful and satisfying professional partnership?

Discussion:

There do seem to be numerous therapist couples who are working together at least part of the time. Other couples who are considering such a joint professional venture are eager to learn from the experiences of those currently in practice. A recent survey conducted by this writer and her spouse cotherapist indicated that married cotherapy teams generally fall into two broad categories: 1) those in which both husband and wife are professionally trained and certified as therapists, and 2) those in which one spouse is professionally trained as a therapist and the other is either informally trained or essentially a layperson. In most cases where there is some disparity between spouses' training and/or credentials, it is the wife who lacks professional training. While each team of married therapists confronts their own particular set of problems and enjoys their own special assets, there are some advantages and disadvantages inherent in this treatment modality for both clients and therapists.

Although there are few research data to substantiate clinical impressions, spouse cotherapy does offer some distinct advantages to clients. First, the cotherapy relationship tends to be more established, and there is less ambiguity or uncertainty concerning the rules of the relationship and the intended permanence of the arrangement. The "older" the marriage, of course, the more certainty and predictability is available in the cotherapy relationship. Married therapists thus have to give less attention to the cotherapy relationship, since the marriage has probably already dealt with many issues which arise in cotherapy, thus the therapists' attention can be given almost exclusively to the clients.

Second, spouse cotherapists have the same kind of ongoing, real relationship to each other as do couples and families in therapy. Thus, clients are able to view the therapists as peers in the sense that the therapists are also partners in marriage. No fantasies are needed to "imagine what s/he's really like with his/her spouse." This authentic marital relationship between the therapists provides a realistic atmosphere for couples and families to work on issues and problems. Additionally, spouse cotherapists can offer a model for clients to learn from. Watching a marital couple who also happen to be therapists as they confront conflict, negotiate developmental stages in their relationship, and share mutual responsibilities provides an opportunity for clients to view firsthand a growing, adapting marriage. The personal examples of interdependent yet individual spouse cotherapists, who obviously care for and value each other, may be one of the most valuable experiences marriage or family therapy has to offer.

But there may be disadvantages as well for clients with spouse cotherapists. If clients or therapists set up the therapists' relationship as "the ideal," or the way marriage "should be," the result will be a restrictive or confining effect on the clients' relationship. All participants must understand that the therapists represent only one of the various ways to be married and that their union, as solid and satisfying as it may be, is subject to the same stresses as are other marriages. Clients and therapists must continually guard against idealizing the therapists' marriage; seeing the spouse cotherapists as perfect marital partners in an ideal relationship is inhibiting to all parties, and therapy within such a restricted setting becomes impossible.

Another disadvantage inherent in the spouse co-therapy modality is that the therapists' interaction is predetermined since it is governed by the same rules that govern the marriage. There is little chance of therapists acting in any way inconsistent or incompatible with the marital contract's rules. A logical assumption, then, is that, if one knows the terms of the marital contract, one can reliably predict the interactions of the cotherapist as well as what issues and problems will be avoided or conflicted if discussed. The freedom and ability of the cotherapists to aid clients with specific problems is dependent in large measure on the degree to which such problems are resolved in their marital relationship.

Spouse cotherapy offers definite advantages to the therapists. Husbands and wives who work together have cited enhanced communication and intimacy as important gains to their own relationship. Sharing common professional experiences and concerns adds another dimension to the marriage. Many therapists say that working with a spouse makes therapy "more fun." Some couples say that cotherapy is a way to spend more time together.

A second advantage is that the therapists do not have to devote as much time and energy to working out the relationship with a cotherapist; they can rely on the tested and proven methods of relating established in the marriage. Most of the problems and procedures which must be worked out in any cotherapy relationship have already been significantly dealt with. For example, they can usually interpret nonverbal messages and communicate effectively. They know something about how to resolve conflict and how to cooperate. They also know each other's strengths and weaknesses. Spouses who have reared children together can draw upon that shared experience in cotherapy as they negotiate differences and disagreements about clients, strategies, etc.

A third advantage for the therapist is that each can be especially helpful to the other as a cotherapist and as a spouse as a result of their working together. The intimate knowledge that a spouse has of the other regarding family of origin, past experiences and current situations enables one as a cotherapist to draw on those in therapy when it is appropriate to do so. It is as though each therapist has the benefit of two perspectives on his/her own experience. Married cotherapists can also help each other by commenting on "blind spots" or compensating for the other; they can consult more easily and freely with each other than other cotherapists because they know each other and their respective histories so well. As spouses, they can be supportive and helpful to one another in times of discouragement or disappointment. One does not have to inquire much about how the day went if s/he was involved in part of it.

The disadvantages of spouse cotherapy to the therapists are less obvious and more insidious than the advantages. First, their professional relationship may encroach upon their personal relationship and eventually dominate it. They may find themselves discussing clients at home in the bedroom, or they may go out for a social evening and end up talking "business." All couples who work together must find some way of demarcating their personal and professional relationships in order to protect the marriage from becoming primarily a business partnership.

Another potential disadvantage is that personal identity and independence may be submerged in the spirit of "togetherness." The likelihood of losing individual identity is directly comparable to the extent to which spouses work together, i.e., those couples who work primarily as cotherapists have a greater chance of losing their individuality than do those who work occasionally together. However, it is not uncommon for one partner to feel more at risk than the other to such a loss of personal identity; a wife who enters the field via her husband's invitation to join him as a cotherapist may feel that she is only a therapist if she accompanies him and that she is not free to develop her own identity.

A third disadvantage of this modality for the therapists is that each may be limited by the experience. If they reinforce each other's blind spots, if they protect each other by not challenging or disagreeing, if they always see things the same way, neither will grow, develop or change as a therapist.

A fourth problem for spouse cotherapists is that difficulties which arise in the professional roles may jeopardize the marital relationship. A provocative question is whether a couple can negotiate successfully the dissolution of cotherapy, for instance, without threatening the marital bond. Disagreements about therapy can and do become personal arguments carried on at home sometimes. Again, establishing the boundaries between marriage and therapy is requisite to the success of both relationships.

It should be apparent by now that the pros and cons of spouse cotherapy are simply opposing views of the same issues. The inherent advantages of this treatment method are also its inherent disadvantages. How, then, can a couple maximize the strengths and minimize the weaknesses of working together as a professional team? The first important step is for each partner to establish him/herself as a professional independent of the other. Whether or not each is established as a professional therapist is probably less important than that each is established separately in some field. If one's identity as a professional person hinges on the support and good will of the other, too great a strain of dependency is placed on the relationship. Such dependency inevitably breeds anger and resentment in both partners.

The second step is related to the first: any disparity in training or credentials between spouse co-therapists must somehow be equalized so that they regard themselves as equals. Each must respect the abilities and trust the judgment of the other. They must be peers in the therapeutic partnership.

Finally, the spouse cotherapy team needs to have supervision, preferably by another team of spouses who are sensitized to the problems of this relationship. The dynamics of the marriage should be scrutinized under the microscope of supervision if the partners wish to maximize their effectiveness as a professional team. While therapy for themselves as a couple may prove helpful, supervision of their joint work will prove invaluable to their growth as therapists.

ANNA BETH BENNINGFIELD, M.A.
Private Practice
Dallas, TX

99. Therapist Adjustments for Adapting Therapy Models to Varied Clinical Settings

Question:

I frequently have opportunities to attend training workshops for therapists in private practice. For the most part these sessions are exceedingly helpful. The extent of application of current theoretical approaches to therapy varies among my colleagues. The type of clients we see would cover the spectrum of possibilities with respect to educational and income levels. Most of us do not operate from high budget multiple-staffed agencies. Single office operations are more common. Where there are cooperative efforts everyone is primarily concerned with his or her own practice. For those of us who see clients day after day there is a necessity for relying on these training programs for keeping up to date. However, many of the innovations in the more current training models of marriage and family therapy seem to require resources which neither I nor most of my colleagues possess, e.g., a cotherapist, a therapy team, a particular level of clientele. Do you have any ideas for adjustments that private practitioners can make to take advantage of some of the new approaches to marriage and family therapy?

Discussion:

One of the frustrating experiences in private practice that seldom gets satisfactorily alleviated revolves around "keeping up to date." Professional organizations are continuing to upgrade their standards, which means there are more and more resources available for continuing education opportunities. The resource faculty tend to operate out of training centers, teaching hospitals and university settings. The probability is, indeed, higher that these contexts will have much greater availability of personnel, equipment and space for more experimental ventures in therapy.

This problem raises an interesting challenge for adapting current therapy models to varied clinical contexts, and the task is one for which training faculty share responsibility. The popular methods for trying to cope with varied clinical needs of therapists in private practice have included more visual presentations, team teaching, more audience participation. Although these have been honest attempts to create more understanding and greater involvement with the models presented, adaptation to varied clinical practice settings has been more or less assumed to be the task of individual therapists.

What may be needed is more direct confrontation with the question of adjustments therapists can make for different families and settings. Some directions to include are as follows:

1) *Adopt a cotherapist.* Cotherapy is often suggested as having particular advantages in clinical settings. Where can a solo therapist get a colleague? One way this can be handled quite nicely is to "adopt" one of the family members to be your "cotherapist." Pick an identified patient whose positive resources may be hidden to all but you, or a peripheral father who needs to be a more central family figure. There are actually advantages to this cotherapy structure: competition between two professional cotherapists is absent, the adopted cotherapist can continue to work at home, and a peripheral figure or "problem-person" is restructured in the family.

2) *Build a more appropriate vocabulary.* One of the inherent problems with progress in theory is the accompanying development of "new lingo." This language eventually filters down to the general populace, but in the meantime its use can create problems. One therapist found he was losing a considerable percentage of high income but lower-educated clients. One eye-opener occurred when when he was talking to a family about "democratic" patterns of childrearing (a recent training session topic) and the family walked out. A useful solution here relies on the sensitive absorption of client vocabulary. For some families words like "democracy" mean permissiveness, and words such as "punishment" are associated with parental respect, order and family stability.

The therapist can give up favorite words without losing their content. He or she can assure the parents that more punishment is needed, and proceed to give guidance for punishment by using democratic content, e.g., "The way to really punish your son is not to let him get by with his behavior. The most effective punishment is for you to pick out two possible choices of consequences and let him decide between the two. If he is not willing to decide then you can say, 'does that mean you want me to decide? You can decide or I will decide. Which do you prefer?' " Changing the clients' definition of punishment and the therapist's vocabulary has been a fruitful avenue for change with this type of clientele.

3) *Color the paradox positive.* The clinical efficacy of paradoxical models in marriage and family therapy makes them increasingly attractive. Because many therapists do not feel comfortable using a paradoxical approach, which is also highly confrontive, they feel they must forego its use entirely. This is another case where creative therapist adjustment can make these resources useful to almost everyone. By positively casting the paradox, the conflict tone is lowered in the therapy session.

A highly ego-centered, selfish individual who had been through one marriage was now in a second marriage. After three years he described himself as unhappy, a terrible person who was consistently critical of his wife and his family and who could not make decisions. This man was told by the therapist that he was a highly caring individual, and that the therapist seldom had the opportunity of working with a client who was so sensitive to others' needs to the extent he was: his criticism of his wife and family showed great caring, i.e., that he wanted their *best* image to be projected. Clients will protest strongly that their criticism is bad. This gives the therapist more ammunition, i.e., the greatest level of caring is one which does not call attention to itself. The therapist insisted that the client needed to be a little more selfish, think a little more of his own long-term needs. This put the client in a positive, therapeutic double-bind. If he resisted the therapist he would have to cease criticizing his wife. If he did not resist he had to see himself in a different light, as one whose "problem" is caring too much and not looking after his own needs enough. This approach is an attractive, positive one for therapists who do not see themselves as strong confronting types.

4) *Create an imaginary therapy team.* A currently popular model for family therapy involves a therapy team who observes therapy behind a one-way mirror and helps construct a paradoxical letter which is read to the family at the end of the session and re-read by the family at home before the next session (Selvini-Palazzoli et al., 1978). Very few therapists in private practice have one-way mirror settings, let alone a team to observe and construct a letter. With only slight therapist adjustments, however, this model can be quite useful to the solo

therapist. The therapist can suggest to the client that he or she would like to provide the advantage of the wisdom of his/her therapy consulting team for this case. Obtaining their consent to "consult," the therapist can in reality talk it over with a colleague and mail the paradoxical letter. Or the therapist can consult an imaginary team, construct the paradoxical letter personally and mail it to the client.

The possible advantages are valuable: The therapist can, at the next session, separate him- or herself from aspects of the letter, to preempt resistance from the client and increase the effectiveness of the therapeutic double bind. For example, if the therapist has been challenging the client family to come to grips with new options, the letter could suggest that the "team" believes the therapist is wrong to push for change now. The therapist can now take advantage of this context at the next session: "I am confused by some of the team's suggestions, but I have great respect for these professional specialists." The client family is caught between the therapist's challenge to change and the "team of specialists" who counsel against change now.

The problem of clinical application of developing models of marriage and family therapy is complex. Training faculty can be more sensitive to varied clinical settings and creative processes for therapist adjustments to compensate for a lack of physical resources and additional professional personnel.

Reference

Selvini-Palazzoli, M., Cechin, G., Prata, G., and Boscolo, L. *Paradox and Counterparadox.* New York: Jason Aronson, 1978.

JAMES F. KELLER, Ph.D.
*Associate Professor and Director
of Supervision for Marriage and
Family Therapy
Center for Family Services
Virginia Polytechnic Institute and
State University
Blacksburg, VA*

100. Keeping the Family Therapist Abreast of Developments in the Field

Question:

As a busy, overscheduled practicing family therapist, I often do not have sufficient time to keep up with the literature, especially the literature pertaining to the emerging schools of family therapy. How can I motivate myself to remain current in this regard, and in essence, help build bridges between the developing theoretical constructs in the family field and my everyday clinical work?

Discussion:

The problem of how an overworked therapist makes connections between the hectic world of clinical practice and the emerging theoretical constructs in the therapy field is far from being new. However, as the saying goes in relation to the weather, everybody talks about it but no one ever does anything. In my own clinical work as well as in my supervision of others, I have discovered a simple activity which not only tends to bridge the gap between theory and practice, but in addition, develops one's own views on the important ingredients in therapy—in essence, developing one's personal theory of family therapy.

All practicing therapists have a least a moderate level of knowledge concerning the key concepts of the family therapy field. Most have had some type of introductory course where the contemporary schools of family therapy were detailed, or at least the major concepts were presented in a non-school-specific manner. It could be said, therefore, that some mean level of theoretical knowledge of the family therapy field could conceivably be determined. However, many training experiences present theory as independent of practice, drawing an artificial boundary between the two. Just as unnecessary distinctions can be made between an individual and his/her social context, the same kind of noninterdependent thinking can occur in relation to theory and clinical practice.

The proposed method for alleviating this dichotomous, nonsystemic dilemma is as follows: After each session, the therapist is to write out on 5 × 9 index cards the major concepts or themes existent in the previous session. Unlike case notes, which often serve as a running process commentary on the cases's evolution, the *concept cards* are intended to have a more precise, deductive focus. The therapist must deduce the salient theoretical constructs or themes and identify them in a definition-generating way. The therapist, then, can make connections between theoretical constructs with which he/she is familiar in the family literature, and relate these constructs in a personally meaningful way through his/her own clinical practice. For example, in a session where parents present a united front, channeling their spousal conflicts through their "sick" child, the structural concept of detouring can be experienced and defined in a personally relevant manner.

The level of involvement in learning family therapy concepts is greatly increased when the concepts can be drawn from the therapist's own practice rather than from textbooks on family therapy. While case books such as Papp's (1976) are quite useful in that they paint a picture of therapeutic process, no text can provide as meaningful and personal a learning experience as can be obtained from your own caseload.

In another session, the therapist repeatedly experienced failure at creating interpersonal enactments between family members. The therapist, however, continually tried the same kind of procedure to create the enactment, and in the same ways. In Watzlawick et al.'s (1974) terms, a "more of the same" situation developed, where the more the therapist tried to create an interpersonal scenario in the room, the more the family resisted. The therapist was not able to effect change of a different order by simply reversing his field or attempting to effect enactment in a different manner (doing less of the same). Again, these kinds of constructs, if they can be identified by the therapist as being a part of his/her everyday clinical world, will hold more personal meaning and longer-lasting professional usefulness.

Here is a final, and conceptually more general, example: Family therapists are taught, hopefully, to think in terms of systems and contexts. Often, however, there is an overemphasis on the family system to the exclusion of important extrafamilial networks of influence. In a case where a probation officer inadvertently sides with the 16-year-old identified patient against frustrated parents who cannot impose necessary and appropriate limits, a therapist can truly learn the importance of considering systems of influence outside of the family context which perpetuate the recursive cycles of symptomatic behavior. In this situation the concept card can be written on the variety of contexts necessary for a family-oriented therapist to consider and in which he/she must effectively intervene to help the family.

Concept cards can be a useful tool in organizing the focus of one's supervisory sessions. Supervision sessions, in addition to having a case-specific, intervention-generating function should also focus on matters relating to the trainee's own developing personal style, as well as issues transcending the particulars of any one case (Liddle, 1980).

The concept cards can be especially useful in this latter regard. Learning the art of family or context-oriented therapy occurs simultaneously at many levels. At the cognitive level, the broadest and perhaps most important learning must be considered the paradigm-shift or capacity to think of human problems in systemic, interpersonal, nonlinear and interdependent ways (Liddle and Saba, 1979). At the next level of cognitive functioning, a language or grammar of family therapy must exist to allow concepts such as conflict-detouring and context to have meaning.

Concept cards can rapidly personalize and organize what can be a confusing and disorienting field, often filled with unfamiliar jargon to the beginning clinician. The cards can thus be useful with supervisors and be ready, specific, and discussion-stimulating devices to aid the training process. One of Bateson's more familiar concepts is deutero-learning, or learning to learn. This seems to have relevance in describing the usefulness of a method such as concept cards. As supervisors, we are not only interested in teaching a trainee the most effective ways of handling Cases A, B, and C, but, of course, are concerned with the issue of generalizability. That is, will the trainee be able to generalize his learnings from Cases A, B, and C to cases D through Z? Identifying the relevant operational constructs from one's own clinical practice can be a step in this direction.

The cards can also be helpful in organizing data for discussion with networks or groups of peers consulting with one another about their cases. A therapist might listen to audio tapes of recent sessions and come up with four or five concepts recurring in his/her sessions. The concept cards, along with the segment of the audiotape exemplifying the theoretical construct, could then comprise the data for the consultant group's discussion.

The cards can be useful in discerning trends in thinking and observation in one's own work. For example, useful information exists if one finds certain concepts overutilized or others noticeably absent from one's developing stack of cards. Feedback from others in this regard can be most useful in identifying conceptual areas of over- and underdevelopment.

Above all else, however, it could be said that the most essential value to an activity such as concept cards is in the area of clarifying what our own operational beliefs, assumptions and conceptual patterns are in relation to the therapy we conduct. It is an activity which forces us to be precise in defining what we believe to be the essential elements of family therapy. Einstein's famous remark, "It is the theory that determines what we can observe" (Watzlawick and Weakland, 1977) has relevance in our case. Our theories, or, less formally, our views about families and their functioning, determine not only what we can observe, but also what we can and will do with these families. It therefore seems important that we devise methods to determine what precisely these theories or views are.

In conclusion, Bateson (1979) defined epistemology as the act of knowing, thinking and deciding. The concept cards activity can assist in what we might call an epistemologic declaration—that is, an evolving statement of how and what we know about families, how we think about them, and what our mechanisms of decision making are in everyday clinical matters.

References

Bateson, G. *Mind and Nature: A Necessary Unity*. New York: Dutton, 1979.

Liddle, H. A. On teaching a contextual or systemic therapy: Steps toward an integrative training model. *American Journal of Family Therapy*. 1980, *8*, in press.

Liddle, H. A., and Saba, G. Teaching family therapy at the introductory level: A conceptual model emphasizing a "Pattern Which Connects" training and therapy. Submitted for publication, December, 1979.

Papp, P. *Family Therapy: Full Length Case Studies*. New York: Gardner, 1976.

Watzlawick, P., Weakland, J. and Fisch, R. *Change*. New York: Norton, 1974.

Watzlawick, P. and Weakland, J. *The Interactional View*. New York: Norton, 1977.

HOWARD ARTHUR LIDDLE, Ed.D.
Director
Family Systems Department
Institute for Juvenile Research
Chicago, IL

PART E

Violence and the Family

101. Treatment and Value Issues in Helping Battered Women

Question:

Recent awareness of the problem of violence in intimate relationships has spurred discussion among family therapists of potential treatment approaches. What treatment and value issues do therapists need to consider when confronting the problem of spouse abuse, especially wife abuse?

Discussion:

I will focus on the physical abuse of women rather than men mainly because women are subject to more serious forms of abuse and because they are trapped to a greater extent in the relationship both economically and psychologically (Straus, 1978). It seems that even minor forms of violence need to be taken seriously because, rather than being a substitute for severe violence, minor violence is associated with it (Straus, 1974) and can drastically change a power balance.

There is currently no consensus regarding the choice of approach when working with battered women and their partners. Several years of research will be needed to answer the empirical questions involved. In the meantime, however, we can explore our beliefs and attitudes as they may influence our selection of treatment methods. Decisions about the extent and type of treatment are probably influenced in subtle ways by our attitudes and beliefs about the problem.

Therapists' Beliefs and Attitudes

Therapists' attitudes toward victims of abuse may parallel our cultural propensity to blame victims. Victim-blaming may arise from a psychological need to see the world as basically just, resulting in a belief that people deserve what they get and get what they deserve. It is easy to see that the tendency to blame increases the more the victim differs from oneself; however, derogation of innocent victims similar to oneself may occur as a defense against thoughts that similar acts of violence might occur to oneself.

Attitudes toward female assault victims deserve especially close scrutiny. Sexist attitudes are associated with the belief that female assault victims are responsible for the assault and with similar negative attitudes toward all victims (Feild, 1978). Some studies indicate that men are more likely than women to withhold assistance from women victims and to have more negative attitudes toward them. Less sympathy may be aroused for battered wives than for battered children or women assaulted by strangers because it is difficult to see the many forces (masochism not among them) holding wives in abusive relationships. Antidotes for victim-blaming include reading the numerous accounts of battered women's lives (e.g., Dobash and Dobash, 1979; Walker, 1979) and participating in consciousness-raising exercises.

Views of violence are also likely to influence treatment approach. Is the violence the result of an instinctive drive or is it a learned behavior? Much empirical literature exists to help answer this question. Questions regarding personal reactions to working with someone who has been violent also need to be explored: Am I fearful of being attacked? If so, how can I best cope with this fear? Does my rejection of violent behavior generalize to the rejection of the person who has been violent?

Some general maxims of family therapy may need to be altered. The family system provides the stage but may not be the source of the violent behavior. The family system operates within the larger social system which oppresses women. In many cases wives become the convenient targets for frustrations the man develops elsewhere. Many of the men seem threatened more by their partner's status and personal resources than by their partner's behavior, and the men often need help in coping nonviolently with these threats.

There are value issues which also require exploration. Our values may be reflected in beliefs about the amount of violence considered justifiable in response to particular situations and about the overall value of marriage to men and to women.

Many battered women describe the added shame and despair they feel when helpers try to take a "neutral" stance with regard to all of the couple's problems, including the violence. Treating the violence as a problem in its own right, rather than as a symptom of faulty communication, does not have to elicit the man's defensiveness, withdrawal or hostility. I will describe briefly some ways of doing this.

Problem Detection. There seem to be no particular diagnostic categories which would signal the need to ask about spouse abuse. The woman will probably show signs of depression but will often seek help for her children rather than herself. The shame which prevents all family members from speaking about the violence indicates the need to ask all distressed families directly about the presence of abuse. (Some battered women have been in family therapy up to three years with no detection of the abuse.) A funneling technique, going from the least to most threatening questions, seems to work well; for example: "How do each of you usually react when you have differences of opinion? During your arguments, do you sometimes raise your voice? Have there been times in your relationship when physical force was used? Who? When? What happened?" At this point separate history-taking interviews may be necessary if the partners have very disparate perceptions of the abusive episodes.

Interventions

As one might expect, the man's motivation for therapy is usually low. Often the threat of losing his partner is the strongest incentive. Several steps can be taken to enhance the man's internal motivation: (a) If he puts himself down for receiving help, he can be aided in constructing some alternative self-statements, e.g., "It takes courage to get help for my aggression." (b) The therapist can empathize with his feelings of anger, hurt and fear while confronting his violence, e.g., Man: "I wouldn't have had to do it if she had heard me out." Therapist: "I understand how frustrated you got when she didn't listen to you, but that's no excuse to hit her." (c) For the man who is less attuned to feelings, prides himself on control, yet says "She made me explode" or "I lost control," I suggest saying that you can help him learn how to control himself better, how to prevent others from the "getting the best of him." (d) It can also help to point out that he may carry violent habits into future intimate relationships.

The men (as well as the women) need to be assessed for suicide risk because the men typically have low self-esteem and periods of strong guilt. Guns increase the risk of homicide and suicide, and the couple may agree to have the police department or a friend keep any weapons. Temporary separation can be explored, and recommended if the violence is frequent. The option of divorce may need to be explored in individual sessions at first because of danger to the woman in discussing it openly. A no-violence contract, with or without contingencies, is often useful. Support and shelter services may be available to the woman in your community and crisis counseling services may benefit both the man and the woman.

Other forms of treatment for aggression include the following: (a) relaxation training and the listing of physiological cues which precede agression; (b) becoming aware of self-talk which generates anger and creating alternative coping statements, e.g., moving from "My wife has a new hairdo—she's probably starting an affair", to "Relax, I need to check out my insecurity" (see Novaco, 1976). These and other interventions are described in more detail elsewhere (Fleming, 1979; Saunders, 1977; Walker, 1979).

After the preliminary interventions which focus on ending the abuse, semi-structured communication and negotiation training is usually appropriate. Most clinicians agree that an emphasis on insight into early causative factors is not productive.

There are other issues which I cannot discuss in the space here, such as how to work with the children in these families and the pros and cons of individual, family and group formats at various stages of treatment. I encourage family therapists to discuss these issues with their colleagues as well as to take responsibility for detecting spouse abuse, confronting it with the family, and inspecting their own beliefs for unhelpful stereotypes.

References

Dobash, R. E. and Dobash, R. *Violence Against Wives*. New York: Free Press, 1979.

Feild, H. Attitudes toward rape: A comparative analysis of police, rapists, crisis counselors, and citizens. *Journal of Personality and Social Psychology*, 1978, *36*, 156-179.

Fleming, J. *Stopping Wife Abuse*. New York: Anchor, 1979.

Novaco, R. *Anger Control*. Lexington, Mass: Lexington, 1976.

Saunders, D. G. Marital violence: Dimensions of the problem and modes of intervention. *Journal of Marriage and Family Counseling*, 1977, *3*, 43-52.

Straus, M. A. Leveling, civility, and violence in the family. *Journal of Marriage and the Family*, 1974, *34*, 12-29.

Straus, M. A. Wifebeating. In *Battered Women: Issues of Public Policy*. Washington D.C.: U.S. Civil Rights Commission, U.S. Gov't Printing Office, 1978.

Walker, L. E. *The Battered Woman*. New York: Harper and Row, 1979.

DANIEL G. SAUNDERS, Ph.D.
Counselor and Social Worker
Family Service
Madison, WI

102. Couple Counseling with Rape Victims

Question:

Some of the referrals I have received from our local community hospital are married couples in which the wife has been the victim of sexual assault (not cases of wife abuse). The husbands seemed more upset about the rape than their wives did. My problem is that I can't seem to find anything in the literature on counseling rape victims and their husbands. What do I tell an enraged husband when his wife refuses to report the rape to the police? How soon should he expect to resume sexual relations with her? Should he wait for his wife to initiate sex? Is it "normal" for a 25-year-old wife to have nightmares, insomnia, lose her appetite and avoid sex because of an assault which occurred when she was a high school senior? As a male therapist, do I need a female cotherapist for couple counseling with rape victims?

Discussion:

The acute response of rape victims has been carefully described by Burgess and Holmstrom (1974) based on their five-year study of 146 rape victims. However, until recently, the victim's husband and his reaction to the assault was overlooked. We now realize that the husband and wife are *both* victims and that the husband's grief reaction which parallels his wife's has a critical impact on her subsequent adjustment—for better or for worse. Likewise, her response significantly affects him and the future of their marriage.

When a husband is called to meet his wife at the emergency room, his first response is likely to be fear for her safety. Was she shot, beaten, stabbed? Will she become pregnant? Will she get V.D.? Once he sees her and is reassured as to the extent of her physical injuries, if any, his next thought is likely to be, "Who did this to her?" He smolders with the urge to punish the rapist so that he will never be able to hurt another woman again. Thoughts of murder or castration are very common. Occasionally, husbands or fathers search for the

497

rapist in order to act out their violent fantasies. This rage response in the male during the acute crisis makes it difficult for him to give his wife the support and understanding she needs.

For the woman, rape is *the loss of control over her body and her life.* In fact, this control was not lost but stolen, often in a random, meaningless way. She may have done something moderately "risky," like walking alone to her car after work. She may have done the same thing a thousand times before without mishap. Or she may have done absolutely nothing, like the client who was raped by a man who broke into the apartment while she was doing the dinner dishes. In any case, the attack was not deserved and she felt powerless to stop it. Now she finds herself in the hospital being examined by strangers in white uniforms and being questioned by more strangers in blue uniforms. Because she has entered the medical bureaucracy, she is usually stripped of her clothes and her identity so that again she has no control over her life or her body.

By the time her husband sees her, she is numb with psychological shock. If she has strength enough to become angry, she may rebel against pressures to identify the attacker or against questioning by curious doctors, nurses or police who want more details than they need. She may try to regain control by refusing to cooperate and by refusing any help that is offered, especially if the help is offered in a patronizing way. She will resent her husband if he insists on being overprotective and treats her like an invalid or sick child. This is a critical time for therapeutic intervention.

Lack of effective communication may well put the relationship in serious jeopardy. Although rape occurs to couples in all degrees of marital adjustment and maladjustment, it may be more likely to happen to couples who are separated, because unescorted women run a higher risk of attack. Thus, the therapist may be seeing a couple who has reconciled recently due to crisis-generated intimacy. Their marital relationship may not be functional enough to endure the added strain of adjusting to the rape. In some cases the husband is interested in rebuilding the marriage, but the wife sees reconciliation as weakness on her part. Reinstating the separation will then seem to be a return to her prerape state—a reinstatement of her control over her own life.

It is essential for the marital therapist to understand that both husband and wife are beginning to mourn the abrupt loss of security and self-determination, as well as the violation of their privacy. However, their grief reactions are not synchronized because of the woman's prolonged fear of retaliation by the rapist. If she can identify him, she assumes that he can identify her. Meanwhile, the husband is preoccupied with his own anger. The emotional distance between husband and wife may be increased if his anger triggers memories of the violence inflicted upon her by the rapist. She may also fear for her husband's safety if he goes looking for the rapist himself. Even men who are ordinarily mild-mannered or intellectual types may be surprised at the intensity of their emotional response. If this is the case, the wife may choose to delay her own grief to help comfort or control him. Miscommunication may also occur if the husband pressures his wife into testifying against her attacker. Since testimony begins with each witness giving his or her complete name and address, her fears of retaliation from the rapist or his friends are not unrealistic. She may also feel that reliving the details of the rape in court with the rapist present would be more than her nerves could stand. It is the therapist's role to comfort the wife while helping her husband to ventilate. The therapist must then help the couple to understand the wife's need to "act normal" and the way in which that pretense may delay or prolong the normal grief response.

The second crisis occurs when the couple goes home. If the attack happened at home or in the vicinity, the wife will most probably find the area aversive. With the exception of adolescent victims living with their parents (from whom they may be keeping the rape secret), the vast majority of rape victims change residence as soon as they can arrange it. For some couples this is financially impossible. For all couples, a precipitous move is a financial hardship. Some clients move in with inlaws until their home can be sold. Unfortunately, moving cuts off the support system provided by friends and neighbors.

The third crisis occurs when the wife's physical wounds have healed and her husband begins to wonder when they can resume sexual relations (Miller and Williams, 1979). Some women see resuming sex immediately as part of their return to normal and may initiate having intercourse whether or not they are sexually aroused. Other women need to wait one to two months and need greater amounts of physical (nonsexual) affection in the interim. As with their communication, the couple's particular response depends on the quality of their prerape relationship. If their sex life was rewarding, intercourse may be a source of mutual comfort and satisfaction. If their sex life was unrewarding or one-sided, the rape may be used as an excuse to avoid sex indefinitely. This pathological response to rape is probably being maintained by other longstanding problems in the relationship.

If the husband wants to know how soon he should bring up the subject of lovemaking, the answer depends on the extent of the wife's physical trauma. With little or no physical damage, she may still be sore for a week from the bilateral shots of penicillin in her buttocks. If there was tearing or cutting of the vaginal or rectal area, she may require suturing which delays intercourse from four to six weeks. Once intercourse is attempted, the flashbacks evoked may prevent adequate arousal so that a lubricant may be needed for a few weeks. In addition to temporary aversion to physical contact by men, physical discomfort during sex due to trauma, and changes in her physical response to sexual stimulation, Holmstrom and Burgess (1979) found that women worried about their partner's reaction to them after the rape. The majority of male partners see rape as an act of violence against a woman, but there remains a minority of men who see rape as unfaithfulness because "she had sex with another man," regardless of how bruised or traumatized she was. They may focus on their own hurt or feel betrayed and repulsed if they feel that she "could have put up more of a fight." When a woman is threatened with a knife, gun, or broken bottle, she may submit passively so as to avoid being maimed or murdered. Since her only scars are psychological, her husband may doubt her role as victim. This problem is compounded if she then refuses to identify her attacker or attackers in court.

Certain events or situations may bring back vivid memories and nightmares many months or years later. Any person, place or thing (e.g., a particular after-shave lotion or the smell of stale beer) present during the attack can evoke an overwhelming emotional response in the victim. Both she and her spouse need to be reassured that this is a normal happening. When the cues are sexual, a lamp may need to be left on during intercourse so that the female partner can reassure herself that she is still safe.

A woman who has been assaulted while a high school student *can* have a long-delayed reaction. For example, if she had been hitchhiking and did not tell her parents or her friends that she was raped, the memories may stay buried until the first time she tries to have sex with her husband or boyfriend. If she has avoided sex until she is 25 years old, the flashbacks can still occur on her wedding night. In other situations, the couple may have a rewarding sexual relationship, but flashbacks may be triggered when the husband asks his wife to experiment with oral-genital or anal sex. Again, the triggering stimulus depends on what she was forced to endure during the assault, which in many cases she has not previously shared with her husband. Other stimuli setting off a delayed response may include: the anniversary of the attack or of the trial; seeing the rapist on the street (or seeing someone resembling him); learning that the rapist has been released from prison; or seeing a dramatization of rape and its aftermath on television. Both partners need to be reassured that her responses are conditioned and can be unlearned. She is neither crazy nor faking.

Finally, a female cotherapist gives a male therapist several advantages in helping rape-victim couples (Williams and Miller, 1979). During the acute crisis, the male therapist can help the husband ventilate his rage and explore his feelings of guilt, shame or betrayal. At the same time the female therapist can comfort the wife and reaffirm her identity and value as a person. During the treatment of chronic rape-related marital problems, the wife may only be willing to describe the incident in detail (necessary for identifying the conditioned aversive stimuli) to another female. One client was unable to explain to a male therapist how ambivalent she had become about being *alone* with her infant son. She knew that if her son's life were again threatened by a rapist, she would again have to submit. She felt that only another woman could understand how vulnerable she still felt two years later.

References

Burgess, A. W., and Holmstrom, L. L. Rape trauma syndrome. *American Journal of Psychiatry*, 1974, *131*, 981-986.

Holmstrom, L. L. and Burgess, A. W. Rape: The husband's and boyfriend's initial reactions. *The Family Coordinator*, 1979, *28*, 321-330.

Miller, W. R., and Williams, A. M. The impact of rape on marital and sexual adjustment. In B. Lakey (Chair), *Women as Victims of Physical Abuse*. Symposium presented at the meeting of the Eastern Psychological Association, Philadelphia, 1979.

Williams, A. M., and Miller, W. R. *Sexual assault victims and their husbands/boyfriends: Presenting complaints and therapy goals.* Paper presented at the meeting of the Society for Sex Therapy and Research, Philadelphia, March, 1979.

ANN MARIE WILLIAMS, Ph.D.
Research Associate
Department of Psychiatry
University of Pennsylvania
Philadelphia, PA

Termination of Family Therapy

103. Termination in
Family Therapy

Question:

I have come to family therapy from a traditional psychodynamic background. I am intrigued by the efficacy and directness of family therapy, but I am having trouble knowing how to end family treatment. And no one seems to discuss termination. Most of the teaching focuses on the beginning phases of treatment—the initial interview and defining or redefining the problem. Hardly anything is said about ending treatment.

When is it appropriate to end treatment? How should the therapist broach the subject of ending treatment with the family? How should the therapist respond if the family wants to leave treatment after some improvement? And, finally, if a family returns to treatment after a "successful" course of therapy, does this mean that the therapy was not so successful?

Discussion:

As you know, not all family therapists think or teach alike about almost every aspect of family treatment. The same is true for the issue of termination. Some therapists who are closer to the psychoanalytic tradition, who expect a longer duration of treatment, and who use the transference in treatment may be thoughtful about the process of termination. Even so, Boszormenyi-Nagy and Spark (1973) do not discuss the practicalities of this phase of treatment in *Invisible Loyalties*. Other family therapists tend to describe ending family treatment more casually. Carter (1977) writes: "When she announced herself definitely in charge of her life, now, she asked to see me at increasingly spaced intervals, and I agreed. This is my usual form of 'termination', in which the client's own work continues with less and finally no need to consult with me regularly."

I think there are several reasons why ending family therapy is not a major didactic or even therapeutic issue. Haley (1971) says that family therapy is distinguished from other therapies by its emphasis on outcome. All family therapists will agree that when you really start to "think family" your thinking changes. Assumptions about pathology, diagnosis and treatment planning change. So does the expectation of "cure." In moving from the concepts of your traditional training to those of family therapy you are changing from a linear, cause and effect thinking, where there is a beginning and an end, to a more intricate, systemic thinking, characterized by sequences, interrelationships and continuities. Though we concentrate much thought and writing on the beginning of family treatment, usually this is because it represents the important process of inducting the family into a new kind of therapeutic process, often dramatically different from their expectations of treatment as represented in the medical model, for example. But once the process has begun it is hard to define an endpoint.

Another reason it is hard to define the endpoint is the increasing awareness in the family field of the human life cycle—the evolution and development of biological systems which extends beyond childhood, affecting individuals as well as the family system as a whole. The family is never definable as "not right" in a certain correctable way. Instead, it is a system in motion, having come from somewhere and going on to somewhere else.

A third problem with defining the termination phase of family treatment has to do with the search for competence and utilization of the client's resources which is inherent in the family model. (It is also characteristic of some of the newer individual therapies.) Using the family members as resources for each other is but one level of application of competence-oriented thinking in family work. Since it is the clients who find "the answers" amongst themselves, the process of disengaging from a therapist and "making it" on their own should be insignificant.

When we talk of ending family therapy, then, we are talking about a time when the family and the therapist, who have for some time participated together in a mutual episode, will go their separate ways, or will at least change the nature of their client-therapist relationship. When is it best to do this? When the chief complaint is resolved or when the family system has been mobilized and restructured in such a way that they can work on the problem—or other problems—in a different and more comfortable manner.

Family therapists look for what Rabkin (1977) calls the "satisfied dropout," the client who got what he or she came for and leaves without much ado. A nice example of such an ending is described by Charles

Fulweiler (in Haley and Hoffman, 1967) as follows: "Just at the end, an amusing thing happened. The father came into the terminating session and declared that there had been an enormous change in the family and that things were great. The reason he gave for this change in the family was not the therapy but their going to hear Billy Graham . . . I felt it was really an accolade because I was completely out of it . . . The goal is to have the (family) equation stay in balance without you. Then the job of the therapist is over" (pp. 95-96).

When the family has made a basic change in the interaction around the symptom area and seems on its way to a new system of managing the problem issues, the therapist should first compliment them on their work. It is important to give them the credit and responsibility for the changes they are making if they are to continue without the therapist. After this the therapist should ask if there is anything more they would like to work on. Often, family members may respond by requesting more time to work on the current problem. The therapist may need to decide whether this is really necessary or whether it is a way to avoid assuming the responsibility. In either case, the therapist may elect to space out the sessions, receiving a phone call in the place of a session, for example, to give the family more time to work on its own. Frequently, family members may raise other problem areas for examination. Here, again, the therapist needs to assess whether these are really different, from the point of view of family functioning, from those which have already been worked on. For example, parents may say, "Yes, we feel that we have the problem with Johnny under control but we would like to work more on problems in our marital relationship." If the therapist had been working all along with changes in the way the parents interacted with each other around Johnny's problem, he/she might not feel it necessary to focus on the spouse system at this point. The therapist might encourage the family to try things on their own, with a suggestion that now that they had got things better with Johnny, they may find things already different between them. On the other hand, the therapist might see this as an opportunity to work on some other family issues—perhaps involving the family of origin. At this point the therapist may make a new contract with the family. Often, too, the family will agree that the problem is resolved or that progress has been significant and that further treatment doesn't seem necessary to them, either.

Frequently the family raises the question first: "What are we doing here? We were wondering if we couldn't stop coming or see you in two weeks or a month?" This is an important message to the therapist. It usually means that the family is feeling a renewed sense of comfort and competence with their issues. The therapist may worry that there has not been sufficient change or that there will not be lasting change. But the family therapist's commitment to client competence will induce him/her to encourage the family to try things out with less frequent sessions, or stopping altogether with an open invitation to call if they wish. As Boszormenyi-Nagy and Spark (1973) state: "The family's goal may be limited to removal of the initial referral problem in the designated patient member. In our years of experience as both individual and family therapists this usually occurs sooner in family than in individual therapy. Although there is no assurance that such individual symptomatic change is proof of a systemic rebalancing and reorientation in family relationships, this goal is a legitimate one and the therapist should be ready to accept termination of therapy at such a point" (pp. 377-378).

Thus, if the family should initiate the desire to leave treatment after some improvement, this is best seen as the family's experience of something beneficial having been discovered, some new-found competent ways of interacting in the problem areas. If the therapist responds this way, the family can continue to work on its own and can also return for more treatment at a future date. To expect that the family will be "cured" imposes a tremendous burden on the therapeutic system and demands that the therapist assume a position which is beyond expertise towards omnipotence.

In summary, in response to your questions about termination in family therapy, I have tried to explain why I think termination is not a useful concept in family treatment. In response to your questions about how to end family therapy, I have offered some suggestions. I would like to end this discussion with a comment by Keith and Whitaker (1977): "Families end casually. Family therapists seldom talk about ending. Families usually close the gestalt on their own away from therapy" (p. 130).

References

Boszormenyi-Nagy, I., and Spark, G. *Invisible Loyalties*. New York: Harper and Row, 1973.

Carter, E. Generation after generation. In P. Papp (Ed.), *Family Therapy: Full Length Case Studies*. New York: Gardner, 1977.

Haley, J. Approaches to family therapy. In J. Haley (Ed.), *Changing Families: A Family Therapy Reader*. New York: Grune and Stratton, 1971.

Haley, J., and Hoffman, L. *Techniques of Family Therapy*. New York: Basic Books, 1967.

Keith, D., and Whitaker, C. The divorce labyrinth. In P. Papp (Ed.), *Family Therapy:*

Full Length Case Studies. New York: Gardner, 1977.

Rabkin, R. *Strategic Psychotherapy.* New York: Basic Books, 1977.

LEE COMBRINCK-GRAHAM, M.D.
Director of Child Psychiatry Training
Philadelphia Child Guidance Clinic;
Clinical Assistant Professor
Department of Psychiatry
University of Pennsylvania
Philadelphia, PA

104. Premature Termination in Marital and Family Therapy

Question:

As a supervisor in a family service agency, I have become increasingly aware that my staff do a good job of maintaining their individual clients but have a higher premature termination rate with couples and families. This often takes place before the end of the first four sessions. Our staff have a variety of training backgrounds ranging from psychodynamic, behavioral, gestalt, through a communication systems approach. There seems to be little relationship between theoretical approach used and ability to maintain clients. If my staff were cold and detached, they would not be able to maintain ongoing therapeutic contact with their individual clients, but this is not the case. I feel they are warm, empathic and relatively skilled workers. Also, in examination of our premature termination data, we seem to have a higher rate with those referred by physicians and clergy than with clients who are self-referred or who are referred to us by past clients. I would appreciate suggestions to sharpen our focus in this area, for if we can't hold our couples and families, we can't do much to help them.

Discussion:

First, it might be important to find out what kind of therapy your staff prefer to do, individual, couple or family. In a research project conducted a couple of years back, I found that those therapists who indicate that they prefer to do individual therapy, whether brief in nature or long term, frequently did not maintain couple or family clients on initial contacts or through to therapeutic terminations. This was in contrast to those therapists who indicated that they preferred working with couples or families. In the same study those therapists who considered their basic theoretical model to be systems (communication or structural) tended to connect and hold couples and families longer than therapists who indicated their theoretical model was psychodynamic, gestalt, transactional analysis, behavioral, etc. Thus, it would seem important to recognize that preferred models of working determine some aspects of premature termination.

I also found that those therapists who had been involved in a long-term individual therapy of their own within the past ten years tended to prefer individual models of working and more of them moved clients from conjoint models of working to individual models within the first four sessions. Therapists who had experienced personal, marital and/or family therapy tended to value conjoint models of therapy and rarely moved clients to individual sessions, except to examine part of the subsystem. Thus, our own personal therapeutic experience also affects our style and how we maintain clients who come to us.

The most important characteristic affecting whether a client feels like therapy is worth staying for is the degree to which the therapist can join each client's own "reality" of how he or she structures his or her world. Thus, a therapist working with more than one client at a time must be able to shift focus and connect emphatically with a variety of persons. People tend to organize their sense of reality around thinking, feeling or doing. So a therapist will need to listen and respond to thinkers with ideas and analogies that enables that person to know that the therapist respects his/her way of thinking. At the same time, the therapist must connect with another family member whose reality is more geared to feelings. Here, empathic feeling responses are vital. Other family members may be more "doing" oriented so the therapist will need to connect at a behavioral level and perhaps create tasks that "get things done." To relate in a joining way at all these levels within the same session takes flexibility. To do it in such a way that enables each to feel heard and joined by the therapist takes a clear usage of content and process that differentiates and yet joins the various members of this family present for therapy. This skill in differentiating and yet establishing "belongingness" is a major step in any conjoint therapy.

Unlike individual therapy, most conjoint sessions need something specific to happen in the very early sessions. There is not time to wait to gather lots of information. Using the process which emerges during the session to create specific tasks for therapeutic work brings the focus to here-and-now change, instead of hearing the clients tell you about past events or feelings. Conjoint therapy needs to be present oriented and future paced so that clients have specific goals they are working on in the relationship during the therapy hour and between sessions. These may be in terms of communication, structural changes, paradoxical interventions or delabelling and/or relabelling behavior.

The establishment of a clear contract with goals that are agreed upon by clients and therapist can also be vital in avoiding premature terminations. I recommend the setting of four-session contracts, to be reevaluated at that time by both parties and recontracted. This tends to keep clients from feeling that they are getting "locked" into something that could go on and on. A clear model or map of how you work as therapist is also helpful.

You indicated that those clients referred by physicians or clergy tend to terminate prematurely more readily than some others. It is very important to understand the nature of your referral contacts with your agency and with the clients. Many individuals who have not been to therapy before have no real understanding of what "should" take place. They may model it after contacts with their physician or clergyman. This may mean that they believe they can use the relationship as they want or need and find it difficult establishing an ongoing contract.

It is also important to understand that if they have a rather dependent relationship with their referral source they may be reluctant to change. Despite the pain experienced in the marital and family context, clients may resist change because that change may appear to necessitate the loss of dependency with a trusted other, that is the referring person. Most therapists do not take seriously enough the past and current interaction of clients with their referral source, and thus do not recognize the double-bind many clients feel. They want to follow their doctor's recommendation and use the therapy to change; yet to change has the potential of losing the vital contact they have built up with that doctor or other referral contact over the past few months or even years. I find that when in doubt as to the nature of the relationship between client and referral source, it is best to bring it clearly into the open and talk it through, for this frequently avoids premature termination.

CLAUDE A. GULDNER, Th.D.
Associate Professor
Department of Family Studies
Coordinator of Marriage and Family Therapy Program
University of Guelph
Guelph, Ontario, Canada

105. Couples Who Do Not Want to Terminate Therapy

Question:

When marital objectives are met, crises resolved, and individual symptoms abated, some couples do not even begin to ask about leaving therapy. I have usually tried to be rather pointed at these times in asking couples if there is anything they can now think of that could justify spending the time and money to continue to see me. Some cannot and say so, and they agree to terminate promptly. Others can and convince me that they are ready to define and pursue a new phase of therapy. A few can do neither but wish to linger anyway. What is going on with the latter couples? Am I being duped by their dependency urges if I continue to see them? Or, are their concerns more substantive but beyond our perception? If I let them stay in therapy, what should I do with them?

Discussion:

The dilemma of the more or less successfully treated couple who is still clinging to therapy is one that used to cause me grave self-doubts but more recently has become a new source of fascination and opportunity. The doubts arose from imprinted exhortations from my early psychotherapy training to examine my own countertransference for the motivation for either prolonging a treatment relationship or questioning prolonging it. Am I too invested in this patient? Is he or she picking up my wish to nurture and pacifying me? Am I fostering an inappropriate dependency? Later, I became more practical but still with the focus on my motivations. Am I doing this to maintain my caseload, generate more income, avoid starting another new case?

Now, I find myself asking radically different questions. What's going on for them? What would it take to help? Can I do it? I still experience a modicum of agonizing self-scrutiny, but I am increasingly willing to give people's judgements the benefit of the doubt. There is something more that they want. Calling it "dependency" may only be the termination phase equivalent of labeling onset phase behavior as "re-sistance." We have learned that ignorance as to how to reach a shared objective and/or expected impotence in dealing with a problem, once defined, often leads to the label, "resistance." I am coming to suspect a similar process when we label behavior as "dependency."

Discovery of a new technique has led me to some surprising and favorable experiences with terminating couples. These are couples who have made significant strides by their own as well as my estimation, have chosen to stay together, and don't want to leave therapy. The technique is Neurolinguistic Programming (NLP)*, developed by Grinder and Bandler and associates (Bandler, 1978). Armed with these experiences, I dared to probe further than I had gone before into the details of what was bothering these lingering, dependent couples. I discovered the obvious. Just being in the presence of one another often triggered unhappiness. In retrospect, this is probably what I had feared I would find all along. The difference was that now I felt I might have a remedy.

I will give an example from one of my cases that clearly illustrates the nature of this type of unhappiness and one way that I found to deal with the "condition." The results, I feel, confirm, at least, that there was a specific, identifiable condition to treat that previously I would have preferred to keep vague (rather than admit that I had no way to treat it yet).

A woman in her forties was referred by her family doctor with the initial complaint of uncontrollable tearful episodes, fitful sleeping and difficulty concentrating at work for several weeks. Only her sleep pat-tern had partially improved on antidepressant medication prior to referral. Her husband had spent the past year working weekdays in another city and commuting home most weekends. Their children were grown and out of the home. Their arrangement had initially been mutually agreed upon by the couple. Shortly before onset of his wife's symptoms, the husband had announced that he was having an affair with a younger woman.

Both husband and wife were asked to come to the first session and most subsequent sessions. We met weekly for nearly a year, though there were numerous breaks for vacation or work-related reasons. As a structural, problem-solving, strategic therapist who also incorporates behavioral marital therapy, transgenerational approaches and more, I drew upon many different techniques at different phases of their therapy.

_____

*Neurolinguistic Programming is a registered trademark of Not Ltd., Inc. of California.

I gave them some rules and a "caring task," courtesy of Stuart (1976), which was followed shortly by the husband's termination of the affair and a mutual commitment to therapy. Individual symptoms and marital distress continued. Their marital contracts, spoken and unspoken, were reviewed in depth, with the aid of Sager's reminder list (Sager, 1976). This process highlighted several "contractual" areas especially related to their post-child-rearing developmental phase that required renegotiation. Subsequently, the wife elected to accept an offer for intensive advanced training, which led to a higher level career beginning a few months later.

They were still in therapy. Individual symptoms were decreased but not gone. There was only a tentative marital commitment and improved but limited satisfaction when together. She had embarked on a serious weight loss program for the first time since becoming obese six or seven years earlier. The couple had also resolved some differences over sexual expectations. Along the way, it had become apparent that the husband was suffering from chronic fatigue and was excessively irritable. A diet and exercise program had successfully altered these conditions.

The next phase involved work particularly with the wife's family of origin. Most of this occurred through assignments to be done at a distance, but her mother also took part in an office session with the wife. Their marriage could be seen as initially consisting of a complementary relationship between an oldest daughter, who could never admit weakness to either mother or husband, and a youngest son identified in his family with a mother who was also a youngest and without weight in her family. These roles were manifest, for example, in her not sharing with him any but her most major concerns and his acceptance of having no say in which chores he must do in the home. By the time of his affair, he had come to feel lonely and put upon at home. Through the cross-generational phase of therapy, their relationship took on a much more symmetrical pattern.

The wife's initial symptoms were completely cured only after the couple was helped to identify and begin to openly and effectively address one of their son's serious psychiatric problems. After ten months of therapy, the wife was no longer depressed or tearful; she had lost 25 pounds; their son was functioning well; and the couple was relating, by their own account, the best they ever had. I told them that they should stop therapy unless they could come up with some good reason for continuing, making it clear that I was unaware of any compelling reason. They said that the marriage was solid but they were not ready to leave therapy. For a combination of vacation and strategic reasons, they were then given a five-week time-out from therapy.

When therapy resumed, all their gains had been maintained; but she admitted to not looking forward to being with him as much as she wanted. She felt "down" about herself, but only in his presence.

By chance, and then design, the therapy in the three sessions that followed, prior to one joint termination session, was with her alone. In the second of these sessions, she was asked to recover, with both an image and a feeling, the experience of feeling down. The precise moment she felt down was identified. It did not have to do with seeing her husband as she had assumed, but rather with hearing a tone of displeasure in his voice. For example, the moment she felt down was not when she saw him in the airport, or when he entered the car, or when he said, "Hi." It was upon his first complaint, however slight and whether about the plane, the weather, work, or her.

This down moment was anchored by a specific touch to facilitate later recall. Explications of "anchoring" and the other NLP technical terms used here may be found in Bandler (1978). She was then asked to recover an experience when she felt the opposite of down. She found a time in her memory when she could "hear" a teacher complimenting her, and she labeled her feeling at that time "warm." Warm was also anchored with a different touch. An overlapping procedure was then used in which both anchors, the touch for warm and the touch for down, were then applied to the auditory experience of husband complaining. It had the desired confusional and, hence, option-broadening effect. The next step was to help her experience warm consistently in the face of the same (still imagined) complaining circumstances that previously generated down. This was accomplished through several brief repetitions of a visual-kinesthetic disassociation process during which she first came to tolerate the mental process of stepping out of herself and observing herself as though somewhat younger and confronted with her husband complaining. Next, she was guided to take warm with her and become the person reacting to the complaining tone. When this was accomplished, it was repeated with and without accompanying anchors to consolidate the change for the future. Technically, this has been called "futurepacing."

One week later she returned, beaming. She reported that she left town to visit her husband rather than his traveling as planned, that she had felt good about herself throughout her approach to him and the visit, and that he had not complained even once, though she knew he had much at work about which he could have complained. She also felt filled with "insight." For example, she concluded that she had more influence on this complaining than she realized, and that her feeling "controlled" by her husband and by her mother led her to eat to assert her individuality. In fact, that week for the first time, she "did not even think about candy," much less buy or eat any.

She saw now only one hurdle, overcoming the strain of dealing with an otherwise welcome visit from her mother. Similar procedures to those just described for the previous session were then carried out with regard to her reaction to the look and sound of disappointment from her mother.

The next and final session took place with the couple two weeks later, right after an eight-day visit from her mother. She reported feeling fully comfortable with both her mother and her husband; and, remarkably, her mother too had "not even given (her) an opportunity" to try out her new behavior. Her husband suggested, with obvious admiration, that her mother must have been afraid to show disappointment because she could see how firmly and well her daughter now deals with him. In addition, she reported renewed weight loss of four pounds, but now without effort. Husband reported that he felt robust and more pleased with himself and with his marriage than ever before, and both agreed to terminate therapy. Incidental contact several months later showed gains were persisting.

The type of experience described here is forcing me to reexamine my own early learning and assumptions. At the very least, I have decided that I will accept that "dependency" which is manifest chiefly by a less than well-defined wish to linger in therapy is simply a statement that an individual or a couple has not yet found a successful way to tolerate their circumstances without help. As in the case of the couple I have discussed here, this can occur after successful intervention with crises and even after achieving more long-term, complicated relationship objectives. I suspect the underlying issue frequently involves some form of automatic, unpleasant response within an important relationship.

No doubt there are and increasingly will be other interventions than NLP techniques to apply to these residual automatic conditions. Couples group experiences with socially comparable, adept couples and well-devised and individually tailored rituals are two that I see as having some similar potential. Having been armed with a little NLP and delving further because of it was a uniquely enlightening experience for me, and I now take more seriously couples' wishes to continue in therapy and the potential of therapy to help them.

References

Bandler, L. *They Lived Happily Ever After*. Cupertino, CA: Meta Publications, 1978.
Sager, C. J. *Marriage Contracts and Couple Therapy*. New York: Brunner/Mazel, 1976.

Stuart, R. B. An operant interpersonal program for couples. In D. H. L. Olson (Ed.), *Treating Relationships*. Lake Mills, Iowa: Graphic Publishing Co., 1976.

DONALD I. DAVIS, M.D.
Director
Family Therapy Institute
of Alexandria, VA;
Clinical Associate Professor
of Psychiatry
George Washington University
Washington, DC

106. Who Should Get Credit for Change Which Occurs in Therapy?

Question:

Sometimes, at the point of termination after successful therapy, a family will begin to shower you with praise for your competence. They will thank you profusely for "all you have done," implying that you deserve total credit for anything good that happened. They may hint or wonder whether they can "make it" in the future without you. Or, they may palpably show their gratitude by giving you gifts. These actions can make you uncomfortable, particularly when you are not sure what to do—how to handle the situation. While Haley (1976) and others have asserted that the therapist is responsible for bringing about change (or failing to do so) in therapy, does this notion apply here? Should you accept the family's thanks more or less unconditionally, openly sharing with them the perception that you were pretty much responsible for the positive outcome?

Discussion:

It is natural for a family to feel indebted to their therapist for helping to bring about improvement. It is also natural for a therapist to relish their praise. However, it is unwise to do this. You should be reluctant to accept credit even if you consider yourself mainly or partly responsible for the outcome. This is an important therapeutic action and one which I have heard emphasized only by strategic and structural therapists (Stanton, 1980a). There are several reasons for it.

First, no matter how much effort and concern the therapist devoted to the therapy, it is a sure bet that he or she in no way had to go through as much pain during the process as did the family. On the way to successful completion of therapy, it is likely that considerable agony was experienced and considerable energy expended by them. Among the family members, *somebody*, at *some* time during treatment,

519

had to take a chance in order to get things going in a different direction. *Everybody* probably went through a period of tension, conflict and anxiety—all of which are part of the creaks and groans accompanying new patterns, behaviors and structures. For the therapist not to recognize this would be naive. In other words, the family members *deserve* credit for the suffering they have undergone and the effort they made to get past it.

Another reason to refuse credit, especially when the index patient is a child or young person, is because not to do so can place the therapist in competition with the parents. It is difficult for parents not to resent a therapist who has done a better job with their child than they have. You have succeeded where they have failed, and this can both undermine their status in the eyes of their children and lessen their views of themselves. Under such circumstances it is not uncommon for parents to subtly encourage their child to become symptomatic again, thereby attenuating the therapist's power and influence. Through their actions, the parents may in a sense be trying both to reassert their authority and "get their child back" from the therapist. Therapists who see children in individual treatment are particularly susceptible to this sort of "rebound" (Montalvo and Haley, 1973). Giving parents credit for the outcom is one way of preventing such a recurrence.

Related to the above, the most important reason for not accepting credit for change is because it increases the chance that the positive effects of treatment will *last*. This applies equally to family, marital or individual therapy. Again, the idea in family treatment is to make the *family* or *parents* feel responsible for the improvement (Haley, 1980). If this is not done, the family members may see themselves as less competent to cope effectively with new situations or future symptom-provoking events. The therapist would be conveying the message that they cannot "hack it" on their own, and they will become both indebted to, and dependent upon, the therapist. Indeed, the task with some families is to get them to stay *out* of therapy, so that it does not continue as a way of life; certain families, especially within the upper middle-class suburbs, can become so "therapized" that they grow very uncomfortable when they are not in treatment, even if their problems have abated.

It should be noted that this is *not* the same as foisting the responsibility for change on the family, in opposition to the dictums of Haley (1976) and others. Clear distinctions should be made here. First, the issue in question usually occurs at termination, when the therapy is essentially over. Second, the responsibility is being apportioned for what has *already happened* in therapy, rather than what should be done in the future. There is a difference between ascribing credit for past accomplishments versus assuming or telling a family at the outset that it is responsible for whether the forthcoming treatment succeeds or fails.

Fostering a sense of accomplishment in the family or parents for having helped or corrected the original problem will provide them with confidence for handling future difficulties. When the next problem comes along they will feel more capable of dealing with it themselves, which, after all, is (or should be) an implicit goal of therapy. Thus, it is tactically wise for the therapist to underscore to them the extent to which their own efforts, ideas and commitment really "turned things around" (Stanton, 1980b). You should disown credit, stating to them that they "did the work." If they thank you for "it" (referring to the change), Thomas Todd (1975) suggests that you become very specific about what is meant by "it," asking questions such as, "Who did what?" "Didn't things start to get better when you did X?" etc. You should challenge them mildly by pointing out the specific contributions of each member, with the most credit going, where appropriate, to the parents. I sometimes find it helpful to chide the family jokingly, stating, "You people are too modest," or perhaps telling a given person, "You are so shy and modest that you would probably turn down the Medal of Honor, even if you earned it." The general idea is to turn the family's praise back on itself, so that in effect they earn their own appreciation. It is unlikely that this technique will either (a) stop the family from returning in the future if they really do get "stuck" again, or (b) make them hesitant to refer to the therapist friends or acquaintances who might also be in need of treatment at some later time.

Acceptance of gifts can be a little more touchy. Every therapist will encounter this at some point, and you must decide for yourself how to handle it. My own practice is usually to accept small gifts, especially if given by a child. However, even in these cases I commonly invoke the responsibility issue, making it clear that credit for change belongs to the family, not to me. Larger gifts, whether given or promised, are more of a problem. When such offers occur, it is usually because I have not done my job properly as far as assigning credit is concerned. My normal procedure is to refuse such a gift with a polite "thank you." This might be followed with a statement such as:

> I wouldn't feel right accepting this. I've been paid for my services. My reward is being able to see you folks pull yourself up by your bootstraps and take charge of this thing. As a matter of fact, I might want to ask you guys (or parents) to come back some time and help some of the other people I see who seem to get stuck with this kind of problem.

The above is a way of countering the gift in proportion to its magnitude. Not only are family members given credit for their work, but they are elevated to the level of "experts" who are so accomplished that they can even help others overcome such difficulties.

In some ways, the above practices could be seen as a "thankless" part of therapy. It is more gratifying to bask in the family's praise than to shift the credit back to them. From an overall view, it might even be seen to backfire, if giving the family credit reduces the chance that they will require treatment again; in other words, this tack could be viewed as operating toward the obliteration of one's profession—a not ignoble goal, but one which does not seem likely for the immediate future. However, for the sake of the family, the therapist must be content with the inherent satisfaction of a job well done. The reward comes from the knowledge that, if a family terminated a successful treatment with the feeling that they, not the therapist, were responsible for beneficial change, the chances for long-term success are increased.

References

Haley, J. *Problem-Solving Therapy*. San Francisco: Jossey-Bass, 1976.

Haley, J. *Leaving Home: Therapy with Disturbed Young People*. New York: McGraw-Hill, 1980.

Montalvo, B. and Haley, J. In defense of child therapy. *Family Process*, 1973, *12*, 227-244.

Stanton, M. D. Family therapy: Systems approaches. In G. P. Sholevar, R. M. Benson and B. J. Blinder (Eds.), *Handbook of Emotional Disorders in Children and Adolescents: Medical and Psychological Approaches to Treatment*. Jamaica, New York: S. P. Medical and Scientific Books (division of Spectrum Publications), 1980a.

Stanton, M. D. Strategic approaches to family therapy. In A. S. Gurman and D. P. Kniskern (Eds.), *Handbook of Family Therapy*. New York: Brunner/Mazel, 1981.

Todd, T. Personal communication. March 1975.

M. DUNCAN STANTON, Ph.D.
*Director, Addicts and Families Program
and Senior Psychologist, Philadelphia
Child Guidance Clinic;
Associate Professor of Psychology in
Psychiatry, University of Pennsylvania
School of Medicine
Philadelphia, PA*

INDEX